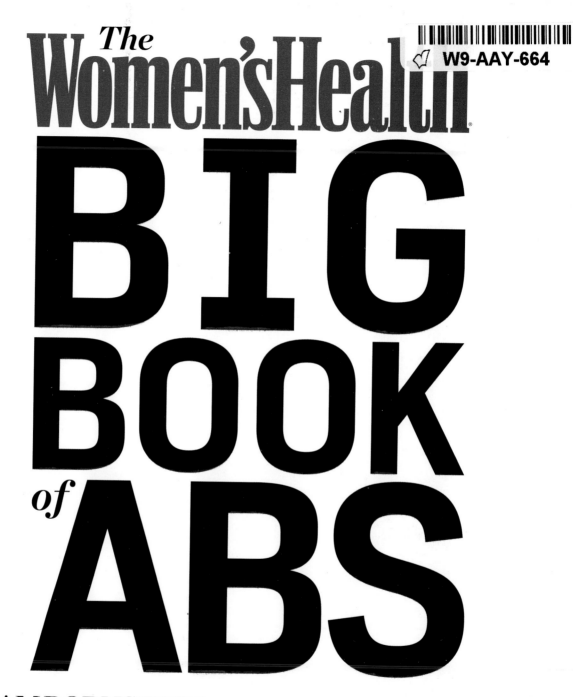

The *Women's Health*

BIG BOOK of ABS

by **ADAM BORNSTEIN** and the Editors of *Women's Health*

RODALE.

Book design by Laura White
With George Karabotsos, design director for *Men's Health* and *Women's Health* Books

Photography by Beth Bischoff

Cover hair and makeup: Robert Huitron
Cover styling: Thea Palad and Allison Richman

Library of Congress Catalog-in-Publication Data is on file with the publisher

ISBN: 978-1-60961-875-9

2 4 6 8 10 9 7 5 3 1 paperback

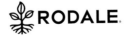

We inspire and enable people to improve their lives and the world around them.
rodalebooks.com

Contents

Acknowledgments

This book would not have been possible without the incredible help, inspiration, and hard work of many talented individuals.

Thank you to Maria Rodale and the entire Rodale family. You've been blazing the path of health and wellness, and continue to find new ways to help millions of people. To *Women's Health* editorial director and brand leader David Zinczenko, thank you for providing endless leadership and your never-ending determination to make health an important topic. Same to Stephen Perrine, publisher of Rodale books. You opened the door and gave me the opportunity to write books, and it's been a life-changing endeavor. Thank you.

Many thanks go out to the editors at *Women's Health* and the brilliant minds at *Men's Health*. It's impossible to thank everyone I've worked with, but I'm eternally indebted to the staff at *Men's Health* for making me a better writer, researcher, and editor.

To the people who brought this book to life: Thank you to Debbie McHugh for your vision and belief that I could make this happen. To Jeff Csatari, your never-ending creative ideas were essential in getting this project off the ground. Mike Zimmerman, there are few men better than you. To my incredible editor, Ursula Cary—I have never sounded better on paper (or made more sense to women). The amazing photography by Beth Bischoff. I can't forget Erin Williams, whose copy editing skills are unparalleled; and Laura White and our design team, led by George Karabotsos. George—I don't think you could design a bad-looking book if you tried.

Special thanks to Alan Aragon and Mike Roussell for their nutrition genius. And John Romaniello—you are first class in every sense of the term, and your fitness programs will make a lot of women very happy.

Neema Yazdani—the dream still lives.

Abby Lerner, Maria Masters, and Naomi Piercey: You don't realize it, but I couldn't have written a book for women without your help.

To my many mentors: Martin Rooney, Alwyn and Rachel Cosgrove, Bill Hartman, Eric Cressey, Mike Robertson, Valerie Waters, Joe Dowdell, Mike Boyle, Jason Ferruggia, Jim Smith, David Jack, Robert Dos Remedios, and Craig Ballantyne—I stand on your shoulders.

To my Demand Media and Livestrong.com family, particularly Dan Brian and Jeremy Reed: Thank you for allowing me to take on this project for the greater good of all people.

A special mention goes out to my mentor, Ted Spiker: You offer the greatest gift anyone could ever offer: unconditional belief and support, and the ability to make anyone believe they are capable of doing more.

To my parents: Mom and Dad, sorry I missed so many calls while I was working too much. Everything I am, I owe to both of you.

My brothers Josh, Aaron, and Jordan: You are my best friends in the world.

And of course, Rachie: You are the heartbeat of my strength and bring out an incredible version of me that I never thought was possible. You are my #1.

I am humbled by all of you. Thank you. Now let's see some abs.

Your New Body Starts with Your Core

FORGET YOUR DIETING PAST—THE NEW WAY
TO YOUR BEST BODY EVER
STARTS WITH PUTTING YOU BACK IN CONTROL.

If you've picked up

this book, you could probably use a little bit of relationship advice. Now, just hear me out. Most women are in a bad relationship and don't even know it—and the problems have nothing to do with cleaning, cuddling, or Sunday night football. No, it's more of a fundamental issue. You want to be in love with each other, but you're stuck in a rut that doesn't have any hope for significant change. By now you probably know I'm not talking about your guy, right? You're at odds with your own body.

You want to look slim and feel healthy and energized. You want a sexy body that sizzles and the confidence that comes with knowing you can have a banging bod without starving yourself. But your body appears to settle for something less. No matter

Your New Body Starts with Your Core

how many diets you try or hours you spend at the gym, nothing changes. Maybe you make a few sacrifices to improve the situation. You eat less, yet still gain weight; spend extra money on a fancy gym membership, but see no return on your investment. Maybe you even avoid the foods you love, like bread or cheese, and still get no results.

You're stuck. But unlike a bad-news boyfriend, you can't break up with your body. It's truly for better or worse. So you're left with two options: Continue to try and make a change, or give in and settle for a miserable relationship.

Contrary to what you might think, your body doesn't want a complicated relationship. It wants to be lean, fit, and happy. And no matter what you have experienced or may think, you are not destined to have a pooch and your metabolism isn't plotting against you to pack on the pounds. You don't have to settle for anything less than your leanest, sexiest body ever! And we're here to help you make that happen.

Trust me, your body is capable of the amazing transformations you read about and see in *Women's Health*. Forget your past failures, frustrations, and confusion—it's all about to change. That's why we created *The Women's Health Big Book of Abs*. You're just a few simple steps away from changing the relationship with your body for good and unlocking the real you. We know that all women can be toned, sexy, and confident—without making dramatic sacrifices. And in a matter of weeks, you'll have the body to prove it.

The Truth about Weight Loss

You're probably wondering how this time will be any different. You've tried the diets, done the exercises, and worked hard. You definitely don't have an issue with effort, so maybe you assume that your body is flawed. Maybe you've watched your friends and family lose weight while you continue to struggle. And there's no shortage of celebrities who flaunt their beautiful bods on a weekly basis in magazines and on TV.

Naturally, you might blame yourself for being unable to banish your belly. You know that exercise works. And eating healthy must do something if Jennifer Hudson can lose all that weight! In fact, you've probably even experienced some success yourself, say around every January. You start a new program and things seem great.

But at some point, your new program spirals out of control faster than an episode of *The Real Housewives of New Jersey*. You cave to a craving, which starts a downward cycle of bad eating habits. In order to compensate for your struggles, you become desperate to add more "calorie-burning" cardio, but your body doesn't change. The scale seems to move in the wrong direction. You continue to exercise more and eat less, and still see no difference. What gives?

Bad genetics? It's possible. Troubled thyroid? It happens. But more likely, you've yet to tap into the natural mechanisms that help your body burn fat fast.

You see, your body actually is designed to incinerate the unsightly chub that covers your sexy abs, firm butt, and lean legs. But the problem is that you've been fed a steady diet of misinformation about what your body needs in order to look its best. And we can tell you that radical, dramatic steps are the last thing your body needs. Sure, those crash diets might provide short-term joy—like a sweet summer fling. But those are usually temporary and end up causing you heartache in the long run. You need something more stable.

The Women's Health Big Book of Abs is a proven plan based on the information provided by the best fitness and nutrition experts and the latest research. You know what we discovered? If you treat yourself right and follow a few simple guidelines, you can literally switch your body into a fitter, healthier mode—it will burn more calories, build more muscle, and look 10 or even 20 years younger.

The best part: You'll be eating foods that you never thought would be on a diet plan. You can drink wine without worrying about how many calories are in a glass. You can even indulge in dessert and still flatten your belly. In fact, Greek researchers found that those who *don't* eat dessert on a healthy eating plan are *more* likely to gain weight. That's the type of digging we've done for creating the most comprehensive guide to unlocking a better you. All you need to do is keep reading, to find out how.

New Plan, New You

Fit, toned bodies don't come from pills. Or drinks. Or miracle slimming bodysuits.

If they did, we'd all look the way we want (and have a more questionable fashion selection than Lady Gaga). Unfortunately, we've all tried the do-whatever-it-takes approach to losing weight. Not only does that lead to a shortage of cash, it also bends our will. In fact, a UCLA study notes that nearly 70 percent of women don't believe that exercise and diet can help them lose weight. That's a scary number for a nation that's already losing the battle against obesity. So it's no wonder scientists estimate that the obesity trend won't slow down until the year 2050! And by that time, it's estimated that nearly half the country will be overweight. Do you want to be a statistic or the one who reverses the trend?

We can tell you that exercise and diet work. Change starts by realizing extreme behaviors are not the solution. Let's go back to the 1980s. That's when dietary fat was identified as the root of all evil and cardio was elevated to the best form of exercise. Next thing you knew, the entire country was gorging on fat-free foods and going on slow jogs.

Fast-forward 30 years and those decades of eating fat-free, sugar-loaded foods have expanded our tummies. And long-slow cardio results in—you guessed it—long, slow weight loss. In a Purdue University study, rats that consumed a mix of low-fat diet chips plus regular high-fat chips gained significantly more fat than rats that only consumed high-fat chips. Why? The researchers speculated that not only did the added sugars add to weight gain, but the low-fat foods tricked

Your New Body Starts with Your Core

the rats' bodies and prevented them from shutting off hunger signals, tempting the rats to eat more. In addition, Louisiana State University researchers found that the average number of calories burned during exercise dropped by 100 calories during the past 20 years, even though people were spending more time in the gym. So it should come as no surprise that the prevailing "best" approach to fat loss resulted in obesity rates skyrocketing to all-time highs.

Fortunately, we've learned a lot during the last 30 years, but people are still relying on the same information of the past. It's time to turn a new page, debunk old myths, and set the record straight: You can have flat, toned abs if you follow the lessons of *The Women's Health Big Book of Abs*. Here's why:

You Have More Control

Most fitness plans are inflexible. They are based on a preset routine that doesn't consider your lifestyle. Work, family, friends, and other obligations can make eating healthy and exercising difficult. So much so, according to the Centers for Disease Control and Prevention, that people who turn these lifestyle tendencies into excuses were up to 76 percent less likely to lose weight than those who figured out ways around them. In other words: You need to find techniques that won't result in failure, or else you're destined to eventually stop trying.

One of the biggest reasons why *The Women's Health Big Book of Abs* works is because you can create your own schedule. We empower you to choose how many meals you want to eat, the days you want to exercise, and when you want to escape for a savory dessert or a night out with the girls.

- **You want to eat six meals a day? Go for it.**
- **Your schedule won't allow you to eat snacks? Just have three big meals.**
- **You don't have an hour to exercise? No worries, we have complete body-shaping workouts that will take 20 minutes or less.**

This is the first program that takes into consideration your priorities and offers the tips you need to look your best.

You Have More Freedom

You want to know the real diet secret? Build your plan around the foods you love! Let's be realistic: If the only things you eat are literally Ho Hos and ice cream, you might have to adjust your plan (for the sake of your health most of all!). For everyone else, we insist that you keep your favorite foods as part of your diet. The truth is, the negativity surrounding most foods is inaccurate. You can eat white rice and white bread and still lose weight. Pasta doesn't trigger any fat receptors that cause cellulite. And gym sessions do not have to last hours upon hours for you to look good in your Lululemon pants.

We'll teach you how to load up—the right way—on the food your body craves. You'll be eating what you like, along with what you need, and have more energy and faster fat loss. It's designed to guarantee that you never become tired of what you're eating. By knowing what you can eat—rather than focusing on what you can't—you'll discover the endless meals that can help you lose weight and keep it off.

You Have a Proven Formula

You can't out-exercise a bad diet. That's the most important rule of any successful plan. But a great diet without an exercise plan is incomplete. Your body needs to be active—both inside and outside the gym. Researchers have found that each 10 percent rise in sedentary time is associated with a 3.1 centimeter increase in the size of your waist. What's more, British scientists found that of the subjects they studied, the waist measurements of people who got up most often were more than 2 inches smaller than those of people who got up the least.

But you need to do more than just use the stairs at your office to blast cellulite and make your body sizzle. *The Women's Health Big Book of Abs* will teach you how to upgrade your workout to the most efficient plan ever created. You'll learn that weight lifting will not make your muscles look bulky—believe me! And how adding just 3 days of resistance training per week is enough to help you eat less and turn your body into a fat-burning machine 24 hours a day, 7 days a week.

Your Fittest Life Starts Here

You'd think that a successful diet and exercise plan would be easier to find. After all, we have more information at our disposal than ever before. But all that information creates a different problem: misinformation—and lots of it. That's why you've found yourself struggling to find the solution. Not anymore. We've done the work for you. We've interviewed the best experts, read all of the research, and found the best way to create real results.

As a bonus, you'll uncover hundreds of additional tips, tricks, and benefits. We've debunked the biggest diet myths, so you'll never veer off track with your eating or exercise. "The Lean Guide to Eating" shopping list (page 40) will make every trip to the grocery store an enjoyable experience. We've even included the most pressing concerns and issues that readers have sent directly to *Women's Health* and included them in the book. It's like having your own personal diet coach answering all of your questions—without the ridiculous cost.

We know that living healthy can seem difficult. We understand that many of you have struggled with your health, whether it's dropping 100 pounds or just trimming the last 10. But no matter who you are or where you're starting from, this book was developed for you. We put our brand behind this title because we know it'll work, using the same winning formula found in the pages of *Women's Health*.

Trust us when we say you'll be more than pleased. You'll eat better, exercise smarter, improve your sex life, and see changes to your overall health. It's the total package. Best of all? When you look in the mirror you'll think, *It's good to be me.*

A Flat Belly for Life

16 INSTANT FIXES THAT WILL
MELT FLAB AND TONE YOUR BODY.

There's one fitness

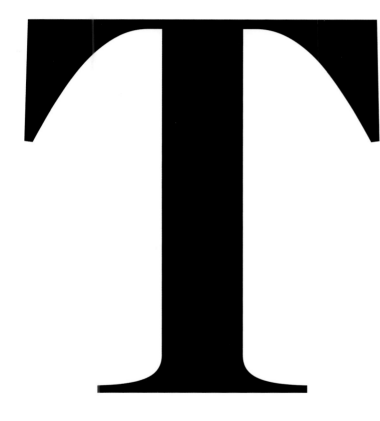

target that's universally understood: abs. No matter how you look at them, a lean, toned midriff represents good health, a fit body, and sex appeal. But flat abs aren't much different than the perfect guy. You want to believe they exist, but no matter what you do to find them, they always elude you! The chase remains, but at some point you start making excuses because of constant roadblocks: bad genetics, a hectic work schedule, Ben & Jerry's Chunky Monkey ice cream. You can let these excuses get the best of you—or you can take control of your destiny. It's easier than you think! Just like finding the perfect partner, the perfect abs are possible once you stop searching so hard for the perfect answer.

A Flat Belly for Life

Just look at Joyce Gochakowski. She struggled for years with her weight. Luckily her weight eventually hit a plateau, but the scale didn't reveal a number she liked. She tried everything from low-carb diets to extreme Spinning classes. Then she tried the program in *The Women's Health Big Book of Abs*. After the initial 4 weeks, she saw noticeable improvement, and in just 6 weeks, she dropped 10 pounds and completely reshaped her body and wardrobe. She changed her approach and saw gains when all hope seemed to be lost.

Like Joyce, you might be trying too hard and overthinking the process. Too many diets and too much exercise have resulted in information overload that probably has you staring wistfully at your skinny jeans, relegated to the back of your closet. It's time to change all of that. Having a great body isn't about making endless sacrifices or following an unbearable plan. It's about understanding how tiny daily changes result in unbelievable transformations. We've seen the overweight become thin, mothers who look great in bikinis, and women who eat, drink, and still shrink.

Sure, some women do seem to be born with a great figure and naturally flat abs. It's about as irritating as those born into megawealth. But you don't have to be born rich to make a lot of money, and you certainly don't need to be born with a six-pack to have a flat stomach and toned abs! Anyone—yes, that includes you—can eliminate their belly and uncover their abs.

The process starts by chucking the misinformation that's been slowing your progress. We're sure you've heard everything by now. Between crunches, planks, weight training, cardio, six-meals-a-day, and weight loss supplements, the process can be overwhelming. So it's time to slow down, hit the Refresh button, and take a new, no-nonsense approach to your body. Just by opening this book, you're well on your way. We've filtered out all the bad information, hunted down the top experts, and compiled only the best tips, tricks, and exercises that will actually help you see your abs.

If you're going to finally transform your body, you're going to need to let go of some previously held beliefs. That starts with your metabolism. No matter how difficult it's been for you to lose weight, your body is not plotting against you. In fact, if you've put on pounds in the last few years, your body is actually working harder to help you become leaner.

Your body is the most sophisticated machine ever created. It burns calories to help you perform all of your daily tasks, like standing up, thinking, and sleeping. This daily maintenance is called your basal metabolic rate (BMR). Everyone has a BMR, but the bigger you are, the faster your metabolism works. Think about that: The more weight you carry, the better your metabolism.

On the surface, it doesn't make sense. After all, skinny people have better metabolisms, right? Well, not exactly. Think about it another way. Say you

THE ABS BENEFIT

57

Percentage by which women with lean bellies are less likely to die of heart disease

have two cars, an Audi and a Hummer. Which needs more fuel? The Hummer does, because it's much larger and has more demands. Your body is no different. The larger you are, the harder your body needs to work and the more calories you burn. Your body wants to be an Audi; you just have to be willing to trade in for a new model.

So how do you become leaner? Surprisingly, it's the small things that really make the biggest differences. And over time, those tiny changes add up to a lean, toned body.

Consider this a refreshing outlook on your transformation: Your metabolism isn't holding you back, and your body isn't hardwired to look a certain way. You can control your ability to lose weight. Simple, small adjustments to your diet, exercise, and other behaviors will make a surprisingly big difference and transform your body.

How easy can it be to see your abs? Here are 15 instant changes you can make that will help your flat belly dreams become a reality.

Sleep more at night
Turns out there's a lot of truth to the term beauty sleep. That's because researchers from Harvard University studied more than 68,000 women and found that those who sleep less than 6 hours a night weighed 5.4 pounds more and were 15 percent more likely to be overweight than those who slept more than 7 hours a night. The weight gain is no coincidence: When you sleep less,

you experience a drop in the hormone leptin, which controls your appetite, and an increase in the hormone ghrelin—which forces you to reach for more food. The result: Those who sleep less eat an average of 220 more calories per day, say researchers from the University of Chicago. What's more, researchers from the Netherlands found that women who were sleep deprived were rated as less attractive and less healthy looking by random observers.

QUICK FIX #1: Want to eat less and look better? Aim for 8 hours a night and don't allow yourself to sleep for less than 7.

Eat the way YOU want
For the past decade, you've heard that you need 5 or 6 meals per day for fat loss. The rationale was simple: When you eat, your body requires energy to burn away the calories from your favorite meals. So the reasoning went that more meals would equal more calories burned. Only one problem—it's not how frequently you eat, but rather what you eat that impacts how many calories you'll burn during mealtime. So if you consume 2,000 calories in a day, it doesn't matter if it's in three, six, or 20 meals. You'll burn the same amount of calories, assuming that the foods you eat are the same.

QUICK FIX #2: There's no need to feel forced to eat more or less frequently. In an attempt to burn more calories, you might have been accidently overeating and sabotaging your weight loss goals. With the diet plan in The Women's Health Big Book of Abs, you'll

THE ABS BENEFIT
40
Percentage by which women are less likely to die of cancer when they are at a healthy weight

understand what you need to eat. Then it's up to you to decide the times and frequency that work best.

Snack smarter

While the number of meals you consume doesn't matter, the size of your snacks do. According to Purdue University researchers, the biggest problem with our snacking behavior is that snacks have become meals, and meals have become feasts. In the last 30 years, snack sizes have increased from 360 to 580 calories. That's a whopping 220 extra calories per snack. And when you consider that the average woman snacks twice a day during the workday, you're looking at almost 500 extra calories per day. That number might seem innocent enough in isolation, but so does online shopping. Just as your credit card bill can skyrocket during a few sessions of retail therapy, so can your waistline. In just 2 weeks, your oversize healthy snacks can contribute to an extra pound of fat.

QUICK FIX #3: Enjoy your food, but do it wisely. The lean, nutritious snacks in the meal plan will help you crush your cravings and whittle down your waist.

Eat more, drink less

Want to instantly drop a dress size? Conduct a quick inventory of what you eat and drink every day, and then remove all of the beverages not named water. Now add up the calories. If you're like most women, you'll find that you can cut your nonmeal calories by more than

50 percent, according to the *American Journal of Clinical Nutrition*. In fact, 65 percent of Americans indulge daily in calorie-rich beverages, and those drinks are oftentimes the real culprit behind your weight loss struggles—not your metabolism.

QUICK FIX #4: Stick to water, coffee (watch the creamers), teas, and calorie-free drinks to help keep your slim-down plan on track. And remember that any sugar drink—whether it's soda or a fruit juice—should be considered the equivalent of a dessert.

Lift weights more often

The calorie tracker on the elliptical might make running seem like a fat loss genie, but all is not as it seems. That's because the more miles you log, the more efficient your body becomes at running and the fewer calories it burns. In other words, running may initially help you drop some pounds, but your progress will flatline as soon as your body adjusts to your exercise regimen. Plus, running long distances on a regular basis takes a physical toll (in the form of injuries, like runner's knee), which can seriously dampen your enthusiasm. Ultimately, all that pain and boredom can cause many people to burn out and give up.

Enter weight training. Pumping iron isn't just for the boys. Just three days a week of resistance training will keep you burning calories and will offer the metabolic boost you need to slash fat and look hot in whatever outfit you choose.

QUICK FIX #5: Head to the gym three times

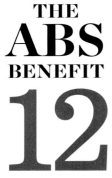

THE
ABS
BENEFIT
12

Percentage by which women are less likely to have a stroke when they lower their body fat

a week—but don't make the cardio room your first priority. Instead, use The Abs Workout in Chapter 7 to put your body on the fast track to rapid fat loss.

Lift heavier weights

Not only should you be lifting weights, you should also be focusing on the larger dumbbells. That's because researchers at Washington University School of Medicine in St. Louis discovered that the more iron you lift, the more fat you burn. Once again, this isn't just a man's world! Women definitely benefit from lifting more. In fact, the researchers found that heavy weights burn more calories during your workout and then increase your sleeping metabolism by 8 percent. That's right. You burn more calories just by lying on your back and pressing the snooze button. That 8 percent isn't much on a daily basis, but it can add up to more than 5 pounds a year.

QUICK FIX #6: When you perform The Abs Workout, don't be afraid to use bigger weights as you get more comfortable and improve your strength. Each time you reach the goal rep range, increase the weights by 5 pounds. As you'll discover in Chapter 2, your hormones will prevent you from becoming big and bulky, and those heavier weights will only help you sculpt gorgeous, lean muscle.

Eat more fish (oil)

There's nothing fishy about fish oil, especially when it comes to your lean body goals. Pennsylvania researchers found that omega-3 fatty acids might be the secret ingredient to burning fat and gaining muscle at the same time. The scientists believe that omega-3s help fight against cortisol—the stress your body produces that makes it easier for you to store fat. By shutting down your cortisol production, you keep the extra weight off your hips, thighs, and stomach, and have an easier time adding lean, calorie-shredding muscle.

QUICK FIX #7: Take fish oil daily, whether it's by a supplement or a whole food source like salmon or sardines. Alan Aragon, MS, a *Women's Health* nutrition advisor, recommends 2 to 3 grams of fish oil per day.

Load up on protein

Every time you eat a meal and don't consume protein, you're telling your body that you don't want to tighten your tummy and firm your tush. Here's why: When you eat other foods—especially carbohydrates—you stimulate insulin, which spikes your blood sugar and makes it easier for you to pack on the pounds. Even so-called "innocent" healthy foods can be dangerous, like a piece of fruit. But protein is your nutrition solution. It controls your blood sugar, keeps you fuller, reduces hunger, and burns more calories during the digestion process so you can stay lean and fit and still enjoy your favorite foods.

QUICK FIX #8: Carbohydrates are not bad. Neither are fats. But when you eat them alone, they set off a series of events that can sabotage your healthy eating habits. So whether you're snacking or eating a meal, include some protein and you'll drop sizes and defeat stress.

WEIGHTS VS. MACHINES— WHICH IS BETTER?

The gym can be a confusing experience—and we're not just talking about the grunting men in tank tops. Your local facility isn't necessarily designed for success. That's because most gyms are filled with machines. And while you can experience a great workout hitting the latest machine circuit, it's an inefficient and dangerous way to exercise, say Drake University researchers. While it's true that you can use more weight with machines, you'll experience greater muscle activation with free weights. You see, free weights work your body harder with less weight. That means you can have a better, more efficient workout, without putting unnecessary stress on your body. Your best path is to use dumbbells and your own bodyweight in exercises, to get back in shape.

A Flat Belly for Life

Don't fear the fat

If science has proved anything during the last 10 years, it's that eating fat helps you become slim. In fact, the Institute of Medicine recommends that fatty foods make up 20 to 35 percent of your total calories. This, of course, isn't an invitation to head over to the nearest fast-food joint. The fats you want to include in your diet are primarily saturated fats—from milk, red meat, and pork products—and monounsaturated fats (MUFAs) like nuts, avocados, and healthy oils.

A report published in the *British Journal of Nutrition* found that a MUFA-rich diet helped people lose small amounts of weight and body fat without changing their calorie intakes. Another report found that a breakfast high in MUFAs could boost calorie burn for 5 hours after the meal, particularly in people with higher amounts of belly fat. What's more, dieters who took a high-fat approach needed 25 fewer days to lose 10 pounds than those who used a high-carb approach, according to researchers at Johns Hopkins. And that was on a diet of 30 percent fat!

QUICK FIX #9: Fat is your friend! As long as you are staying away from fried foods, trans fats, and partially hydrogenated oils, the healthy fats you eat will make you leaner. Still not sure what to eat? Here are 5 fatty foods that are good for your body:

- **Beef (top round and sirloin)**
- **Pork**
- **Eggs (including the yolks)**
- **Sour cream**
- **Cheese (full fat or low-fat)**

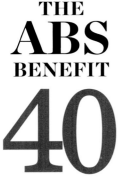

THE
ABS
BENEFIT
40

Percentage by which women are less likely to develop arthritis of the hips or knees when they have less belly fat

Want more options? Be sure to check out "The Lean Guide to Eating" shopping list (page 40).

Eat real foods

Despite their low-calorie, low-carb, or low-fat claims, the "diet" foods at your grocery store might be the worst thing for your body if you're trying to lose weight. The reason is quite simple: Diet foods try to trick your brain. They provide you with the taste of a high-calorie meal without all the calories but are filled with chemicals, artificial sweeteners, and preservatives. Unfortunately, your brain isn't fooled, and it leaves you craving more food, which causes you to overeat. Diet foods are also usually devoid of any nutritional benefits. So not only are you gaining weight, you're also depriving your body of the necessary nutrients that protect your general health. Even worse, diet sodas and artificial sugars may increase your risk for metabolic syndrome, which includes higher levels of belly fat, blood sugar, and cholesterol, according to scientists at the University of Minnesota.

QUICK FIX #10: Stick to whole, unprocessed foods. As a general guideline, try to shop around the perimeter of your grocery store. That's where you'll find more fresh produce and fewer prepackaged items. For all your shopping needs, use "The Lean Guide to Eating" shopping list (page 40).

Enjoy your food!

It's not just what you eat—the way you eat might be the best way to curb your hunger.

Eating fast makes you gain weight, according to Japanese researchers. In their study, they found that people who ate faster gained more weight than those who didn't. But if you want to flip the switch on your insatiable appetite, all you need to do is slow down and enjoy. It takes your stomach about 20 minutes to process food and then signal to your brain that you're full. The slower approach will not only leave you more satisfied, but will also help you eat less food, say University of Rhode Island researchers.

QUICK FIX #11: We don't expect you to bring a timer to your meals, so instead focus on how much you chew your food. Chewing releases more flavor to your tastebuds, which will make all of your meals more savory and enjoyable. The more you chew, the longer it'll take you to eat and the more full you'll feel. Plus it's a much nicer, calmer ritual to actually enjoy your food instead of gulping it down in one bite!

Worry less, eat less

Take a deep breath before you head into the kitchen to cook your next meal. As you know, the more stressed-out you are, the more comfort food you crave. But now scientists have figured out why: Stress activates ghrelin, a hormone that makes you feel hungry. When you're stressed before you eat, it alters the levels of dopamine, suggest researchers from the University of Texas Southwestern Medical Center. The result: You don't achieve satisfaction from your meal, which leaves you craving more food.

QUICK FIX #12: While a stressful day may feel impossible to overcome, the stress in your body is like a light switch: It turns on and off very easily. Simply find a distraction that calms you down—watch TV, listen to music, call a friend—and within 5 to 10 minutes, your stress levels will decrease so you can enjoy your meal, without doubling back for more.

Enjoy dessert

Go ahead, treat yourself—keep it small and frequent. When you're trying to lose weight, the worst thing you can do is ban all indulgences, which creates a feeling of withdrawal. German researchers discovered that this mentality makes it harder to stick to a plan and more likely to pack on the pounds. A more effective approach is one that allows you to satisfy your cravings in controlled portions. Recent research from the University of Alabama found that when overweight women ate small desserts four times a week, they lost 9 more pounds than those who enjoyed a larger splurge whenever they wanted. The small sweets provide the psychological edge that allows you to stay motivated, without derailing your eating plan.

QUICK FIX #13: Within any diet, 10 to 20 percent of your calories can be directed toward a little treat, says nutritionist Alan Aragon. The key is watching the portion size, so that a cup of ice cream doesn't turn into an entire bowl. You'll learn more about how to make dessert a regular part of your diet in Chapter 4.

Eat with your gym crew

People who work out together should dine together. Eating with those who

THE ABS BENEFIT

69

Percentage of decrease in development of type 2 diabetes when you have lower body fat

A Flat Belly for Life

have a similar goal helps you lose pounds faster, according to a study in the journal *Obesity*. Once again, it's all mental. When you're with people who are also trying to lose weight, the social expectation creates a different attitude toward food (for example, you won't have to worry that everyone will be ordering chocolate lava cake for dessert!). It's like weight loss osmosis. The good intentions of your fellow eaters rub off on you, and it makes the entire dietary process easier, say scientists in Rhode Island.

QUICK FIX #14: **Go out to eat but only with the right crowd! Try to make plans with buddies on a similar track to weight loss success. Reward yourself with a trip to a fun new restaurant, with those who will encourage you to make the right menu choices.**

Shake up your diet

The stuff you see in the window of your local GNC isn't just for jocks or serious weight lifters. Those big jars of protein powder can actually help you flatten your belly. While the appearance might be intimidating, it's exactly what your body desires: an efficient source of protein that is low in calories, helps maintain your hard-earned long and lean muscle, and helps you lose more fat and not just pounds. The most efficient kind of protein is whey. According to a study in the *Journal of Nutrition*, participants who took whey protein for 23 weeks had less body fat and a smaller waist than those who consumed soy protein. In fact, dieters who included whey protein in their eating plan doubled their fat loss

compared to those who ate the same number of calories but didn't drink any shakes. Consider protein powder the little bit of extra magic that will finally reveal your abs.

QUICK FIX #15: **Include a whey protein shake once a day or at least a few times a week. But don't feel that you can only have a shake before or after your workout. You can also substitute a shake for breakfast or a snack. Just make sure that shakes are always a secondary option to whole food sources. You'll find some great shake recipes in Chapter 5.**

If these changes seem a little too easy, it's because having the body you've always wanted isn't as unrealistic as you've been led to believe. The real key to a successful diet and exercise plan is cracking the consistency code. Once you find a way to turn these small changes into an overall lifestyle, that's when the fun begins. You'll eat more, curb hunger, and finally start whittling your waist down to a sexy, slim silhouette. Forget high-priced personal trainers and controlling nutritionists. Let *The Women's Health Big Book of Abs* be your coach to your best body ever. Your life-changing journey begins here.

Wake Up to Coffee

This might come as a surprise, but the *least* beneficial aspect of your morning cup of coffee is its ability to provide a sudden jolt and make you more alert. When it comes to improving your health, there are few foods or drinks that offer

---

THE ABS BENEFIT

21

Percentage by which women are less likely to experience arousal dysfunction when they exercise

more universal benefits. The jack-of-all-trades has been shown to improve your workouts by allowing you to push longer and harder and fight off fatigue. But that's just scratching the surface.

Coffee actually contains more antioxidants than most fruits and vegetables, and that helps you fight against the aging process. Harvard researchers also found that the magical bean can lower the likelihood of depression by triggering neurotransmitters in your brain that elevate your mood. What's more, women who drink coffee every day reduce their risk of skin cancer by more than 20 percent. To top it all off, research published in the *Archives of Internal Medicine* found that daily coffee consumption decreases the likelihood of type 2 diabetes, and the American Heart Association reported that coffee reduces the risk of having a stroke by up to 25 percent. All of which is to say, the smartest—and healthiest—way to wake up is with some coffee in your cup.

QUICK FIX #16: **Go ahead and pour yourself a cup of coffee each morning. But don't feel limited to just one serving. Harvard researchers found that the sweet spot is actually 2 to 3 cups for the most benefits, and the American Heart Association noted that up to 5 cups of coffee can still help your health—assuming you can handle all the caffeine. If you don't like the buzz, you can still experience all the positives of coffee in the decaf version.**

All of Your Questions Answered

THE WORST FOODS FOR YOUR ABS,
THE TRUTH ABOUT ARTIFICIAL SWEETENERS,
AND THE FASTEST WAY
TO FIT INTO YOUR SKINNY JEANS.

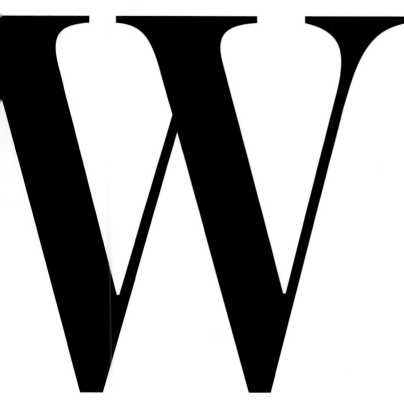

What's the fastest way

to lose weight?"

It's the one question that is asked repeatedly at *Women's Health*, and for good reason. For many women, the answer seems like a puzzle. Whether you're an apple or a pear, it can feel very frustrating trying to find the right program for you. But no matter which fruit you identify with, the right program should empower you to successfully drop excess weight, look great in your clothes, and feel confident about your reflection in the mirror.

The truth is, there's no one "fastest" way. It really depends on your lifestyle, food preferences, and how often you make health a priority. The simple answer is a combination of diet and exercise, but that's the type of answer that has frustrated you in the past.

All of Your Questions Answered

Here's what you need to know for your future: You deserve to lose weight. You work hard, and you should reap the rewards. So savor this answer: Anyone can eliminate their belly and jump onto the body transformation highway. Even better? The road isn't as bumpy as you think, but it does require a few changes, and requires you to throw out some old tricks and habits. To put you on a fast track to a flatter belly, we posed the most common abs-related questions to the *Women's Health* fitness and nutrition experts. They're here to eliminate your confusion, end your frustration, and provide a perfect road map to looking and feeling better now. These aren't just answers—they are the secrets you need to banish your former body and replace it with the one you've always wanted.

I'm losing pounds but not inches. What's wrong?

Usually this means you're not weight training or eating enough protein, says Alan Aragon, MS, a nutritionist in Westlake Village, California. Doing both is the key to eliminating fat and building muscle—as opposed to just losing weight. That's the real key to looking like you have a new body, rather than just seeing a different number on the scale. Resistance training burns calories during your sessions and stimulates your metabolism afterward. Make sure you get enough protein after a workout by adding either 6 additional ounces of meat or 2 scoops of protein powder; each option yields about 40 grams of protein.

How often do I need to exercise to lose fat?

It might sound surprising, but you don't *need* to exercise to lose fat. You can shed your unwanted pounds by making sure you eat fewer calories than you burn, says Aragon. (This should show you the importance of a good diet.)

However, if you avoid exercise, **y**ou won't retain as much muscle, which means it'll be harder for you eliminate your muffin top and have flat, sexy abs. You can lose weight without exercise, but if you don't retain or build muscle, your metabolism won't be as efficient, which means you'll have to eat even *less* food to see the same results.

So how much exercise should be done to help with fat loss? Take note, gym haters, it's really not that huge of a commitment. With just 30 minutes a day, 3 days a week, you can eat the foods you want and fast-track your weight loss. You'll find all the exercises you need starting in Chapter 7.

Do I need to count calories?

Counting calories is mainly a way of staying consistent with an eating plan that will allow you to lose weight, says Aragon. But that doesn't mean you need to do it to be effective. In fact, we've created a no-calorie counting method that sparks fat loss. The foods in this diet are flexible so that you can choose your meals. But they also focus on foods that are energy dense, such as protein-filled foods, fruits, vegetables, and grains. You'll be able to eat more of these foods and feel full without expanding your waistline. You'll eat better, and, without realizing it, you'll be dropping pounds, too.

Do carbs give you a belly?

In a word, no. Your belly is formed by eating too many unused calories. If you overeat, you'll store fat, regardless of where those calories are coming from, says Aragon. French and Swedish researchers have examined many different populations, including Asian countries, New Guinea, Uganda, and Northern Cameroon. The leanest and healthiest populations typically eat more carbs than protein or fat. Controlling weight gain is more about total calorie balance than any particular food. With that said, some people find it easier to control their weight when they reduce or avoid carb-heavy foods that they have a tendency to overindulge in, adds Aragon. But if you can control your intake, enjoy the carbs. The best way to prevent overeating is to make sure most of your carbs come from raw fruits and vegetables, while leaving a minor proportion for desserts.

Are protein shakes only for men?

No way! Don't be fooled by the big-muscle guys pictured on protein containers. Women can absolutely benefit from protein shakes, especially if they have a tough time hitting their protein requirement through regular whole foods. There's nothing sex-specific about protein shakes—but I bet you'll feel a whole lot sexier after incorporating them into your plan and seeing the results.

Will eating smaller meals control my hunger?

Your meals are like your fashion sense: It's all personal preference. Some people do great with a grazing pattern, while others prefer more substantial meals with less frequency. But there's a catch: When people are eating fewer calories than they're used to, they tend to prefer eating two to three larger meals rather than four to six small ones throughout the day, says Aragon. As for more frequent meals being better for your metabolism? That's just a myth that's been recently disproved by science. Canadian researchers proved this in 2010 when they compared three meals versus six meals.

How do I know what fat is okay to eat?

There's no need to avoid any particular type of fat, except for partially hydrogenated vegetable oils, which contain the harmful type of trans fat. Recent research has shown that saturated fat is actually good for you and isn't linked to heart failure or cardiovascular disease, says Aragon.

In fact, your diet probably doesn't include enough fat. The standard American diet lacks omega-3 fatty acids, which can be found in fish like salmon and sardines. Aside from that, the majority of the fats you eat should come from whole, minimally processed foods

All of Your Questions Answered

like meats, dairy, eggs, vegetables, fruits, nuts, seeds, avocados, grains, and olive oil.

Should I take supplements to see my abs?

Most fat loss supplements are a waste of money, and most of them have risks that outweigh the small edge toward the goal of fat loss, says Aragon. The most potent fat loss supplements contained caffeine and ephedrine, but that combination was banned from the market due to too many reports of adverse, dangerous effects. The truth is, the actual fat loss caused by any supplement is minor and is even *less* significant in people who are overweight or have a substantial amount of weight to lose, says Aragon. Bottom line: The best and only real way to see your abs is to focus on two things: what you eat and how you exercise.

Can I just do cardio, or do I need to lift weights to see my abs?

We can't stress this enough: Lifting a little bit of iron isn't just for the boys. When you add resistance training to your routine, it can speed up the weight loss process by making your muscles more efficient fat-burning furnaces, says Aragon. What's more, it's also good for your bone health and cardiovascular health, as well as optimizing glucose control so your body processes carbohydrates better. Plus, in addition to flattening and sculpting your abs, you'll gain definition in your arms and legs. Imagine yourself slipping on a little black dress and turning heads all night. Can you think of better motivation to pick up a dumbbell?

Can I have dairy and still lose my belly?

There's nothing wrong with a little moo juice. In fact, researchers from the University of Tennessee found that dairy might help the loss of belly fat when you're on a diet. You can even enjoy higher-fat cheeses and yogurts if you prefer. The trick is, make sure you don't eat too much. Cheese and milk are both high in calories, so keep a close eye on your portion size—and enjoy!

What are the worst foods for your abs?

Your focus shouldn't be on the worst, but instead on what's best. A great diet—like the one you'll find in this book—highlights the healthy, nutritious foods that make dropping pounds as effortless as texting. It's impossible to judge foods in isolation from the rest of your diet. What matters most for shedding belly fat boils down to calories in versus calories out. It might be tempting to call a certain food, like a candy bar, "bad" for your abs. But if that candy bar is part of a diet that's dominated by whole and minimally processed foods, it could actually be "great" for your abs. Those small indulgences are often what helps you adhere to your program. This is why cheat meals actually work: Virtually no foods are off-limits as long as they're a small portion of what you eat.

I sit at a desk all day. Is there anything that I can do at work to improve my abs?

Get up from your desk as often as you can. A minimum of every half hour, try to at least stand up and stretch, then walk around, take a trip to the restroom, or take a lap around the office, says Aragon. This process is important because it increases your non-exercise activity thermogenesis (NEAT). Your NEAT plays a big role in the number of calories you burn, so even small movements like fidgeting or tapping your heels can contribute to your overall transformation. This will also help prevent your desk job from altering your posture, which can play a role in your slowed metabolism (not to mention an aching back!).

Won't gaining muscle make me look bulky?

Weight training can be very deceiving. When you see men lifting huge, heavy dumbbells, it's easy to assume that's the reason why their muscles are popping out of their T-shirts. But you have to understand that it's tremendously challenging for women to gain muscle like a man, says Eric Cressey, MA, CSCS, strength coach, and owner of Cressey Performance in Hudson, Massachusetts. The reason: Women have far less testosterone than men, which makes it an uphill battle to add significant muscle mass, let alone enough size to make you look bulky. That alone is enough reason to not worry about any negative impact of pumping a little iron. What's more,

putting on major muscle mass is a struggle for many women because it takes a high volume of strength training in combination with lots of extra calories. On this plan, you'll be eating just the right amount of calories and doing just the right amount of reps to achieve long, lean muscles—not a bulky, bodybuilder bod.

Is it okay to have artificial sweeteners?

This is an area of big debate among nutritionists, but there's no scientific evidence that artificial sweeteners make you fat. That said, make sure you don't abuse diet soft drinks, which are filled with fake sugars, says Aragon. As a good rule of thumb, you should limit your intake of artificial sweeteners to 3 to 4 servings per day at most, whether it's from a diet soft drink or some other artificially sweetened product. If your diet consists mainly of real foods, you can enjoy a little sugar, whether it's artificial or not!

Isn't running the fastest way to lose weight?

Running is a great form of exercise, and it can be very good for your overall cardiovascular health. But the way that most women approach running— with long, slow jogs—is not an efficient way to blast away your fat, says Cressey. If running is your preferred form of exercise, then stick to interval training. This form of exercise has you working at a high level of intensity for short periods

All of Your Questions Answered

of time, followed by quick rest periods. Overall, your cardio workouts will be shorter but much more effective.

However, if you want to shed pounds fast, you'll want to spend the bulk of your exercise time performing resistance training. As we already mentioned, lifting weights won't make you bulky (promise!), but it will give you great definition and shape. And adding that lean muscle tone helps you burn more calories, even when you're not exercising. Bottom line: Resistance training doesn't just take body fat off—it keeps it off.

Can I get flat abs without doing any crunches?

You want to lose belly fat as fast as possible, right? In order to do that, you need exercises that activate the most number of muscle fibers, says Cressey. Crunches simply don't cut it. When you perform multi-muscle and multi-joint exercises, you're actually working your abs whether you realize it or not. This is why movements like squats, deadlifts, lunges, chinups, and pushups are so effective. They work the muscles you feel (legs, arms, chest, back, shoulders) and your abs simultaneously. Any workout that incorporates these moves will keep your core working overtime and ensure that you'll see a flat belly in no time.

These compound exercises allow you to do more in less time. They stimulate greater fat loss, and they also carry over to a healthier overall lifestyle. Whether it's picking up a toddler or reaching to put something up on the top

shelf, compound movements prepare you for what life throws your way. And a little bit of strength goes a long way in making your life easier, such as preventing nagging issues—like throwing out your back or having sore knees— that occur naturally when you avoid these types of exercises. These exercises will create such incredible changes to your body that you'll not only be happy with your newfound strength, you'll also be thrilled every time you walk past a mirror.

I've been told not to eat late, but usually I'm starving after my shift. What should I do?

Your body isn't on a 24-hour clock. What counts is whether you burn more calories than you ingest by the end of the day (or better yet, the week), says Aragon. If your cravings surface at night, any combination of fruit, nuts, nut butter, or dairy (such as milk, yogurt, or cheese) makes a perfect pre-bed snack.

If I sit on an exercise ball instead of a chair at my office, will I lose weight?

Sitting on a ball might help strengthen your core, but it won't help you shed significant calories. The misconception comes, in part, from studies on non-exercise activity. Fidgeting, a common example, is often cited as a way to help burn extra calories. Mayo Clinic researchers found a significant increase in energy expenditure if you fidget while standing. But that effect is not as pronounced if you fidget while seated, says Aragon. So any difference between ball sitting and chair sitting is probably too small to have a real impact. But there are other little ways to move around that do keep you more active: walking over to a co-worker's desk instead of e-mailing, standing up while talking on the phone, or just taking a brief lap around your office every so often.

I always gorge after a workout. Bad habit?

Postworkout is actually the best time to have the largest meal of your day—as long as it's a reasonable size and not a full-on gorge. That's because you've just reduced your body's fuel reserves, and food can help aid your recovery. Also, when your body is in a recovery state, incoming calories and nutrients stand a better chance of being absorbed by muscle tissue instead of being stored in fat tissue.

If your goal is to curb uncontrollable hunger after a workout, make sure you're filling up on beef, poultry, or fish. Solid foods are more filling than liquid foods, and protein is the most filling of all. Pair some of that meat with whole food, high-fiber carbohydrate sources, such as beans, because fiber can also help you feel fuller faster.

I love pasta. Will it be impossible for me to lose weight?

Believe it or not, you can eat carbs and still drop pounds with ease. As you'll find out, every food is fair game on the eating plan you'll use in this book. But there are exceptions to every rule, and eating plate after plate of pasta is a recipe for disaster for anyone. Your easy fix? Try spaghetti squash, which has almost the same consistency as the traditional Italian fare, but with only a fraction of the calories. (We promise, you will be *shocked* how good this tastes).

Just cut the squash in half and microwave for 6 to 8 minutes. Then, use a fork and run it through the squash—from top to bottom—to create spaghetti-like strands. Add a sauce or some veggies or meatballs, serve and enjoy.

What's the fastest way to jump-start my weight loss?

Eat more food. Seriously—but make sure your selections are more nutrient-dense foods that will leave you more satisfied with fewer calories. A great example of this is a technique known as carb-swapping, says Aragon. The process is simple: Replace any processed food you eat (think rice, pasta, and bread) with fruits and vegetables. While there's nothing wrong with those original foods, they tend to be higher in calories and don't leave you satisfied, which means you're forced to eat more than you probably want.

That's why fruits and vegetables are the perfect speedy weight loss replacement. These natural foods are not only filled with vitamins and minerals, they're also lower in calories. That means you can eat more without overindulging. What's more, fruits and vegetables are

All of Your Questions Answered

also loaded with belly-filling fiber that will keep you satisfied longer and fight off your hunger pangs. And the sugar in fruit will satisfy your sweet tooth, without impacting your insulin levels and thus avoiding fat storage.

Three Abs Myths, Busted

If you listened to all the flawed abs advice out there, you'd be doing upside-down crunches until you passed out. After all, some people tell you to do crunches, some say planks, and others insist that you avoid them entirely. The truth is, there's a place for almost every type of abdominal training, but not all of them will help you look great in a bikini. Here's the truth about how you can make the most of every rep.

Myth #1: High-rep workouts make your abs grow.

Reality: Your progress will plateau if you do the same exercises, regardless of reps.

You need to intensify your workouts to teach your abs to stabilize your body-weight. Add either one of the following: more challenging variations of body-weight exercises, or weighted abdominal exercises once the unweighted versions become too easy. Matt McGorry, CFT, a trainer at Peak Performance in New York City, recommends the triple plank. This combo—a front plank followed by a left-side plank and a right-side plank—forces you to contract your abs for long intervals, which helps carve your mid-section. Start by maintaining each plank for 15 seconds and work up to 60 seconds. When you hit that level, start adding sets, resting only 30 seconds between them. If planks on the floor are too easy, put your feet on a small box.

But don't forget: "No amount of abs work can take the place of a well-planned diet and a total-body workout," McGorry says. Abs won't magically appear as you work out; they show when you've built all the muscles in your body and cut the fat around your midsection.

Myth #2: Abs workouts involve a lot of movement.

Reality: Exercises that require steadiness are best.

When you bend your spine during crunches or situps, you risk injuring it, says Stuart McGill, PhD, a professor of spine biomechanics at the University of Waterloo in Ontario. Doing those exercises isn't the best way to target your abs anyway, because you're really just repeatedly bending the disks in your back, not forcing your abs to resist motion. That's why McGill suggests exercises that encourage spinal alignment and stability, such as planks. Your abs do all the work to keep you stabilized *and* lower your risk of back injury. (If you have back pain, see a physician before starting any abs regimen. Some abs exercises can make back problems worse.)

Exercises that prevent movement are especially good for building lateral abdominal strength, which is what helps your body stay in proper form under pressure (like when you play sports or do squats and deadlifts). McGill suggests the suitcase carry: Hold a heavy dumbbell in one hand and then walk increasingly long distances while maintaining perfect posture. This actually burns more calories than crunches do—and isn't nearly as tedious!

Myth #3: Rotational exercises are best for building your obliques.

Reality: Rotational exercises don't build obliques well at all, and can harm the spine in some cases.

Your obliques surround and accentuate your abs and protect them from damage when you rotate your body quickly. So while exercises like twisting side to side while holding a weight can help you build your obliques, they may not be the best way to build foundational strength, and they can force your spine to rotate under stress, says McGorry.

Instead, use heavy compound exercises—like squats and deadlifts—to make your obliques work harder to keep your spine aligned. For more challenge, add unbalanced moves such as the single-leg lunge or a deadlift with one dumbbell. These types of exercises require your body to adjust to uneven stress while your spine is in its neutral position, which further stabilizes your core and builds your obliques (as long as you maintain proper form).

■

The World's Greatest 4-Week Diet and Exercise Plan

THE NEW WEIGHT LOSS RULES THAT WORK.

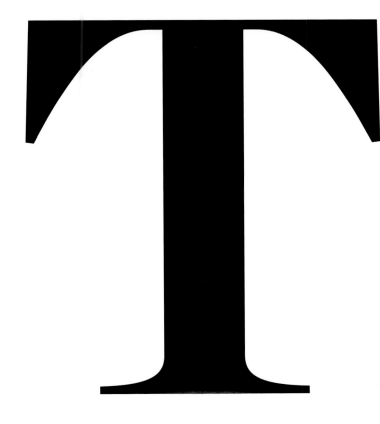

The fix to all of your dieting woes can be solved in three words: Stop counting calories. That was the message of a 20-year study on weight loss conducted at the Harvard School of Public Health. The researchers concluded that dieters who only focused on how much they ate—rather than the types of foods they consumed—were more likely to fail at losing weight.

The reason: Counting calories isn't sustainable and causes stress, which increases the likelihood of long-term failure. That's not to say that counting calories doesn't work. It does. In fact, it's so effective that a Kansas State University professor proved that by counting calories, he could eat a diet consisting of Twinkies and chips and still lose 27 pounds—in just 2 months! (Take that, Slim-Fast!)

The World's Greatest 4-Week Diet and Exercise Plan

The experiment showed that how much food you consume is still the most important factor in the weight loss equation. It also proved that any food—if you can call Twinkies food—can be part of a weight loss plan. And while the empty-calorie diet might leave you feeling full, it won't help you live longer or improve your skin, hair, or nails (see "The Truth about Processed Foods" on page 32). Your goal isn't to minimize how much food you eat. It's to make sure you're filling your body with quality foods that will help you lose weight.

Even though the numbers game works, it's not something that easily fits in to your lifestyle. You don't need scientists at Harvard to tell you that counting calories is more annoying than Joan Rivers. And we know that studying nutrition labels and carrying a scale to every meal isn't exactly great for your social life. Knowing what to eat should be simple and shouldn't create any stress. So, we devised a series of simple rules that offer all the benefits of counting calories—without the math!

If you want to experience success like never before, all you have to do is make these four simple rules your mantra. They're specifically created to blast fat, let you enjoy food without the guilt, and help you look and feel younger than ever. Say them out loud a few times. Learn them by heart. They are the "Lessons of the Lean." And pretty soon they'll become as much a part of your daily routine as checking out your hot new reflection in the mirror!

"I will not be afraid of lifting weights!"

When it comes to weight loss, you can't out-exercise a bad diet. But when you combine the best workout strategies with good eating habits, you can transform your body in ways you never thought imaginable. Since the beginning of time, cardio has been touted as the best way for women to strip away pounds. The weight room was for only guys (and for women who look like Russian powerlifters). Problem is, while running on the treadmill might burn a lot of calories, it's *not* the most efficient way to burn fat. If your goal is to tighten your tummy and firm up your legs and tush, fat loss—not just the number on the scale—is what really matters. And for maximum fat loss, lifting weights is the only way to go.

Need proof? Scientists at the University of Connecticut found that dieters who lifted weights lost nearly 40 percent more fat than those who did traditional cardio, even though the total amount of exercise time was the same. Here's why: Weight training keeps your internal furnace burning for days after you complete your last rep. According to the National Center of Health Statistics, just three sessions a week of strength training can reduce your body fat by 3 percent in just 10 weeks—even if you don't change anything in your diet. It might not seem like much, but that can translate to 3 inches off your hips and waist. What's more, your new muscle will literally transform your body into a fat-burning furnace. A study in *Medicine & Science in Sports & Exercise* found that after 6 months of lifting weights—just 3 days a week—the participants boosted their metabolism by 7 percent.

To really understand the body-transforming impact of weight training, consider this groundbreaking study in *The Journal of Strength and Conditioning Research*. Researchers found that women who completed strength training programs—like the one you'll find in this book—burned an average of 100 more calories in the 24 hours after their workout than they did when they hadn't lifted weights. At three sessions a week, that's 15,600 calories a year, or more than 4 pounds of fat—without having to move a muscle. (It doesn't even count the hundreds of calories you scorch *during* your exercise routine.) That means you're losing weight just sitting around doing nothing! That's something that even the longest run or most restrictive diet can't offer.

Of course, that should be reason enough to pick up a dumbbell. But the benefits of weight training are even sweeter: Not only do you have to work out fewer times per week (we'll recommend a minimum of three times), you also have shorter sessions. That's because intensity is much more important than duration for eliminating fat. So you can spend a fraction of the time in the gym and still kiss your tummy good-bye. In fact, 8 to 12 minutes of intense intervals can burn as many calories as 25 to 30 minutes of constant moderate

exertion exercise. Don't be surprised when you abandon the cardio machines, pick up a few dumbbells, and suddenly find yourself sexier than ever.

These facts are simple, so you might be wondering why cardio has remained so popular. The reason is that the gym is filled with liars. You know them better as the treadmill, elliptical, and stairclimber. While these machines are great forms of exercise, they make you feel like you're working harder than you are. Canadian researchers discovered that cardio machines can significantly overestimate your caloric burn—sometimes by hundreds of calories.

Right now, you might be thinking, "Why run?" If you enjoy it, that's reason enough. Traditional cardio is still good for your body and your heart, and it does burn calories. So if you have time, you can make it a part of your workout routine. In fact, we recommend it! (Of course, if you're training for a marathon or are active in sports, your plan will require more cardio than others.) But if you're tight on time (and we know you are), and you want the most bang for your workout buck, then weight training should always be your priority. Think of your exercise as a prioritized list: As long as weight training is at the top and *always* crossed off, you'll be one step closer to your new body.

We recommend that you lift weights 3 days a week, which will work your muscles, stoke your metabolism, and give you the body you want faster than ever. Researchers at Ball State

The World's Greatest 4-Week Diet and Exercise Plan

IGNITE YOUR WEIGHT LOSS

Science shows that it's not *how* often you eat but *what* you eat that makes the biggest difference. And as long as you're fueling up with the right foods, your metabolism doesn't know the difference between three meals or six in a day. The best plan of attack is to find what works for you. If you want six meals one day and three the next, go for it! As long as your choices are in line with the Lessons of the Lean, eat as frequently—or infrequently—as you'd like.

In this plan, you'll eat three main meals per day (breakfast, lunch, dinner) plus additional snacks. You can eat the snacks as separate meals, or you can add them to any of the main eating times to create a bigger meal. Finally—a diet where you are in control!

Breakfast
Breakfast is designed to get you started off on the right food. That means a plentiful offering of dairy options like yogurt or milk, protein from eggs or a protein smoothie, and your choice of grains or fruit.

University compared participants who performed cardio to those who used resistance training as their primary form of exercise. While both groups lost the same amount of weight, the group that lifted weights burned nearly 5 pounds more fat than the aerobic group. Why? Because the group that used weights burned almost pure fat, while the cardio group was losing lean muscle. Your workout will be structured the same way. In just 30 to 45 minutes per workout, you'll unlock the secret to a long, lean body.

"I will make green my new favorite color."

Here's a rule you probably never thought you'd hear suggested in a diet plan: Eat as much as you want! But that's exactly what we want you to do with vegetables. Whether you prefer spinach, peppers, asparagus, or exotic offerings like bok choy and kale, pack your plate high with as many colors and varieties as you like. Vegetables are packed with so many supernutrients that they have been linked to almost every health benefit imaginable—heart health, cancer prevention, a boost in mood and energy, even revving up your sex life!

But the biggest benefit is weight loss. A study in *The American Journal of Clinical Nutrition* found that women who included veggies in every meal were able to eat 25 percent more food but lose an additional 3.5 pounds. How? Vegetables rev your fat burn and keep you more satisfied, so you're less likely to overeat. (And they have fewer calories.)

What's more, a 20-year review of dietary behavior by the *New England Journal of Medicine* found that people who added just one serving of veggies daily made a positive impact on weight loss. And Penn State researchers found that when participants made sure to include vegetables in every meal, the study participants cut their caloric intake by 11 percent and lost more weight. Need more proof? You'll experience it yourself in The World's Greatest Flat Belly Plan. So enjoy, and if possible, we recommend that you eat your vegetables at the beginning of each meal for the biggest effect. Just choose your favorite vegetables from the list on page 40, and you'll lose more weight and never feel hungry again.

"I will become best friends with protein."

When it comes to a thinner waist, protein is your BFF. When you consider that Johns Hopkins University linked a high-protein diet to lower blood pressure, better cholesterol levels, improved triglycerides, and the prevention of diabetes, obesity, and osteoporosis, it's no wonder we're in favor of protein. But if you're like most women, you're not doing a good enough job using this crucial weight loss tool. According to the U.S. Department of Agriculture, more than a third of women between the ages of 20 and 40 don't get enough protein in their diet.

This is why you'll want to include at least a little bit of protein in every meal and snack. Focusing on protein fights off hunger and makes your stomach unlikely to bulge since protein is less likely to be stored as fat. That's because protein is harder to digest, so you burn more calories just eating the food. This process also helps ensure you eat less. Women who made sure their diet was at least 30 percent protein ate almost 450 calories less per day and lost 11 pounds *more* than those who ate less protein, according to a study published in *Nutrition & Metabolism*.

So whether it's fish, eggs, Greek yogurt, your favorite soy product, or cheese, you'll be eating a constant source of nature's ultimate abs superfood. Need more convincing? British researchers found that emphasizing protein in each meal leaves you feeling fuller, accelerates fat loss, and spares your muscle mass, which is key to shedding pounds and revealing your hottest, most sculpted shape ever.

"I will trade empty calories for *real* carbs."

If there's one food group you should avoid on this plan, it's sugar. But why must it taste so good? Your fix: Eat more fruit. Fruit—nature's sweet reward—provides plenty of carbs for energy, but has less impact on your blood sugar than processed sweets and other carbohydrates. This is crucial to help you avoid the cravings and binges that occurs when your blood sugar rises quickly and then crashes. Ideally, the majority of your carbs will come from fruits. That doesn't mean you won't have grains, beans, or other carbohydrate sources and the occasional treat, but they will be a secondary source. Limit yourself to just a couple servings daily of sugars and processed carbohydrate sources, and consume the rest of your carbs from fresh produce. You'll soon find you don't even miss your old sugary snacks!

Lunch
The foundation of lunch is a source of lean protein like chicken or tuna. Combine that with your favorite vegetables or a side salad to help you power through your afternoon.

Dinner
Your evening meal is packed with more protein, but this time you can go for something a little fattier, like steak, salmon, or trout. These fats will help you stay full. Once again, pile your plate high with veggies, such as grilled zucchini, asparagus, and squash, or sauté some spinach and broccoli.

Snacks
This is where the fun begins and you really take control of your daily menu. Remember, snacks can be eaten separately at any point in the day, or they can be added to any meal. Each day, add healthy fats like nuts, a small source of protein such as deli meat, a piece of fruit, or some grains such as a bowl of cereal.

Special Section:

THE TRUTH ABOUT PROCESSED FOODS

Stop us if this sounds familiar: "All calories are equal, so it doesn't matter what I eat."

It's a mantra that's older than Betty White, and it's a diet fallacy that causes nutritionists to lose their minds.

Processed foods (like cakes and cookies) that are high in refined carbohydrates and sugars can make you crave more food. As a result, you eat more than you need at your current meal—and the next, say Syracuse University researchers. It's dietary double jeopardy: You eat more than you need, and you don't receive any nutritional benefit.

This is why fruits and vegetables need to make up the majority of your carbohydrates. They do what food is supposed to—leave you satisfied. These natural sugars don't play tricks on your mind or your body, and as a result you'll be able to eat to your heart's content without any guilt or the fat to show for it.

Like anything in life, moderation is the key to balance. "You don't need to completely remove processed foods from your diet, but keep them to a maximum of 10 to 15 percent of your daily calories," says nutritionist Alan Aragon, MS. When you eat more than that, you risk creating a diet that doesn't provide you with the vitamins, minerals, and nutrients your body needs. While it might not seem that important, research has found that a diet high in processed foods increases your risk for cardiovascular diseases and metabolic syndrome, says Aragon.

What's more, eating processed foods actually slows down your metabolism, which is why you want to follow our suggested guidelines. Researchers from Pomona College found that meals consisting of processed foods burn significantly fewer calories than a less processed meal. In fact, a 20-year review conducted by the *New England Journal of Medicine* unlocked the reason why so many people gain weight: processed foods. The researchers found that processed foods—like potato chips, cookies, and french fries—cause people to gain up to 17 pounds over a 20-year span. If your plan is to eat, drink, and still shrink, then replacing the processed snacks in your diet can be the small change that finally helps you have flat, toned abs.

How often do I need to eat?

More nutritional information is available to us today than ever before, yet we still can't seem to figure out the most basic question—how often do I need to eat to lose weight? We know that you stress enough about what you eat; there's no need to also worry about how often. So here's a waist-trimming tip that you might find soothing: It doesn't really matter how frequently you eat. All that matters is what you eat.

The multiple meal concept started with a simple premise: When you eat food, you burn calories. As you'll find out, protein helps you burn the most calories, but carbs and fats do the same. Researchers wondered, if we burn fat when we eat, why don't we just eat more often to burn even more calories? In principle, the idea was great. But once more numbers were crunched, the reality painted a different story. Assuming that the foods you eat are the same and the number of calories aren't any different, you won't get a metabolic boost from eating more often.

Now that's not to say multiple meals don't help you lose weight. They do—but not because of some metabolic magic. It works because you feel like you're eating more, without actually taking in more calories.

But snacking can also lead to an expanding waistline. Researchers from the University of North Carolina examined eating habits from the last 30 years. They found that people eat, on average, 500 calories more per day and that the majority of those calories come from overeating on snacks. In fact, people eat more calories as a result of snacking than from increased portion sizes at mealtime.

Even more surprising, researchers from Kansas found that people on a diet who eat less frequently increase their feelings of fullness, while those who snack feel hungry more often. The researchers believe that more frequent meals might make it harder to break the overeating habits and that focusing on better food choices, at fewer meals, is an easier change.

Your best strategy is to follow the guidelines we've provided in The World's Greatest 4-Week Diet and Exercise Plan, meals to keep you grazing all day long.

Don't overthink the eating process. Your body will process foods the right way as long as you are making sure that the majority of your foods come from proteins, vegetables, and fruits. Remember, extreme plans don't work! Take control of the situation and you'll find that your years of weight loss struggles will disappear almost as fast as your belly.

YOUR DIET, YOUR WAY

We've provided you with the ultimate 4-week flat belly eating plan. But that doesn't mean you can't make substitutions and eat your way, every day. Here's a quick cheat sheet that you can use to fuel your body with any food choice. Use "The Lean Guide to Eating" (page 40) and apply your favorite foods. Enjoy!

Meal 1
1 serving protein
1 serving dairy
1 serving fruit or grain
Unlimited vegetables

Meal 2
1 serving protein
1 serving fruit
Unlimited vegetables

Meal 3
1 serving protein
1 serving healthy fat/nuts
Unlimited vegetables

Snacks
(eat separately or add to any meal)
1–2 servings protein
1 serving healthy fat/nuts
or 1 serving dairy
1–2 servings fruit or starches/grains

The World's Greatest 4-Week Diet and Exercise Plan

4 Weeks to Flat Abs

Follow this eating plan, which incorporates all of the Lessons of the Lean and the foods you need to fill up and slim down.

Week 1

Monday	Tuesday	Wednesday	Thursday	Friday	Saturday	Sunday
Meal 1 1 cup plain Greek yogurt ½ cup blueberries ¼ cup granola	**Meal 1** Strawberry-Banana Protein Smoothie (page 398)	**Meal 1** Mexican scrambled eggs (3 eggs, chopped tomatoes, onions, spinach, bell peppers, ½ cup shredded cheese, ¼ cup salsa) 1 orange	**Meal 1** 1 slice whole grain toast 1 tablespoon almond butter 1 cup 1% milk	**Meal 1** Egg and cheese sandwich (2 eggs scrambled, melt 1 slice of cheese, and place onto toasted English muffin)	**Meal 1** Strawberry protein pancakes (Mix 1 scoop vanilla protein powder with 1 egg, ½ cup milk, ½ cup oats, 1 teaspoon salt, 1 teaspoon baking powder. Blend and pour on a griddle. Slice up 1 cup of strawberries and place atop the pancakes after removing them from the griddle.)	**Meal 1** Lox and bagel (mini bagel, 3 ounces smoked salmon, 2 tablespoons cream cheese) Grapefruit
Meal 2 4–6 ounces sesame-crusted ahi tuna served over a bed of mixed greens, drizzled with balsamic vinaigrette	**Meal 2** 6 ounces baked salmon with peach-mango salsa 1 cup sliced cantaloupe Spinach salad	**Meal 2** ½ cup shirataki noodles with 4 ounces ground turkey, roasted spinach, and mushrooms	**Meal 2** 4 ounces grilled chicken with arugula, baby spinach, walnuts, cucumbers, mint leaves, and mandarin oranges	**Meal 2** 4–6 ounces tuna steak marinated in 2 tablespoons soy sauce, 2 teaspoons wasabi, and 1 tablespoon rice wine vinegar Side salad with mixed greens, broccoli, and bell peppers	**Meal 2** Tuna melt sandwich (1 can tuna, 2 slices multigrain bread, ½ sliced avocado, 1 slice Cheddar cheese)	**Meal 2** 4 ounces seared trout topped with herbs and drizzled with olive oil Side of steamed broccoli
Meal 3 4 ounces Cajun-rubbed top sirloin with grilled zucchini, onion, and steamed spinach	**Meal 3** 4 ounces grilled chicken breast, cooked in olive oil, topped with ½ avocado Side of grilled asparagus and squash	**Meal 3** Kebabs with 2 ounces shrimp, 4 ounces chicken, onion, and red and green bell peppers Kale and ¼ avocado salad	**Meal 3** 4–6 ounces grass-fed burger (less than 10 percent fat) with sautéed bell peppers, onions, and mushrooms	**Meal 3** Turkey chili (6 ounces lean ground turkey, diced tomatoes, black beans, corn, dried chili mix, ground flaxseed, ¼ cup water)	**Meal 3** 4–6 ounces grilled chicken and steak skewers, mixed with bell peppers, onions, and zucchini	**Meal 3** 4 ounces broiled salmon topped with lime, slow roasted Roma tomatoes, and Broccolini Spinach and kale salad
Snacks Banana and peanut butter on 1 slice whole grain bread	**Snacks** 1 apple 2 hard-cooked eggs	**Snacks** 1 cup cottage cheese Handful of almonds	**Snacks** 3 strips turkey jerky 1 stick mozzarella cheese 10 crackers	**Snacks** 1 cup vanilla Greek yogurt 1 handful walnuts 1 apple	**Snacks** Chocolate–Peanut Butter Smoothie (page 398)	**Snacks** 1 cup ice cream 1 cup mixed berries

Week 2

Monday	Tuesday	Wednesday	Thursday	Friday	Saturday	Sunday
Meal 1 2-egg omelet with spinach, mushrooms, onions, bell peppers, and Cheddar cheese 1 slice toast 1 tablespoon butter	**Meal 1** 1 strip bacon and 2 fried eggs Grapefruit	**Meal 1** Supercereal (cereal of choice with more than 3 grams of fiber, topped with sliced bananas and 1 tablespoon flaxseed) 2 hard-cooked eggs	**Meal 1** ½ cup oatmeal, cinnamon, ¼ cup raisins 2 links chicken sausage	**Meal 1** Breakfast burrito (2 eggs scrambled, 1 whole grain tortilla, shredded mozzarella cheese, sliced tomato, onions, bell peppers, avocado)	**Meal 1** Protein berry smoothie (1 scoop vanilla protein powder, 6 ounces almond milk, strawberries, blueberries, blackberries, 1 tablespoon chia seeds, 1 cup spinach, 4 ice cues. Blend and serve.)	**Meal 1** Mexican scrambled eggs (3 eggs, chopped tomatoes, onions, spinach, bell peppers, ½ cup shredded cheese, ¼ cup salsa) 1 orange
Meal 2 4 ounces grilled chicken breasts marinated in 3 tablespoons teriyaki sauce and 1 tablespoon water Side of roasted butternut squash	**Meal 2** Chicken fajitas (3 ounces sliced chicken breast, onion, green and red bell peppers, 1 jalapeño chile pepper, cilantro, cumin, 1 whole wheat tortilla)	**Meal 2** 4 ounces grilled salmon with a spinach and arugula salad	**Meal 2** Soba noodle chicken pad thai (¼ cup soba noodles, 4 ounces chicken, peas, carrots, water chestnuts, and ¼ cup diced peanuts. Add a sauce of 2 teaspoons Sriracha and 2 tablespoons soy sauce when finished cooking.)	**Meal 2** 4 ounces roasted halibut with ½ cup fava beans, yellow squash, and shallot sauce	**Meal 2** Spinach wrap filled with 4 ounces sliced chicken breast, bell peppers, black olives, arugula, sundried tomatoes, feta cheese, and ¼ cup hummus	**Meal 2** Tuna melt sandwich (1 can tuna, 2 slices multigrain bread, ½ sliced avocado, 1 slice Cheddar cheese)
Meal 3 6 ounces pork chops glazed with Dijon mustard Side of sweet potatoes and broccoli	**Meal 3** 4 ounces cedar plank salmon seasoned with salt and pepper, and drizzled with olive oil Side salad with cucumber, artichoke, broccoli, sprouts, and tomatoes	**Meal 3** Turkey meatballs (4 ounces extra-lean ground turkey, 1 clove garlic, 4 saltine crackers, ¼ onion, ¼ cup tomato sauce) Grilled bell peppers, butternut squash	**Meal 3** 2 ounces calamari and 2 ounces shrimp grilled and served over sautéed Swiss chard and shallots	**Meal 3** Spicy beef and chicken stir-fry (2 ounces lean steak, 2 ounces chicken, spinach, bell peppers, onions, mushrooms, snap peas, bean sprouts, 2 tablespoons soy sauce, and as much Sriracha as desired)	**Meal 3** Spaghetti squash with 2 ounces scallops and 2 ounces shrimp topped with ½ cup garlic-infused marinara) Side of steamed peas and carrots	**Meal 3** 4 ounces Cajun-rubbed top sirloin with grilled zucchini, onion, and steamed spinach
Snacks 1 cup plain Greek yogurt with ½ cup blueberries and blackberries	**Snacks** Chocolate–Peanut Butter Smoothie (page 398)	**Snacks** 1 cup plain Greek yogurt ½ cantaloupe Handful of almonds	**Snacks** 1 kiwi 1 cup plain Greek yogurt	**Snacks** Apple and 2 tablespoons peanut butter 1 cup milk	**Snacks** 2 hard-cooked eggs 1 stick cheese 1 apple	**Snacks** 1 cup cottage cheese Handful of almonds

The World's Greatest 4-Week Diet and Exercise Plan

Week 3

Monday	Tuesday	Wednesday	Thursday	Friday	Saturday	Sunday
Meal 1 Power protein oatmeal (½ cup oatmeal, 1 scoop protein powder, 1 cup berries) 1 cup almond milk	**Meal 1** Spicy omelet (2 eggs, spinach, 2 mushrooms, 2 tablespoons Cheddar cheese, ½ cup salsa) 1 slice 100 percent whole wheat bread with 1 tablespoon low-sugar jelly 1 cup V8 juice	**Meal 1** Strawberry-Banana Protein Smoothie (page 398)	**Meal 1** Spinach, mushroom, and cheese omelet (2 eggs, 1 teaspoon salt, 1 teaspoon black pepper, ¼ cup Cheddar-Jack cheese, spinach, mushrooms)	**Meal 1** 2 scrambled eggs 1 strip bacon 1 cup mixed berries (strawberries and blueberries)	**Meal 1** Pineapple-banana breeze (1 scoop vanilla protein powder, 6 ounces almond milk, ½ cup pineapple chunks, 1 banana, 1 teaspoon vanilla extract, 4 ice cubes. Blend and serve.)	**Meal 1** 1 cup plain Greek yogurt 1 cup fresh cherries 1 hard-cooked egg
Meal 2 Wild salmon salad (4 ounces wild salmon, arugula, romaine, cherry tomatoes, ¼ cup pecans, mandarin oranges)	**Meal 2** Portobello and tofu kebabs mixed with onions and red, yellow, and green bell peppers Steamed kale and cauliflower	**Meal 2** Chicken spinach Parmesan (4 ounces chicken breast, 1 tablespoon Parmesan cheese, 1 clove garlic, ¼ cup marinara sauce, spinach) Side of ¼ cup quinoa	**Meal 2** Tuna melt (4 ounces canned tuna, 2 slices sprouted grain bread, 1 slice cheese, 1 teaspoon ground red pepper, tomato, lettuce, chopped celery)	**Meal 2** Romaine lettuce, 1 hard-cooked egg, 3 ounces sliced chicken, cherry tomatoes, small handful of sliced almonds, 1 teaspoon rice wine vinegar	**Meal 2** 6 ounces grilled chicken breast, ½ avocado Grilled asparagus and zucchini	**Meal 2** 4 ounces grass-fed burger on a bed of kale
Meal 3 Chicken stir-fry (6 ounces chicken, snow peas, spinach, scallions, mushrooms, chestnuts, ¼ cup peanuts) Serve over ½ cup brown rice	**Meal 3** 4 ounces broiled flank steak Mixed salad with baby spinach, carrots, cucumber, radish, and sprouts	**Meal 3** 4 ounces grilled steak with chimichurri sauce (1 tablespoon water, 2 tablespoons red wine vinegar, 2 minced cloves garlic, 1 teaspoon salt, ground red pepper, black pepper, olive oil)	**Meal 3** 4 ounces chicken, ½ cup black beans, ½ cup salsa, and a small flour tortilla	**Meal 3** 4 ounces grilled chicken sautéed in lime-butter sauce (2 limes, 1 tablespoon butter) 1 cup steamed spinach 1 cup mashed butternut squash Steamed asparagus	**Meal 3** Grilled shrimp and scallops (2 ounces shrimp, 2 ounces scallops) ½ cup cooked quinoa Steamed broccoli and carrots	**Meal 3** Fish tacos (4 ounces grilled halibut, 2 small corn tortillas, ¼ sliced avocado, 2 tablespoons salsa, ½ cup shredded romaine, 1 cup red and yellow bell peppers, sliced onions, ½ sliced jalapeño chile pepper)
Snacks Handful of almonds 1 slice cheese 1 apple	**Snacks** Protein pudding (1 tablespoon almond butter, 1 scoop protein powder, and 3 ounces almond milk; freeze for 1 hour and serve) 1 banana	**Snacks** 1½ cups grapes 1 slice mozzarella cheese 3 ounces ham, sliced	**Snacks** 1 cup cottage cheese 1 cup sliced strawberries	**Snacks** 3 ounces beef jerky 4 celery stalks with 1 tablespoon peanut butter	**Snacks** 1 stick cheese Handful of walnuts	**Snacks** Berry bliss smoothie (4 ounces almond milk, 4 ounces water, 1 scoop vanilla protein powder, ½ cup blueberries, ½ cup strawberries, ¼ cup blackberries, 4 ice cubes. Blend and serve.)

CHAPTER 3

Week 4

Monday

Meal 1
Smoked Salmon and Scrambled Eggs on Toast
(page 390)

Meal 2
Peruvian Seafood Stew
(page 392)

Meal 3
Asian Salmon Burgers
(page 395)

Snacks
Mixed Fruit Breakfast Smoothie
(page 398)

Tuesday

Meal 1
Huevos Rancheros
(page 390)

Meal 2
Berry Goat Cheese Salad
(page 393)

Meal 3
Chicken Lettuce Cups
(page 396)

Snacks
High-Protein Blueberry Yogurt Shake
(page 398)

Wednesday

Meal 1
Flat Green Chile and Goat Cheese Omelet
(page 391)

Meal 2
Tangy Turkey Ciabatta
(page 392)

Meal 3
Chili-Spiced Fish Tacos
(page 395)

Snacks
Mint Chocolate Chip Smoothie
(page 399)

Thursday

Meal 1
Spinach and Feta Frittata
(page 390)

Meal 2
Chipotle Glazed Steak with Black Bean Salad
(page 394)

Meal 3
Beef, Vegetable, and Almond Stir-Fry
(page 395)

Snacks
Chocolate–Peanut Butter Smoothie
(page 398)

Friday

Meal 1
Peanut Butter Strawberry Wrap
(page 390)

Meal 2
Grilled Chicken and Pineapple Sandwich
(page 393)

Meal 3
Chicken with Walnuts and Spinach
(page 396)

Snacks
Strawberry-Banana Protein Smoothie
(page 398)

Saturday

Meal 1
Egg and Avocado Breakfast Sandwich
(page 391)

Meal 2
Special Shrimp Salad
(page 392)

Meal 3
Hoisin-Orange Glazed Chicken
(page 397)

Snacks
1 apple

2 hard-cooked eggs

Sunday

Meal 1
Egg and cheese sandwich
(2 eggs scrambled, melt 1 slice of cheese, and place onto toasted English muffin)

Meal 2
Better-for-You Egg Salad
(page 393)

Meal 3
Pork Gyros
(page 396)

Snacks
1 cup cottage cheese

Handful of almonds

The World's Greatest 4-Week Diet and Exercise Plan

Bonus Menus

Healthy eating doesn't just stop after the 4-week plan! Here are 2 extra weeks of flat-belly meals that you can mix and match to stay slim and satisfied.

Bonus Week 1

Monday	Tuesday	Wednesday	Thursday	Friday	Saturday	Sunday
Meal 1 Egg and Avocado Breakfast Sandwich (page 391)	**Meal 1** Spinach and Feta Frittata (page 390)	**Meal 1** Flat Green Chile and Goat Cheese Omelet (page 391)	**Meal 1** Huevos Rancheros (page 390)	**Meal 1** Smoked Salmon and Scrambled Eggs on Toast (page 390)	**Meal 1** 1 cup plain Greek yogurt ½ cup blueberries ¼ cup granola	**Meal 1** Mexican scrambled eggs (3 eggs, chopped tomatoes, onions, spinach, bell peppers, ½ cup shredded cheese, ¼ cup salsa) 1 orange
Meal 2 Better-for-You Egg Salad (page 393)	**Meal 2** Special Shrimp Salad (page 392)	**Meal 2** Peruvian Seafood Stew (page 392)	**Meal 2** Berry Goat Cheese Salad (page 393)	**Meal 2** Rice Bowls with Shrimp and Bok Choy (page 394)	**Meal 2** Grilled Chicken and Pineapple Sandwich (page 393)	**Meal 2** 4 ounces baked salmon with peach-mango salsa 1 cup sliced cantaloupe Spinach salad
Meal 3 Roast Salmon with White Bean Compote (page 397)	**Meal 3** Hoisin-Orange Glazed Chicken (page 397)	**Meal 3** Chicken with Walnuts and Spinach (page 396)	**Meal 3** Beef, Vegetable, and Almond Stir-Fry (page 395)	**Meal 3** Chili-Spiced Fish Tacos (page 395)	**Meal 3** Chicken Lettuce Cups (page 396)	**Meal 3** Kebabs with 2 ounces shrimp, 2 ounces chicken, onion, and red and green bell peppers Kale and ¼ avocado salad
Snacks Strawberry-Banana Protein Smoothie (page 398)	**Snacks** Chocolate–Peanut Butter Smoothie (page 398)	**Snacks** High-Protein Blueberry Yogurt Shake (page 398)	**Snacks** 1 cup ice cream 1 cup mixed berries	**Snacks** 3 strips turkey jerky 1 stick mozzarella cheese 10 crackers	**Snacks** Apple and 2 tablespoons peanut butter 1 cup milk	**Snacks** 1 cup ice cream 1 cup mixed berries

Bonus Week 2

Monday	Tuesday	Wednesday	Thursday	Friday	Saturday	Sunday
Meal 1 Breakfast burrito (2 eggs scrambled, 1 whole grain tortilla, shredded mozzarella cheese, sliced tomato, onions, bell peppers, avocado)	**Meal 1** Power protein oatmeal (½ cup oatmeal, 1 scoop protein powder, 1 cup berries) 1 cup almond milk	**Meal 1** Spicy omelet (2 eggs, spinach, 2 mushrooms, 2 tablespoons Cheddar cheese, ½ cup salsa) 1 slice 100 percent whole wheat bread, 1 tablespoon low-sugar jelly 1 cup V8 juice	**Meal 1** Spinach, mushroom, and cheese omelet (2 eggs, 1 teaspoon salt, 1 teaspoon pepper, ¼ cup Cheddar-Jack cheese, spinach, mushrooms)	**Meal 1** Supercereal (cereal of choice with more than 3 grams of fiber, topped with sliced bananas and 1 tablespoon of flaxseed) 2 hard-cooked eggs	**Meal 1** Strawberry protein pancakes (Mix 1 scoop vanilla protein powder with 1 egg, ½ cup milk, ½ cup oats, 1 teaspoon salt, 1 teaspoon baking powder. Blend and pour on a griddle. Slice up 1 cup of strawberries and place atop the pancakes after removing them from the griddle.)	**Meal 1** Mixed Fruit Breakfast Smoothie (page 398)
Meal 2 4 ounces sesame-crusted ahi tuna served over a bed of mixed greens, drizzled with balsamic vinaigrette	**Meal 2** 4 ounces grass-fed burger on a bed of kale	**Meal 2** Romaine lettuce, 1 hard-cooked egg, 3 ounces sliced chicken, cherry tomatoes, small handful of sliced almonds, 1 teaspoon rice wine vinegar	**Meal 2** Wild salmon salad (4 ounces wild salmon, arugula, romaine, cherry tomatoes, ¼ cup pecans, mandarin oranges)	**Meal 2** 4 ounces roasted halibut with ½ cup fava beans, yellow squash, and shallot sauce	**Meal 2** 4 ounces tuna steak marinated in 2 tablespoons soy sauce, 2 teaspoons wasabi, and 1 tablespoon rice wine vinegar Side salad with mixed greens, broccoli, and bell peppers	**Meal 2** 6 ounces grilled chicken with arugula, baby spinach, walnuts, cucumbers, mint leaves, and mandarin oranges
Meal 3 Roast Salmon with White Bean Compote (page 397)	**Meal 3:** Pork Gyros (page 396)	**Meal 3** Hoisin-Orange Glazed Chicken (page 397)	**Meal 3** Chicken with Walnuts and Spinach (page 396)	**Meal 3** Beef, Vegetable, and Almond Stir-Fry (page 395)	**Meal 3** Asian Salmon Burgers (page 395)	**Meal 3** Chicken Lettuce Cups (page 396)
Snacks Mixed Fruit Breakfast Smoothie (page 398)	**Snacks** High-Protein Blueberry Yogurt Shake (page 398)	**Snacks** Chocolate–Peanut Butter Smoothie (page 398)	**Snacks** Strawberry-Banana Protein Smoothie (page 398)	**Snacks** Mint Chocolate Chip Smoothie (page 399)	**Snacks** Protein pudding (1 tablespoon almond butter, 1 scoop protein powder, and 3 ounces almond milk; freeze for 1 hour and serve) 1 banana	**Snacks** 1 kiwi 1 cup plain Greek yogurt

The Lean Guide to Eating

PROTEIN SOURCES	DAIRY	STARCHES AND GRAINS	FRUITS	NUTS AND FATS	VEGETABLES
(serving size = 4 ounces)	*(with serving size)*	*(with serving size)*			*(unlimited)*
Canned tuna	Cheese *1 stick or slice*	Black beans *1/2 cup*	Apples	Avocado *1/2 tablespoon*	Artichokes
Chicken breast	Cottage cheese (2% fat) *6 ounces*	Bread (with 3 grams of fiber or more) *1 slice*	Bananas	Nut butters (Almond, Cashew, Peanut) *2 ounces*	Arugula
Eggs			Blueberries		Asparagus
Fish (all types)	Milk (2% fat) *1 cup*	Cannellini beans *1/2 cup*	Cantaloupe	Nuts (Almonds, Brazil nuts, Cashews, Pecans, Pistachios, Walnuts) *a handful (1 ounce)*	Bell peppers
Lean ground beef	Plain low-fat yogurt *6 ounces (one single serving of prepackaged)*	Cereal (with 3 grams of fiber or more) *1 cup*	Grapefruit		Bok choy
Lean pork (ham, bacon)			Grapes		Broccoli
Lean turkey		Corn tortillas *1 tortilla*	Kiwi	Sour cream *2 tablespoons*	Cabbage
Shrimp		Flour tortillas (with 3 grams of fiber or more) *1 tortilla*	Oranges		Carrots
			Peaches		Cauliflower
		Garbanzo beans *1/2 cup*	Pears		Celery
		Oatmeal *1/2 cup*	Pineapple		Cucumber
		Pasta *1/2 cup (cooked)*	Raspberries		Green beans
		Pita bread *1 pita*	Strawberries		Kale
		Potatoes (regular or sweet) *1 medium-size potato (size of your fist)*	Watermelon		Leafy greens
					Leaks
					Lettuce
					Mushrooms
					Onion
					Spinach
					Sprouts
					Squash
					Zucchini

7 Days of Abs

British psychologists recently uncovered how your mental approach to exercise can lead to greater physical changes. Instead of focusing on monthlong goals, they found that boiling your goals down to week-by-week plans, and not weight loss benchmarks, actually builds consistent behaviors that create long-lasting fat loss. That's why we've created a 7-day exercise guide for you to follow. Don't worry about the scale or how your clothes fit. Just do your best to stay on track and accomplish your exercise goals. Check each of these items off your weekly list, and you'll scorch thousands of calories and score abs in just 4 weeks!

Monday
Perform Workout A of The Abs Workout on page 68. The program should take 45 minutes.

Tuesday
Today is a rest day. Focus on your diet, and if you're not too sore or tired, perform any type of cardio you'd like. This can be a run, your favorite sport, or just a walk around the block. We recommend that you limit your activity to 30 minutes.

Wednesday
Perform Workout B of The Abs Workout. Once again, 45 minutes of training and you're done for the day.

Thursday
Today is another rest day. You don't need to do any exercise, but if you'd like, you can again add some light or active cardio. Keep it to around 30 minutes max.

Friday
Perform Workout A of The Abs Workout. Once you're done, you've completed your resistance training for the week.

Saturday
Saturday is a free day. You can take the day off and relax, or you can take on your most difficult cardio task of the week. Run sprints and push yourself as hard as you want.

Sunday
Today is an off day. No exercise whatsoever. Rest, relax, and let your body recover for the start of a new week.

THE EXERCISE PLAN

It doesn't matter if you've been exercising for 10 years or never stepped foot in a gym—you've never experienced a workout like this. We've created a fat-scorching plan designed specifically to uncover your abs. It's the perfect combination of time-tested exercises that tone your muscles and innovative movements that challenge your core and keep your workouts fun and engaging. The program is so effective that you'll only work out for 45 minutes a day, just three times a week! That's because the exercises will exhaustively work all the muscles in your body, and you'll need the rest of the week to recover so you can continually improve. As you get in better shape, the workouts become even shorter—making this the greatest flat belly workout plan ever created.

On Monday, you'll restart the week of workouts, but this time you'll begin with Workout B.

Just remember, prior to every workout, make sure you perform a 5- to 10-minute warmup to prepare your body and prevent injury. We recommend "The Total Body Jump-Start" (page 250).

The Secret to Flat Abs

**THE 4-STEP PLAN THAT
WILL STRIP AWAY POUNDS IN DAYS.**

You can have flat abs.

That's the first thing you need to convince yourself of before you start this plan. Like most women, you probably find it hard to believe that you can flatten your belly without starving yourself or removing a few ribs. After all, it's not like you haven't tried to eliminate your pooch in the past. Do marathon cardio sessions and Pilates sound familiar? How about diets that forbid you from eating after 6 p.m.? Maybe you've even made a few purchases of so-called toning equipment from QVC that are now hiding under your bed. To score the sizzling body you want, you need an approach that doesn't require a complete lifestyle makeover and isn't full of empty promises.

The Secret to Flat Abs

Consider this the last solution you'll ever need. This diet and exercise plan is based on cutting-edge university research that utilizes the most effective fat loss strategies. In fact, the foods you'll eat on this program have been found to boost fat loss by more than 30 percent compared to the standard American diet. And when combined with The Abs Workout, you'll transform your body into a calorie-burning machine that even works as you sleep.

Best of all, by following these tips, you'll eliminate the reason why most diets fail: frustration. Most diet and exercise plans tell you exactly what to do and when. Suddenly your flexible lifestyle is trapped in concrete. Between teaching yourself to like new foods and trying to find hours to exercise each day, you burn out. The supposed healthy plan becomes a threat to your comfort zone. This plan is different. The exercise and diet were designed around simple strategies that put you in charge of owning the body you want.

The Diet

There's a secret among the top nutritionists in the world. Most diets are created for short-term results. It's a cruel trick that has created the endless cycle of deceptive weight loss and depressing weight gain. Your body is very good at losing weight—until it adapts and makes it seemingly impossible to burn off another pound. It's why each of your ex-diets ended in a messy breakup. Atkins? Sure, he was great, but you've always been a bread-and-pasta girl, and you just couldn't commit. South Beach? It had its thrills, but you're not into math and counting all your meals. Paleo? The caveman thing was retro, but we progressed passed the Stone Age for a reason.

If you want to keep eating the foods you like—and losing weight—you need to understand how the body processes food and work with it, not against it. We understand if you want to swear off diets forever, but there's something else the nutritionists tell their clients: Diets work. That's why it's time to eliminate your fears about the dreaded D-word and show you how to make food work for you.

The nutrition experts at *Women's Health* understand the adaptation process and know how to prevent you from hitting the dreaded plateau that has been the beginning of the end for all your previous diets. This plan fills your body up with the right kinds of foods, so you burn calories more efficiently. The payoff: You can eat more food, burn fat faster, and still indulge in some of your favorite treats. If it sounds too good to be true, we don't blame you. But we've already seen the results. In fact, dieters in a study at UCLA followed a plan that included similar foods to what you'll find in this book. Not only did they lose more weight compared to a traditional diet, they also consumed more food and felt more satisfied from their meals. Sounds like your type of plan, right?

So dig in and enjoy this new approach to eating. It's a proven road map to tone up all your trouble spots and scorch belly fat, regardless of your shape, size, or age. We've created a plate that represents what you should consume at each meal. Your job: Simply select the foods you enjoy from each category and see results that last. That's it. No counting calories. No removing foods completely. Follow each of these guidelines, and science will prove that the pounds will melt off in no time.

The Guidelines

The key to a good diet is remaining satisfied. That's why The World's Greatest Flat Belly Plan is all about filling your plate. But sometimes it's difficult to know how much to eat without overeating. So we searched for a simpler way to fill your plate without having to count calories and created a system that's as easy as counting to four. Literally. These four steps, when utilized for each meal, will have you on the fast track to a flat belly. Follow these simple guidelines to ensure that you're always eating enough, seeing results, and never having to count calories again!

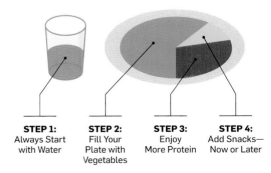

STEP 1: Always Start with Water

STEP 2: Fill Your Plate with Vegetables

STEP 3: Enjoy More Protein

STEP 4: Add Snacks— Now or Later

Always Start with Water

Few dieters realize that it's the small, simple tactics that create the greatest changes. Food is habitual, so it's best to determine the daily changes you can make that can become a part of your lifestyle. Few weight loss strategies are as easy—and effective—as drinking water. Everyone knows that a little H_2O is good for your body. But drinking water at the right time does more than hydrate. It can actually set you up for a day of fat loss without any effort.

In a recent study in the journal *Obesity*, dieters lost an additional 4.5 pounds when they drank 2 cups of water before each meal. That's why the leanest individuals start every meal with two glasses of water and continually drink throughout the day. A study in the *Journal of the American Dietetic Association* found that having 2 cups of water before breakfast can cut your daily food intake by 13 percent.

Additional research performed by German scientists revealed that 6 cups of cold water per day (think just 2 cups before breakfast, lunch, and dinner) can raise your resting metabolism 50 calories a day. Although 50 calories probably doesn't have you thinking, "Skinny jeans here I come!" they add up to 5 pounds in one year. Sounds a little better, right? Though the extra calories you burn drinking a single glass don't amount to much, making it a habit can add up to pounds lost without any effort.

Drinking water also means that you're not dehydrated—another stealthy

The Secret to Flat Abs

roadblock in your fat loss journey. Scientists at the University of Utah found that when you don't drink enough, your metabolism burns up to 2 percent fewer calories per day. When you're trying to fight back against a stubborn metabolism, the last thing you need to do is give your body any reason to store fat.

Abs Secret #1
Before each meal, consume 16 ounces (2 cups) of water. The water can be cold or hot. Feel free to mix your water with tea, preferably one without any calories or sweeteners. We recommend green tea because of its extra metabolism-boosting benefits.

Fill Your Plate with Vegetables
It doesn't take a doctor to tell you to eat your vegetables. You know that greens are good for you, but they possess enough weight loss and health benefits to fill an entire medical encyclopedia. Vegetables are packed with so many supernutrients that they have been linked to improving heart health, fighting off nearly every disease imaginable (including cancer), increasing positive emotions, creating more energy, and even revving up your sex life.

We know what you're thinking. "Great. A diet based on salads. Original." We might not be the first to suggest vegetables, but on this plan your veggies are just the appetizer, not the main course. Here's why: A 20-year review of dietary behavior by the *New England Journal of Medicine* found that people who added just one serving of veggies daily had a positive impact on weight loss. And Penn State researchers found that when the study participants included vegetables before every meal, they cut their caloric intake by 11 percent and lost more weight.

But that's just the beginning on why it's great to go green. Leafy greens happen to possess special nutritional qualities that allow you to eat as much as you want without gaining weight. After all, no one ever became fat on a diet of spinach, bell peppers, and mushrooms. In fact, a study in the *American Journal of Clinical Nutrition* found that you can eat more and still slim down. The researchers compared women who needed to lose weight. One group followed a reduced-calorie diet, while the other followed a similar approach but feasted on vegetables. The veggie group ate 25 percent more food (by volume) but lost more weight. How? They were loading up on vegetables, which decreased their hunger, but they actually ended up eating fewer calories.

That's why we suggest you start every meal with vegetables. It guarantees that you won't forget to eat this weight loss superfood, and eating them early in the meal can potentially make your fat loss more potent. Research has shown that high-fiber vegetables can rev your fat burn by as much as 30 percent. So by kicking off your meal with your favorite variety, you improve satiety and ignite more caloric burn during your meal. Whether you eat a starter salad or mix vegetables with your main course, this will be one of the most important steps in keeping you satisfied and helping the pounds vanish.

Abs Secret #2

Pile your plate high with veggies and enjoy them before you begin your main meal. Remember, green veggies, bell peppers, onions, and a host of other options are "free food." That means you can literally eat as much as you want—but that doesn't mean you can pour as much salad dressing as you want. Start with 1 to 2 cups of steamed broccoli or spinach, a side salad, or some bell peppers, onions, and mushrooms drizzled lightly in olive oil.

Enjoy More Protein

It's time for you to admit something to yourself: You probably don't eat enough protein. Sure, you might sneak a can of tuna or toss some tofu in your stir-fry, but women are notorious for significantly undereating the most powerful abs-friendly food group. Maybe it's because of your fear of growing bulging muscles or the mysterious nature of protein smoothies. But your body could use more of nature's most potent nutrient. According to British researchers, emphasizing protein in each meal leaves you feeling fuller, accelerates fat loss, and spares your lean muscle mass.

Look at some of the fittest women in the world. All seem to possess a lean body secret—and it's not just because they can afford trainers and live-in chefs who prepare their meals (although that helps, too). Fit women understand that high protein intake is critical to losing fat and having a rocking body. Perhaps the biggest benefit of a high-protein diet is that you burn calories by eating. Your metabolism is increased when you eat. This process is known as the thermic effect of food (TEF). Every type of food affects your metabolism differently, but nothing is as powerful as protein. The TEF of protein is about 30 percent, meaning more than a quarter of the calories this nutrient provides are burned during digestion and processing. Carbohydrates have a TEF of 8 to 10 percent, and fat's TEF is just 3 to 5 percent. This is why consuming protein at each meal can keep your metabolism elevated and prevent larger meals from storing too many calories.

No matter what, we don't want you to worry about protein turning you into Suzy McBulky. Adding muscle mass to your body is the result of your hormones and eating a significant amount of calories. So unless you decide to start injecting yourself with testosterone or consuming 5,000 calories a day, your high-protein diet will make you look more like Mila Kunis than The Rock. In fact, as you build more muscle, your body will burn more fat, which makes every dietary slipup (we know you love the occasional slice of cheesecake) a nonfactor.

While you might not be thinking in

THE DAILY DESSERT

So how does dessert fit in to all of this? Simple: Your daily desserts will come from your snack allotment. Remember, you can enjoy one small indulgence every day, whether it's a small candy bar, a scoop of ice cream, or maybe a cocktail. For the first two weeks, we'd recommend that you limit dessert to every other day (if you choose to eat it). This isn't necessary, but if you struggle controlling your junk food urges, this should help you adjust to the smaller portions.

Here's your guide to keep you lean and satisfied.

---

1 glass wine
=
2 servings grains

½ cup ice cream
=
1 serving fat

---

2 party-size candy bars
=
2 servings starches/ grains

---

1 small slice of cake/ pastry
=
2 servings starches/ grains

The Secret to Flat Abs

terms of saving your muscles, that's the difference between your bikini body and looking "skinny fat." Think about it: As you lose weight, you want to make sure you reveal a sculpted, hot body. Eating protein helps makes this possible, especially when it's consumed before and after your workouts. University of Syracuse researchers found that when you down protein around your weight training session, you blunt the effects of cortisol, the stress hormone that tells your body to store fat. As a result, you burn more fat not only during your workout, but for an additional 24 hours afterward.

Focusing on protein also keeps your stomach more satisfied and keeps it lean. When you overeat carbohydrates or fat, both nutrients are easily soaked up by your body and stored as fat. But protein is different. That's not to say protein can't make you fat, but when you need a little food therapy after a rough day, a high-protein meal is less likely to make you fat.

Abs Secret #3
Here's where you can go a little crazy. There are lots of flavorful protein options just waiting to be enjoyed. Grill yourself a steak. Bake some chicken. Crack eggs or pan-sear your favorite fish. If you're a vegetarian, create your favorite soy variety or try seitan (called the wheat meat). Even if your favorite form of protein has some fat on it, don't worry (see "Eat Fat to Lose Fat"). However, if you select a form of protein that's high in

EAT FAT TO LOSE FAT

Everything you need to know about the dangers of consuming a diet that's high in fat can be summarized in one sentence: The health scare surrounding saturated fat and cholesterol was overblown.

That was Walter Willett's conclusion after reviewing 21 studies on high-fat diets. Willett, MD, DrPH, the chairman of the department of nutrition at Harvard University, published a study that showed there is no evidence that dietary saturated fat is associated with coronary heart disease, stroke, or cardiovascular disease. This was the defining moment in a 30-year battle to determine if eating fat makes us fat. The confusion began in the 1980s when obesity rates began to climb. The low-fat craze took over, and the next thing you knew, we all became fatter. The number of overweight people increased by 30 percent while the amount of fat consumed decreased by 11 percent. So clearly, fat wasn't the problem. What people didn't realize is that not only is fat not bad, it's actually an incredibly potent weight loss tool.

Research now indicates that as much as 20 to 35 percent of your calories should come from fats. Not only do the fat-filled meals keep you full, they also burn calories. Researchers from Georgia Southern University found that eating a high-protein, high-fat snack increases your resting calorie burn for up to 3.5 hours. When it comes to understanding fat, your options can be broken down into two main groups: saturated and unsaturated fats. Both of them are good, and both possess a variety of benefits.

Monounsaturated fats—MUFAs
(pronounced MOO-fahs), for short—come from the healthy oils found in plant foods such as olives, nuts, and avocados. A report published in the *British Journal of Nutrition* found that a MUFA-rich diet helped people lose small amounts of weight and body fat without changing their calorie intakes.

Another report found that a breakfast high in MUFAs could boost calorie burn for 5 hours after the meal, particularly in people with higher amounts of belly fat. And a study in the *American Journal of Clinical Nutrition* showed that people who swallowed 1.9 grams of omega-3s daily (you'd find twice that in a 4-ounce portion of salmon) reduced their body fat, lowered their triglycerides, and raised their HDL cholesterol.

Saturated fats—like those found in
red meat, eggs, and milk—used to be avoided. But now they are an essential part of a healthy diet. No food represents the benefits of fat better than eggs. If you're skipping out on the yolks, you're missing out on one of the best fat loss foods. A study in *Nutrition Research* showed that the fat in eggs helped reduce appetite for up to 24 hours. And British scientists discovered that dieters who ate eggs for breakfast instead of a bagel lost 65 percent more weight—without any negative consequences to their cholesterol or triglycerides. Research has also found that consuming calcium dairy foods, such as milk and yogurt, may also reduce fat absorption from other foods, which makes it easier to stay lean.

Abs Secret #4
Embrace fats in the form of avocados, butter, nuts and seeds, as well as olive, canola, and coconut oil. Cook your foods in these healthy fats, or add them to your meals for additional flavor, nutrition, and fat loss benefits.

The Secret to Flat Abs

fat, make sure you limit how much additional fat you add to your meal.

Add Snacks—Now or Later

The time has come to reinvent weight loss. Rather than repeating the mistakes of so many diets, we want to accommodate the most overlooked aspect of every weight loss approach: YOU. An eating plan should revolve around your preferences, your busy lifestyle, and your need to adjust to daily demands. And let's be honest, while all diet plans expect some give-and-take, few provide real flexibility required for long-term success. It's expected that you'll have to make changes to how you eat, but that doesn't mean you need to give up your favorite foods or be forced into an eating schedule that doesn't work for you. We're all familiar with late-morning starts altering our breakfast plans, unscheduled business lunches disrupting an anticipated meal, or nonstop travel making it seem impossible to eat healthy. That stops here.

We already mentioned that you'll choose how frequently you'll eat. Whether you want six smaller meals or three big meals, you decide what you need, without having to worry that one option will be better for fat loss. This all becomes possible with snacks. These are flexible foods that you can eat at any point in the day—and they are usually the foods that you enjoy the most. Think pasta, bread, and even dessert. As long as you follow the Lessons of the Lean, you can have some fun with your diet.

You might be wondering what makes this approach to snacking any different than other plans. Simple: We've created a diet where you'll only eat a snack when it's needed. Because the foods you'll be eating will keep you satisfied longer, you'll find that you need to eat snacks less frequently. And when you do, they won't be sabotaging your weight loss plan. You see, the snacks have been strategically designed to only take up a small portion of your daily calories. It's enough to leave you satisfied and not craving some of your favorite foods—but not so much that you'll derail your diet faster than you can say "Ho Ho."

Here's how it works: Breakfast, lunch, and dinner will be the foundation of your eating plan. You decide when to eat them, and structure each meal around the Lessons of the Lean. That means start by drinking water, then consume veggies and fill your plate with protein and healthy fats. From there, the fun and flexibility begins with "floating meals."

Ever feel like you needed just a little more food on your plate? Or you were curious about how much you could graze without gaining weight? Snacks, or floating meals, solve all of these issues. These are foods that you can add to any meal (breakfast, lunch, or dinner), or you can use these foods as daily snacks. That means if you want to add two or three mini-meals during the day, you simply select the foods you want from the floating meals allotment to keep yourself satisfied. If you're not much of a snacker but would prefer a bigger meal, you can take the floating meals and eat them in addition to one of your main meals. This way, you can eat more without taking a step back.

The plan is designed to always leave you feeling satisfied, and it takes into consideration that sometimes your hunger is unpredictable and the demands of your day can control how you eat.

Abs Secret #5

Add the following foods as snacks during the day or in addition to your main meals. These additions are optional, so if you're satisfied by breakfast, lunch, and dinner—or by just a few of the snacks— you don't need to eat more. The idea is that these foods will fuel your body, not your fat cells. So you can eat them if you're hungry, but keep in mind you only need to consume them if you're not satisfied. And always remember the first three rules: Drink water first, begin your plate with veggies, and stack up on protein. And if your protein source is high in fat (like pork or a rib eye steak), try to avoid adding nuts to the meal.

Your Snack Allowance
Unlimited servings: vegetables
1 serving: healthy fat/nuts or dairy
1–2 servings: fruit or starches/grains
1–2 servings: protein

The Truth about Late-Night Meals

Breakfast has long been touted as the king of all meals. In fact, many researchers have hypothesized it's the most important meal of the day. A University of Massachusetts medical school study found that people who routinely skipped breakfast had a significantly higher incidence of obesity than those who ate eggs and an English muffin. But just because one meal is good doesn't mean the others are bad. Yet, somehow the importance of breakfast turned into a dietary game of telephone that condemned dinner as a meal that packs on pounds. Fortunately for you, nothing could be further from the truth.

Cutting-edge research from scientists all over the world appears to have finally cracked the weight loss code. And the solution is late-night eating. If you're serious about changing your body, these findings might be the key to unlocking new fat loss pathways. That's because your body's ability to gain weight is mainly about what you eat and how much, not when you eat. Your body isn't on a 24-hour clock. What counts is whether you burn more calories than you ingest by the end of the day (or better yet, the week).

Researchers from Israel wanted to test whether eating more at night actually led to more weight gain. What they found was groundbreaking. In the 6-month study, the scientists compared people who ate their largest meal at breakfast to those who ate their largest meal at dinner (8 p.m. or later). The participants who satisfied their late-night munchies not only lost more fat, they also experienced more fullness throughout the entire 6 months and saw more favorable changes to their fat loss hormones.

Consider some of the impressive findings. Compared to the morning eaters, those who ate at night:

- **Had less hunger cravings and were more satisfied with their meals**
- **Lost 11 percent more weight**
- **Had a 10 percent greater change in abdominal circumference**
- **Lost a whopping 10.5 percent more body fat**

What's more, a study conducted by the U.S. Department of Agriculture also showed some convincing evidence for nighttime feasts. When dieters ate 70 percent of their calories after 7 p.m. compared to earlier in the day, they preserved muscle mass and lost more body fat.

So how did we come to fear late-night meals and, even worse, carbs? It was a classic case of misunderstanding. Many people eat at night out of boredom or other emotions instead of hunger, and they wind up consuming more calories than they need for the day. Remember when we said that counting calories works? Well, nighttime eaters typically bust past their calorie goal, leading to fat storage. But that doesn't mean your body processes food differently at different times of day. In fact, late-night meals actually do a better job of priming your hormones for fat loss and improving sleep.

If you've ever experienced a stressful week at work or in your home, you know that a lack of sleep appears to instantly add pounds to the scale. And researchers from Wake Forest University discovered why: Too much or too little shut-eye causes weight gain. People who slept 5 hours or less each night gained nearly 2.5 times more abdominal fat than those who logged 6 to 7 hours. People with sleep deficits tend to eat more (and use less energy) because they're tired, say the researchers. And if you're sleep deprived and not just groggy, University of Chicago researchers report that lack of sleep can torpedo weight loss by slowing metabolism, increasing appetite, and decreasing the number of calories burned. All the more reason to eat late, sleep better at night, and watch the pounds melt—and stay—off your body.

But the best reason to eat late at night has nothing to do with losing fat or sleeping better. It's a decision that's best for our social life. How many times have you gone out and sabotaged a perfect day of eating with a few drinks or a big celebratory meal? On this plan, you can eat out without the guilt. Simply save your carbohydrates for the last meal of the day and indulge. Not only will these carbs help you sleep better, they'll also fuel more fat loss. This doesn't mean you can't have carbs earlier in the day, but most people prefer a big dinner to a big lunch. And on this plan, we encourage this approach for amplified results.

Abs Secret #6

It's time for you to let loose and have some fun with your eating plan. If you've been following The Abs Secret guidelines, you should be free to enjoy your final meal of the day. If you haven't used up your floating meals, this is where you can squeeze in more calories to help you sleep better and improve your metabolism. We recommend that you save 1 to 2 servings of your grain allotment for dinner. Remember, carbs at night can be a great thing for your weight loss goals. But if that's not your preference, your results won't be slowed.

Abs for Every Eater

WHETHER YOU'RE LACTOSE INTOLERANT,
A VEGETARIAN, OR DON'T EAT GLUTEN—
THIS IS THE SOLUTION FOR YOUR SPECIAL DIETARY NEEDS.

Dieting can make the

weight loss process feel like high hurdles. Rather than simply running toward your goal, you're constantly forced to jump over obstacles that you can't avoid. Don't eat this, limit that. The rules don't seem like they were made for a human. We understand that the worst part of your diet isn't necessarily what you can eat—it's what you can't. And we're not talking about cookies, cakes, and Cokes. Those are tasty indulgences that have their place but can lead you astray. This is more about the hurdles you face as a result of personal health practices or health limitations.

In today's society, more and more people have dietary restrictions. Whether you're a vegetarian, lactose intolerant, or practicing gluten-free

Abs for Every Eater

eating, most diet plans don't account for the restrictive nature of your eating approach. And it doesn't matter if your habits are by choice or necessity. When you aren't given options that work within your food confines, it's hard to create an effective weight loss plan.

For example, we've shown you that eating a high-protein diet is a great way to burn body fat and maintain muscle. But what happens if you're a vegetarian? Most high-protein food suggestions include some sort of animal protein. Does that mean you can't follow a high-protein approach? Of course not.

Vegetarians aren't the only ones frustrated by limited suggestions. Milk and cheese are commonly included as meals and snacks because calcium has been scientifically shown to shrink your gut and help fight against the aging process. However, if you're lactose intolerant, those foods could destroy your insides before making your outsides look better. The same can be said for those who have to follow a gluten-free diet.

There's no reason your dietary preferences should stand in the way of your goals. We turned to Mike Roussell, PhD, founder of Naked Nutrition, to ensure that your unique relationship with food isn't a hindrance to uncovering your abs. After all, the reason this diet works is because it complements your lifestyle. Dr. Roussell created this guide to help you navigate some of the most common and complicated diet scenarios that can make it seem impossible to follow a healthy plan. These tips and tricks offer a solution that will make your eating headaches a thing of the past.

THE HURDLE:
You're Lactose Intolerant

If no one suffered from lactose intolerance, odds are we'd all be a little healthier and trimmer. That's because research suggests that the calcium you consume from dairy is a stealthy way to eat more food and still lose weight—because the calories you eat from dairy are more likely to provide energy than be stored as body fat. More surprisingly, avoiding dairy makes you more likely to pack on the pounds. According to a study in the *American Journal of Clinical Nutrition,* reducing the amount of dairy you eat sends a signal in your body to make more fat cells.

The process might seem a bit magical, but it's nothing more than your body reacting to a primary need. When you don't have enough calcium in your body, you try to hold on to what you have. This triggers a reaction where your body releases a compound called calcitriol, which increases the production of fat cells. If you want fewer fat cells, eating extra calcium suppresses calcitriol, which breaks down fat and makes your fat cells leaner and your tummy flatter.

Fortunately, being lactose intolerant and avoiding dairy doesn't need to get in the way of you finding your abs. It is important to remember that if you're lactose intolerant, there are different levels of severity. Being lactose intolerant simply means that your body does not produce sufficient amounts of the enzyme lactase. Lactase is responsible for chopping the dairy sugar, lactose, in half so that your body can use it for energy. If lactose goes undigested, you're left feeling bloated and uncomfortable.

Some people can tolerate small amounts of lactose, while others cannot tolerate any. Figure out which one you are and then apply these tips accordingly, to help ignite more weight loss.

Add the Missing Ingredient

Sometimes the best approach is the simplest: Eat dairy. For those who don't have severe intolerance, taking a lactase supplement with a dairy-filled meal can help you experience all the benefits of milk and cheese. By supplementing with the enzyme, you're giving your body what it is missing. A diet high in dairy has been estimated to boost weight loss by as much as 70 percent, so using the supplement might be the extra kick you need, says Dr. Roussell.

Choose a "Better" Protein Powder

Whey is the most common protein used in protein powder, but there are different ways that whey is purified and processed in order to extract it from milk. Some of these processes leave small amounts of lactose that can cause you to bloat and cramp. If your protein powder is causing these symptoms, switch to a powder that only contains whey protein isolate, suggests Dr. Roussell. This is the purest form of whey, in which all the lactose is removed.

Eat More Probiotics

Dairy products such as kefir and certain brands of cottage cheese and yogurt contain good bacteria called probiotics. These cultured dairy products contain lower levels of lactose because the probiotics break down the lactose sugar for you, making it easier on your stomach, says Dr. Roussell. Oftentimes people who can tolerate low levels of lactose can eat these products without any problems. Cottage cheese and plain yogurt are both high in protein and serve as good snacks on a weight loss diet. Kefir is a great milk substitute for smoothies, and its high concentration of probiotics can help ease your intestinal discomfort.

Remove Dairy Entirely

If your lactose intolerance is severe or you have trouble achieving a sleek midsection with sexy lines, your best option might be to remove dairy entirely. While restrictive, this will eliminate the cause of your intestinal problems completely, while also reducing the total amount of sugar that you consume in your diet. While the sugar from dairy is not a bad thing, it does serve as a hidden source that could put you over the edge and further away from your hard body.

THE HURDLE:
You're a Vegetarian

Being a vegetarian poses dietary challenges that can hinder your weight loss. It's not that a plant-based diet is bad for you. That's why one of our Lessons of the

CALCIUM CONTROL

Just because you're not eating dairy doesn't mean you can't have calcium in your diet. Remember, not enough calcium triggers the release of fat-friendly calcitriol. Because calcium-rich diets are essential in treating and managing many conditions, it's imperative that you maximize your opportunities to supplement calcium with other options. These include dark leafy greens (spinach, kale), almonds, sesame seeds, salmon, and fortified foods (orange juice).

Abs for Every Eater

Lean focuses on greens. Eating meals rich in vegetables provides nutrients that can help you fight off every disease from cancer to cardiovascular breakdown, as well as slow the aging process and help you supercharge your body with energy. But vegetarians have a tendency to eat less protein. And as you know, eating protein not only burns more calories during the digestion process, it also helps you build more muscle and improve your metabolism.

Another issue: Vegetarians eat a diet that tends to be excessively high in carbohydrates. While eating carbohydrates is part of a balanced eating plan, they are not as filling as protein. This means that in order to feel satisfied, vegetarians eat more and more carbs in order to satisfy their hunger.

Unintentionally, this leads vegetarians to underestimate how much they eat, consume more calories than they should, and put on weight. With a few small adjustments, any vegetarian can maintain a green-based approach while accelerating fat loss.

Use Protein Powder

If you want to make sure that you lose fat and not muscle, you need to include more protein in your diet. For vegetarians, hitting daily protein goals without overeating carbohydrates can be difficult. That's because many of the best vegetarian protein sources such as beans, legumes, and higher protein grains contain more carbohydrates than protein (per serving). Your solution: protein powder. These powders are a convenient way to boost your protein intake without adding excess carbohydrates to your meals or snacks. Add a scoop to the foods you bake or to carb-based meals such as oatmeal, or blend as a smoothie.

Go Nuts

One of the best foods for vegetarians is also one of the most effective snacks for any diet. Nuts, such as almonds, cashews, and walnuts, are loaded with fat-fighting benefits. Adding 1 to $1\frac{1}{2}$ ounces (about a handful) of nuts each day is a great carbohydrate-controlled way to fuel your body while continuing to shed fat and eliminate hunger. Nuts contain fiber, protein, and fat, all of which will keep you fuller longer while also slowing digestion. What's more, nuts can help control rises in your blood sugar. This is essential for optimizing your fat loss hormones and age-proofing your body against weight gain.

Take Strategic Supplements

While eating whole foods is always the foundation of any good eating plan, vegetarians should add a few supplements to fill gaps created on a plant-based diet. Creatine and docosahexaenoic acid (DHA) are two supplements that most women don't take, but are essential for vegetarians concerned about weight loss and their general health, says Dr. Roussell. Creatine is typically viewed as a muscle-building formula for men, but it has many additional benefits for vegetarians. Supplementing with 5 grams of creatine following each of your workouts will help you maintain your lean muscle and improve brain function.

DHA is an omega-3 fat found in fish oil supplements that will potentially boost weight loss by stopping the growth of fat cells. If you don't eat fish, you can still add the vegetarian (or vegan) version of the supplement to your diet. DHA is produced by algae, and when fish consume the algae, they become a concentrated and potent source of the powerful, healthy fat. Vegetarians should take at least 1 gram of DHA per day from an algae-based supplement.

THE HURDLE:
You Follow a Gluten-Free Diet

A funny thing happened to the wheat industry thanks to the low-carb movement: People stopped eating breads and grains. And that wasn't all that happened. Lots of dieters who made the change lost weight and felt better than ever. But the reason wasn't what everyone assumed. While a lower carb diet can help you lose weight, it's not that carbs are the enemy. In fact, they are a vital nutrient that will help you get lean fast and keep you energized for your workouts. The reason the diet changes made such a difference was because many people were overeating carbs, and the change in diet meant they were eating more protein and vegetables. The shift also shed light on a growing medical problem: gluten intolerance. Turns out,

thousands of people are sensitive to gluten, a compound that is found in most grains, breads, and wheat products. So when the foods were removed, people improved their digestive health, which aided in weight loss.

Even if you're not allergic to gluten, removing the by-product from your diet is one of the best ways to lose weight. That's because gluten-containing foods are packed with faster-acting carbohydrates, which can hinder your weight loss, says Dr. Roussell. Whether you're gluten free by choice or necessity, use these suggestions to make that approach work for you.

Don't Overdo Gluten-Free Foods

Gluten-free eating is very popular right now, but as a result there are myriad gluten-free food substitutes available in your local supermarket, such as gluten-free pretzels, bagels, and breads. Much like the low-fat craze of the 1980s and '90s, and the low-carb movement in the early 2000s, just because a food is low in gluten (or fat or carbs) doesn't mean it's a health food. You should approach these foods as you would any other meal. Make sure that they fit into your dietary needs, and buy accordingly. These foods—gluten free or not—will hinder your weight loss by adding unnecessary sugars and calories to your diet. Starchy (rice, potatoes) and grain-based (breads, pasta, bagels) foods should be limited if you're trying to get your abs to shine through. Eat them in smaller quantities first thing in

Abs for Every Eater

the morning or directly after you exercise for the best return on your weight loss efforts.

Watch Out for High-Protein Foods

We've made it more than clear that you need to eat more protein to see your abs and maximize weight loss. But when you go gluten free, you must be wary of high-protein foods that aren't naturally loaded with protein. This includes foods like granola, cereal, and high-protein grains that have been engineered to boost your protein intake. While great in theory, the protein in these foods are usually fortified with pure gluten and can be a stealthy nightmare on your cleaner-eating approach.

THE HURDLE:
You Always Eat Out

Making a home-cooked meal is the easiest way to ensure better nutrition. You buy the ingredients and know exactly what went into your meals. Unfortunately, most people don't have the time or confidence to cook on a daily basis. In fact, the number of calories that Americans consume outside of their homes has doubled since the late 1970s—and that number is directly linked to our increase in weight gain. A study in Spain found that people who ate at restaurants two or more times per week were 33 percent more likely to become overweight or obese. What's more, those same people were also 40 percent more likely to be at least 4 pounds heavier at the end of the year than those who rarely dine out, says Dr. Roussell.

The easy solution would be to cook more meals at home. That's why we created a cookbook full of recipes, which will provide easy-to-make, nutritious meals that fit our instant abs eating plan. But we know you'll still want to eat out. And since the best diet plan is all about flexibility, we've provided a crash course in navigating a restaurant menu, so that you can lose weight without losing your favorite place to eat.

Control Your Environment

When you eat out, no one is going to control calories for you, and you shouldn't be expected to count calories for yourself. But these are the facts: You are likely to eat 36 percent more calories when you eat out than when you're at home. So you need to take steps that help limit your overindulgence.

Calorie Saver #1: Ask your server to remove the bread basket from the table.

Calorie Saver #2: Tell your server what you would like on your plate. If your meal comes with french fries or chips, ask for those to be left off your plate.

Calorie Saver #3: Ask for sauces or salad dressing to be brought on the side. This way you can add them in the amounts you need (not in the excess amounts that most restaurants provide).

Calorie Saver #4: It's very hard to overeat vegetables, but rice, potatoes, pastas, and breads are carbohydrate- and calorie-dense foods that can sabotage your weight loss.

FIVE TIPS FOR AVOIDING GLUTEN

Many unexpected foods could be secretly sabotaging your efforts.

If you have a gluten allergy (i.e., celiac disease), then staying away from gluten is very important. Celiac disease in an inflammatory condition, and high levels of inflammation run counter to your weight loss efforts. If you are having trouble breaking through a weight loss plateau, make sure that you are truly gluten free. Foods like soy sauce, deli meats, marinade and sauces, meal replacement shakes, and oats (which don't contain gluten but a similar compound that many people with celiac disease don't respond well to) may be adding gluten to your diet without you knowing, says Dr. Roussell.

TIP 1
Read foods labels carefully to make sure that gluten or wheat isn't being added as a binding or thickening agent to marinades or sauces that you are using.

TIP 2
Look for oat- and gluten-free hot cereal to replace your morning oatmeal.

TIP 3
Make sure you are buying soy sauce that is specifically labeled gluten free.

TIP 4
Skip the deli meats; instead cook and slice your own. If you like using deli meats for convenience, choose a brand that doesn't contain additives or preservatives. This will limit your exposure to hidden sources of gluten.

TIP 5
Meal replacement shakes oftentimes contain oat and/or barley fiber to enhance the fiber content of the shakes. These are ingredients you should avoid if you are gluten free. Instead make your own. In a blender, combine 1½ scoops vanilla protein powder, 3 tablespoons walnuts, 2 tablespoons ground flaxseed, ½ cup blueberries, 1 teaspoon powdered green tea, 1½ cups water, and 3 ice cubes for a gluten-free, carbohydrate-controlled, 400-calorie meal replacement shake.

ABOUT THE EXPERT

Mike Roussell holds a doctorate in nutrition from Penn State University. He is a sought-after nutrition consultant known for his evidence-based approach that transforms complex nutrition concepts into practical nutrition habits and strategies for his clients. "Dr. Mike" works with a range of clientele that includes professional athletes, executives, food companies, and top-rated fitness facilities. He is a widely published author, and his work can be seen regularly on newsstands, on leading fitness Web sites, and at your local bookstore. To learn more, check out Facebook.com/nutritionphd.

CHAPTER 6

The Ultimate Abs Workout

SCULPT YOUR BODY FROM HEAD TO TOE
WITH THIS CHALLENGING TOTAL-BODY WORKOUT.

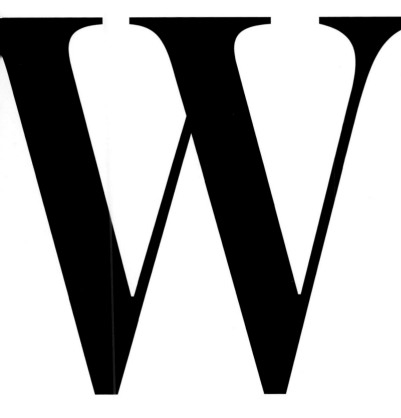

hen you visit the gym, you probably make your way into one of two areas: the cardio room or Spinning class. Both offer stress relief, burn calories, and will improve your overall health. And while we'd never suggest that you completely ignore an activity you enjoy, using either of these methods is not the best way to see rapid results—especially when your biggest challenge is simply finding time to exercise. You need an exercise plan that guarantees every second of your gym time will result in a flatter tummy.

That's why we created The Abs Workout. It doesn't matter if you've been exercising for 10 years or never stepped foot in the gym—you've never experienced a workout like this. We created a fat-scorching plan

The Ultimate Abs Workout

designed specifically to uncover your abs. It's the perfect combination of time-tested exercises that tone your muscles, and innovative movements that challenge your core and keep your workouts fun and engaging. The program is so effective that you'll only lift weights 3 days a week. That's because the exercises will exhaustively work all the muscles in your body, and you'll need the rest of the week to recover so you can continually improve.

The Fall of Machines

This workout offers everything you'll ever need to transform your body as efficiently as possible. But as you check out your new workout, you might think you notice a flaw: There are no machines. That's not by mistake. If you want some insight into why so many people struggle to lose weight, just step into any cookie-cutter gym. There, in the big open space, you have a template for obesity: lots of cardio equipment lined up in front of televisions. Rows and rows of beautiful exercise machines, strategically organized to help you work every single muscle in your body.

The gym owners aren't stupid. They built these facilities to make you feel at home and comfortable. Machines are welcoming, convenient, and enjoyable. But there's nothing worse than spending hundreds of dollars on a membership, hours and hours in a gym, and still not see results from your hard work. And while there might be several reasons for your struggles, the machines deserve some blame. After all, machines—for all their convenience—are less effective at

making changes to your body, say Canadian researchers.

In fact, both dumbbells and body-weight resistance are a better alternative and can help you burn more calories, say researchers from Columbia University. They found that free weights activate more muscle fibers, which results in more calories burned. While you won't notice a difference, your body will. That's because the nonmechanical approach allows you to perform your entire workout in fewer exercises. Think about it: Machines target each body part specifically, whereas it's much more efficient to select exercises that work multiple muscles at the same time. So instead of doing leg curls, leg extensions, and the thigh machine, you could just do lunges—and see better results in a fraction of the time.

Faster results are one thing, but aren't machines safer? That's the general feeling among most people who train at a gym. After all, you're much more likely to drop a dumbbell than experience a machine falling apart while you're using it. However, a review of physical therapists discovered that machines are actually more likely to cause injuries than dumbbell and barbell exercises. That's why we've outlined a new plan that removes machines from the equation and, at times, removes all equipment entirely so you can do your entire workout at home. Your bodyweight can help you score the ultimate body.

Don't take it from us. We reached out to the top fitness experts, and they insisted that a machine-free approach is not only cheaper, but also better at helping you bust out of a slump and putting you on the fast track to shed sizes and shrink your belly.

Your Abs—Revealed

By now you might feel that you have a pretty good idea of what it takes to flip the switch on the ultimate body makeover. So let's try a little pop quiz.

Which of the following is true:

(a) **Your abs are the key to a flatter belly.**
(b) **Gimmick devices and supplements will help you eliminate your muffin top.**
(c) **Crunches are the worst exercise for your abs.**

So what'd you pick? Hopefully you were waiting for **(d)** **None of the above.**

You see, the Lessons of the Lean are not what they used to be, which means the methods of changing your body are not what you commonly see in the gym. So let's start with the basics: The terms core and abs are not interchangeable. Crunches work your abs. But for the biggest benefits, you need to work your entire core, which is made up of the four layers of the abs (rectus abdominis, external and internal obliques, and the transverse abdominis), hip flexors, spine extensors, hip adductors (inner thigh muscles), hip abductors (including gluteus medius) and multifidus (a series of muscles that connect and support your spine; they are activated first to

protect your spine from injury).

That's the real purpose of your core: to prevent movement. So when you are focusing on doing crunches—or creating movement—you're doing the opposite of what was intended for your body. While crunches feel like they're doing something, they're actually one of the last exercises you want to include in an ab-revealing routine. Not only do they put your back at risk for injury, they also work your muscles significantly less than other alternatives. In fact, a study published in the *Journal of Strength and Conditioning Research* found that crunches create a 64 percent activation of your six-pack muscles. That sounds great until you realize that Canadian researchers found that a variation of the basic plank achieves 100 percent activation of the same muscles.

The message is simple: The more you train your abs for stability—with planks, side planks, and other exercises that activate your entire core—the better you'll look. The best part: You'll barely have to move, which should eliminate your strains and pains. Just beware. The exercises in this program are deceptively difficult but surprisingly effective at finally uncovering your abs.

Your program

Your plan consists of two workouts: Workout A and Workout B. Alternate between Workout A and Workout B three days a week, resting for at least a day between each session. So if you plan to exercise Monday, Wednesday, and

The Ultimate Abs Workout

ABOUT THE EXPERT

The Abs Workout was created by John "Roman" Romaniello, a fat loss specialist and creator of the Final Phase Fat Loss training program. He is the founder of Roman Fitness Systems and a New York City–based trainer, coach, writer, and model. He works with clients of every stripe—from overweight teenagers to professional athletes to media and literary sensation Gary Vaynerchuk. John has been featured in *Men's Health* and has appeared on *Good Morning America*. You can find out more about him at romanfitnesssystems.com.

Friday, you'd do Workout A on Monday, Workout B on Wednesday, and Workout A again on Friday. The next week, you'd do Workout B on Monday and Friday, and Workout A on Wednesday.

Before you begin

Start each workout with a 10-minute warmup. Or, you can hop on the treadmill, elliptical, or stairclimber. Make sure you push yourself hard enough during your warmup. Your heart rate should be elevated, and you should have light perspiration before you begin.

What you need

This workout only requires a few pairs of dumbbells, a stability ball, a chinup bar, and a step or bench. Start with lighter weights to assess your comfort level, and then increase the weight as your strength increases. Remember, don't be afraid of using bigger weights and becoming bulky. As you gain strength, you'll build more lean muscle that will melt fat and allow you to eat the type of foods you enjoy without feeling guilty.

Extra credit

All you need is three days a week of exercise, and you'll completely transform the way you look. You don't need to do any other form of exercise. However, if you want to do additional activity, such as cardio, perform it on the days you're not schedule to work out. For instance, if you exercise Monday, Wednesday, and Friday, you could do cardio on Tuesday and Thursday. Just make sure you give yourself at least 1 full day off every week.

DIRECTIONS

Each workout consists of four groups. Complete all of the sets and exercises in a group before proceeding to the next group. You should always perform the exercises in the order shown. When you see a number with a letter next to it, such as 1A, it means that the exercise is part of a group circuit. Perform 1 set of the first exercise (1A) and then do a set of the next exercise in the group (1B). Continue this process until you complete 1 set of each exercise in the group. Once you complete a set, repeat the process until you've completed all sets. Then move on to the next group.

For example, if a group consists of four exercises and requires three sets, you'll perform 1 set of all four exercises, rest, and then repeat the entire process two more times before beginning the next group of exercises. Use the specified number of repetitions, sets, and rest periods included with each exercise description.

RECTUS ABDOMINUS

The most well-known, these are your six-pack muscles. They help support your spine and keep your back healthy when you're bending over or picking up any weight—whether it's a dumbbell or your child.

SERRATUS ANTERIOR

This muscle is essential to your shoulder health and helps improve your posture and eliminate pain.

TRANSVERSE ABDOMINUS

Research shows that you can't "isolate" this muscle, but by bracing your abs during exercise (squeeze like you're about to be punched in the gut), you can help engage your transverse abdominus and prevent lower back pain.

EXTERNAL OBLIQUES

These aren't just flashy muscle on the side of your abs, they also help your rotate and bend sideways without pain.

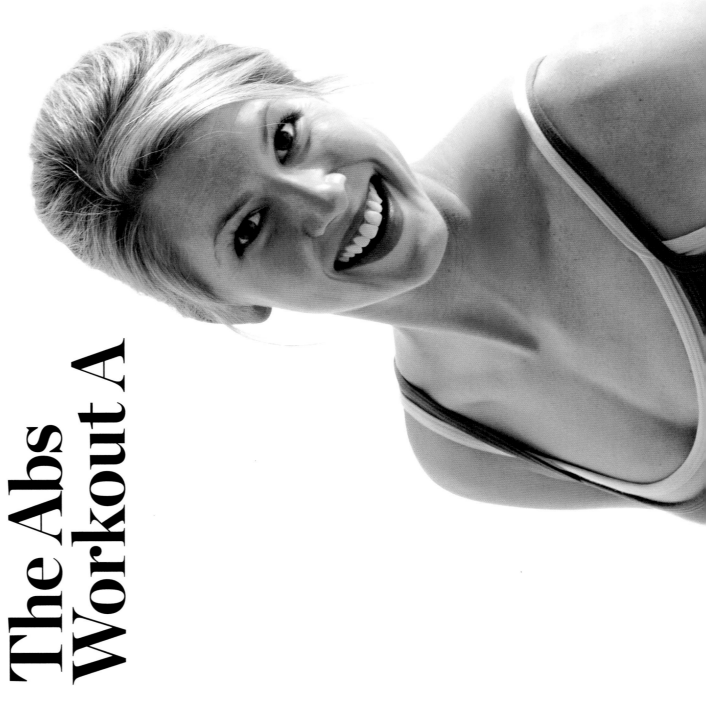

The Abs
Workout A

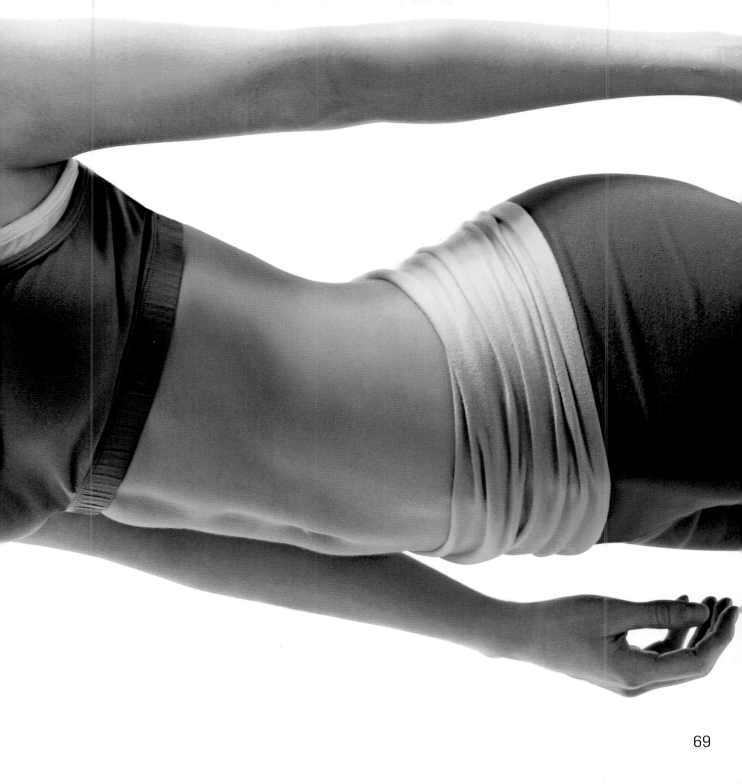

The Abs Workout A

HOW TO DO IT

This workout is made up of four groups, each consisting of three exercises. Try to rest as little as possible between all exercises within a group. Once you complete 1 set of all exercises in a group (1A through 1C, for instance), rest 2 minutes. Repeat this process two more times (for a total of 3 sets). Then rest 2 minutes and move on to the next exercise group (Group 2).

1A
Alternating DB Chest Press on Swiss Ball

A
- Grab a pair of dumbbells and lie on your back on a Swiss ball.
- Raise your hips so that your body forms a straight line from your knees to your shoulders. Your arms should be straight and above your chest. Your palms should be facing out but turned slightly inward.

B
- Without changing the angle of your hands, lower one dumbbell to the side of your chest.

C
- Press it back up to the starting position, then repeat with your other arm.
- Continue alternating arms until you complete all reps.

REPS 12/side **SETS** 3

1B
Swiss Ball Jackknife

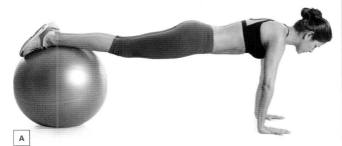

A

- Assume a pushup position with your arms completely straight. Rest your shins on a Swiss ball. Your body should form a straight line from your head to your ankles.

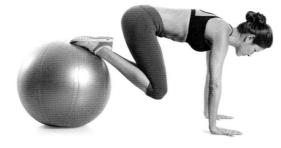

B

- Without changing your lower back posture, roll the Swiss ball toward your chest by pulling it forward with your feet.
- Pause, then return the ball to the starting position by rolling it backward.

REPS 10 **SETS** 3

1C
Unsupported One-Arm DB Row

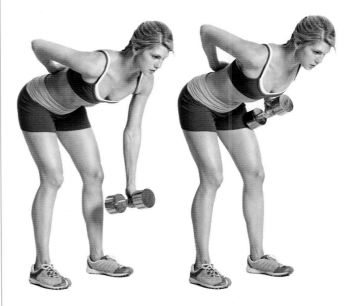

A

- Stand with your feet shoulder-width apart. Grab a dumbbell in your right hand, bend at your hips and knees, and lower your torso until it's almost parallel to the floor. Let the dumbbell hang at arm's length from your shoulder.

B

- Pull the dumbbell to the side of your torso, without rotating or lifting your torso as you row the weight. Make sure you keep your elbow tucked close to your side.
- Pause, then return the dumbbell back to the starting position.
- Do all reps, then repeat using your left arm.

REPS 15/arm **SETS** 3 **REST** 2 minutes

The Abs Workout A

2A
Squat Thrusts

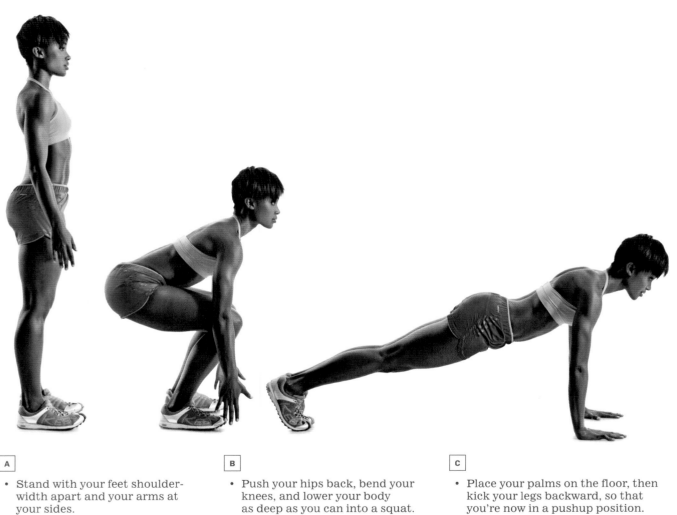

A

- Stand with your feet shoulder-width apart and your arms at your sides.

REPS 10–15 **SETS** 3

B

- Push your hips back, bend your knees, and lower your body as deep as you can into a squat.

C

- Place your palms on the floor, then kick your legs backward, so that you're now in a pushup position.
- Quickly bring your legs back to the squat position and jump up quickly back to the starting position. That's 1 rep.

2B
Single-Leg Dumbbell Deadlift

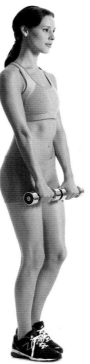

 A

- Grab a pair of dumbbells with an overhand grip and hold them at arm's length in front of your thighs. Stand with your feet hip-width apart and your knees slightly bent.
- Raise your left foot slightly off the floor.
- Without changing the bend in your knees, bend at your hips and lower your torso until it's almost parallel to the floor.
- Pause, then raise your torso back to the starting position.
- Do all reps and then switch legs.

REPS 12/leg **SETS** 3

2C
Jump Lunges

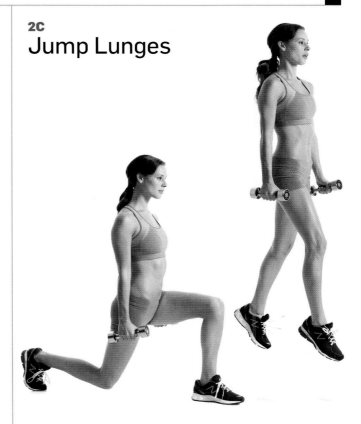

 A

- Hold a pair of dumbbells at arm's length next to your sides, your palms facing each other. Stand in a staggered stance, your left foot in front of your right.
- Lower your body as far as you can, or until your rear knee nearly touches the floor.

B

- Quickly jump into the air with enough force that you can scissor-kick your legs so you land with the opposite leg forward.
- Repeat, alternating back and forth with each repetition.

REPS 20 **SETS** 3 **REST** 2 minutes.

The Abs Workout A

3A
Dumbbell Pullover

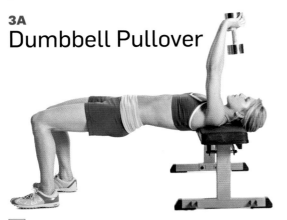

A

- Grab a pair of dumbbells and lie faceup on a bench so only your head, neck, and upper back are supported by the bench. Your feet will be flat on the floor. (If this is too difficult, lie on top of the entire bench).
- Hold the dumbbells straight over your chin with your arms extended.

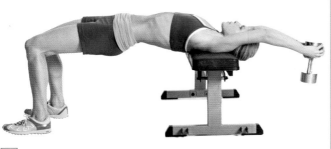

B

- Without changing the angle of your elbows, slowly lower the dumbbells back beyond your head until your upper arms are in line with your body or parallel to the floor.
- Pause, then slowly raise the dumbbells back to the starting position.

REPS 10–12 **SETS** 3

3B
Dumbbell Overhead Triceps Extension

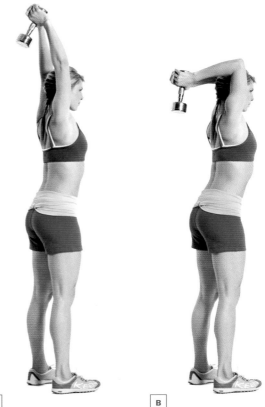

A

- Grab a dumbbell and stand tall with your feet shoulder-width apart.
- Hold the dumbbell at arm's length above your head, your palms facing each other.

B

- Without moving your upper arms, lower the dumbbell behind your head.
- Pause, then straighten your arms to return the dumbbell to the starting position.

REPS 6–10 **SETS** 3

3C

Single-Leg Squat

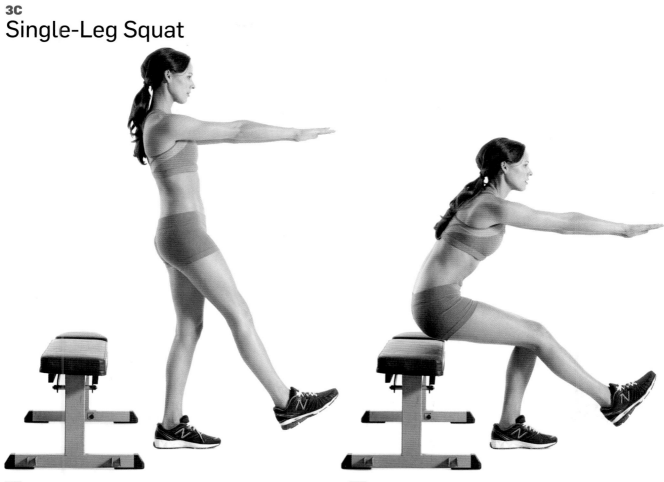

A

- Stand on your left leg in front of a bench or box that's about knee height. Hold your arms straight out in front of you.

REPS 10/leg **SETS** 3 **REST** 2 minutes

B

- Balancing on your left foot, bend your left knee and slowly lower your body until your right heel lightly touches the floor.
- Pause, then push yourself up.
- Complete the prescribed number of reps with your left leg, then immediately do the same number with your right. If this is too hard, lower your body as far as you can, pause, then press back up.

The Abs Workout A

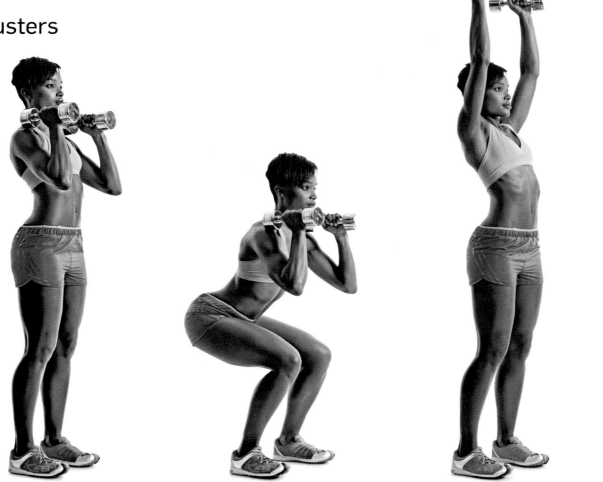

4A
Thrusters

A
- Grab a pair of dumbbells and hold them next to your shoulders, your palms facing each other. Stand tall with your feet shoulder-width apart.

B
- Lower your body until the tops of your thighs are at least parallel to the floor, while keeping your torso upright.

C
- Push your body back to a standing position as you press the dumbbells directly over your shoulders.
- Lower the dumbbells back to the starting position and repeat.

REPS 10–12 **SETS** 3

4B
Swiss Ball Plank with Feet on Bench

A

- Place your forearms on a Swiss ball and your feet on a bench. Your body should form a straight line from your shoulders to your ankles.
- Brace your core by contracting your abs as if you were about to be punched. Hold this position for 60 seconds.

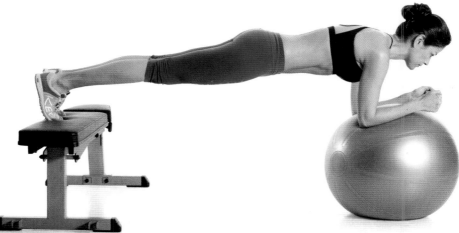

REPS 60 sec **SETS** 3

4C
Bodyweight Squat

A

- Stand as tall as you can, with your feet shoulder-width apart.

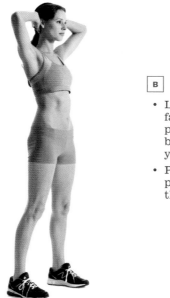

B

- Lower your body as far as you can by pushing your hips back and bending your knees.
- Pause, then slowly push yourself back to the starting position.

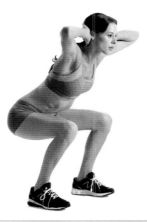

REPS 10–15 **SETS** 3

The Abs
Workout B

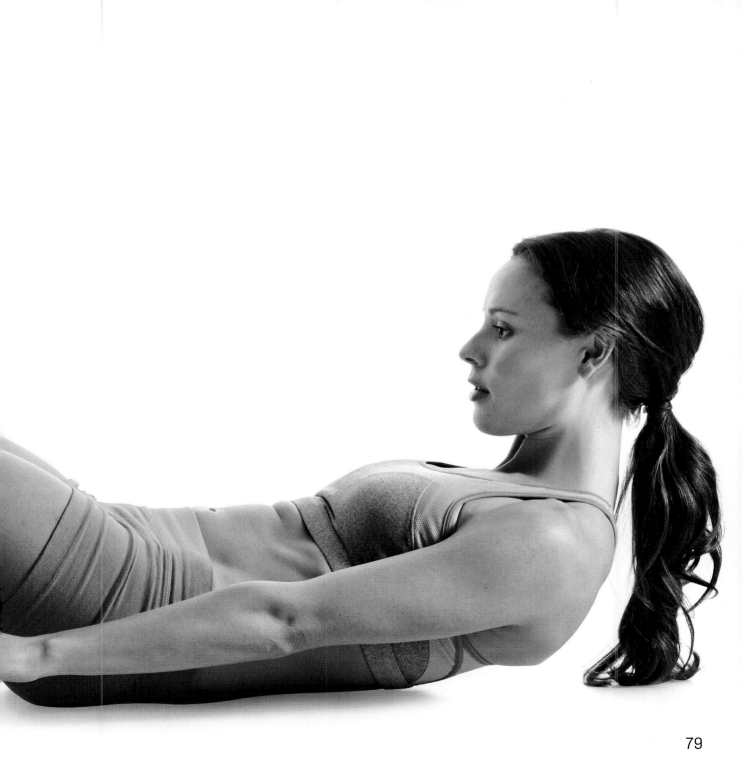

The Abs Workout B

HOW TO DO IT

Perform 1A to 1E sequentially, resting 30 to 45 seconds between exercises and 90 seconds after you complete a set of all the exercises in the group. Perform this circuit a total of four times. After your last circuit, rest 60 seconds and proceed to Group 2.

1A
Offset Dumbbell Lunge

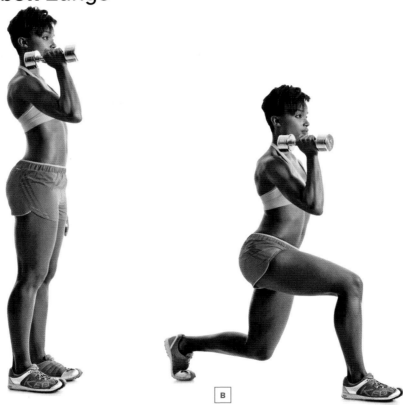

A

- Stand with your feet slightly closer than shoulder-width apart. Hold a dumbbell in your right hand next to your right shoulder with your arm bent.

REPS 10/side **SETS** 2

B

- Step forward into a lunge with your right foot. Hold for a second and return to the starting position.
- Complete the prescribed number of reps on that side, then switch arms and lunge with your left leg for the same number of reps.

1B
Mountain Climbers

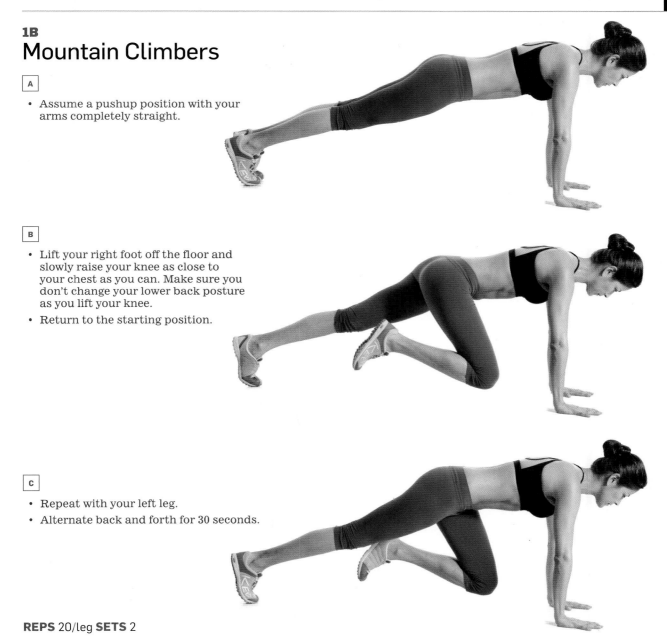

A

- Assume a pushup position with your arms completely straight.

B

- Lift your right foot off the floor and slowly raise your knee as close to your chest as you can. Make sure you don't change your lower back posture as you lift your knee.
- Return to the starting position.

C

- Repeat with your left leg.
- Alternate back and forth for 30 seconds.

REPS 20/leg **SETS** 2

The Abs Workout B

1C
Swiss Ball Rollout

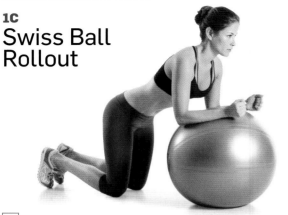

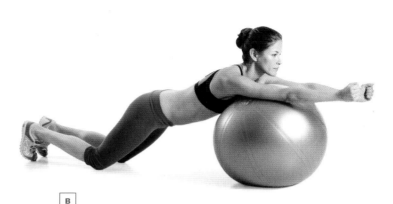

A

- Sit on your knees in front of a Swiss ball and place your forearms and fists on the ball. Your elbows should be bent about 90 degrees.

REPS 10–15 **SETS** 2

B

- Slowly roll the ball forward, straightening your arms and extending your body as far as you can, without allowing your lower back to collapse.
- Use your abdominal muscles to pull the ball back to your knees.

1D
Swiss Ball Jackknife

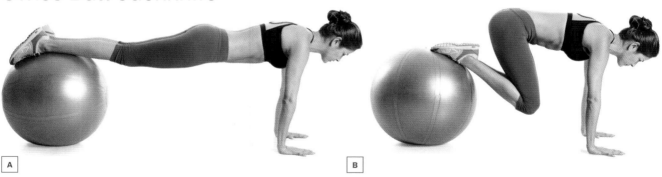

A

- Assume a pushup position with your arms completely straight. Rest your shins on a Swiss ball. Your body should form a straight line from your head to your ankles.

REPS 8–10 **SETS** 2

B

- Without changing your lower back posture, roll the Swiss ball toward your chest by pulling it forward with your feet.
- Pause, then return the ball to the starting position by rolling it backward.

1E

Underhand Grip Rear Lateral Raise

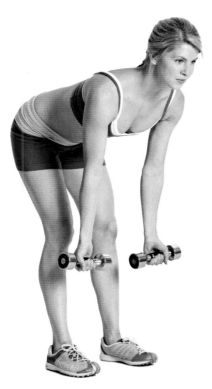

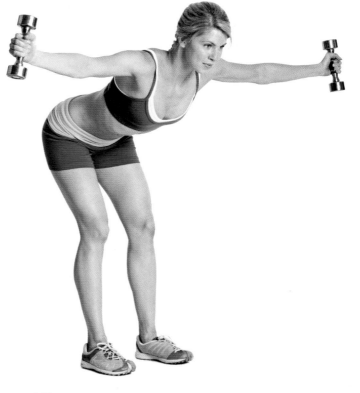

A

- Stand with your feet shoulder-width apart. Grab a pair of dumbbells and bend forward at your hips until your torso is nearly parallel to the floor. Let the dumbbells hang straight down from your shoulders, your palms forward.

B

- Without moving your torso, raise your arms straight out to your sides until they're in line with your body. At the top of the movement, your thumbs should be pointing up.
- Pause, then slowly return to the starting position.

REPS 10 **SETS** 2

The Abs Workout B

HOW TO DO IT

Perform 2A to 2D sequentially, resting 30 to 45 seconds between exercises and 90 seconds after you complete a set of all the exercises in the group. Perform this circuit four times. After your last circuit, rest 60 seconds and proceed to Group 3.

2A
Negative Chinup

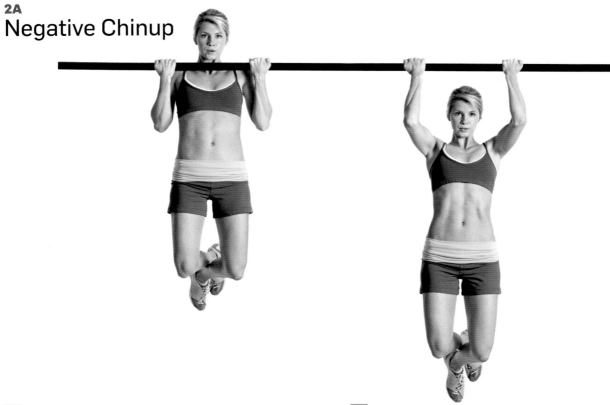

A

- Set a bench under a chinup bar, step up on the bench, and grasp the bar using a shoulder-width grip.
- From the bench, jump up so that your chest is touching the bar.

B

- Cross your ankles behind you, and try to take 5 seconds to lower your body until your arms are straight. If that's too hard, lower yourself as slowly as you can.
- Jump back up to the starting position and repeat.

REPS 10 **SETS** 4

2B

Dumbbell Romanian Deadlift

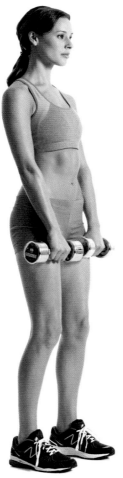

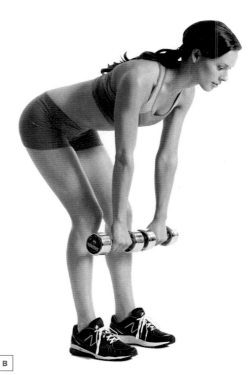

A

- Grab a pair of dumbbells with an overhand grip, and hold them at arm's length in front of your thighs. Stand with your feet hip-width apart and your knees slightly bent.

REPS 15 **SETS** 4

B

- Without changing the bend in your knees, bend at your hips and lower your torso until it's almost parallel to the floor.
- Pause, then raise your torso back to the starting position.

The Abs Workout B

2C
Jump Squat

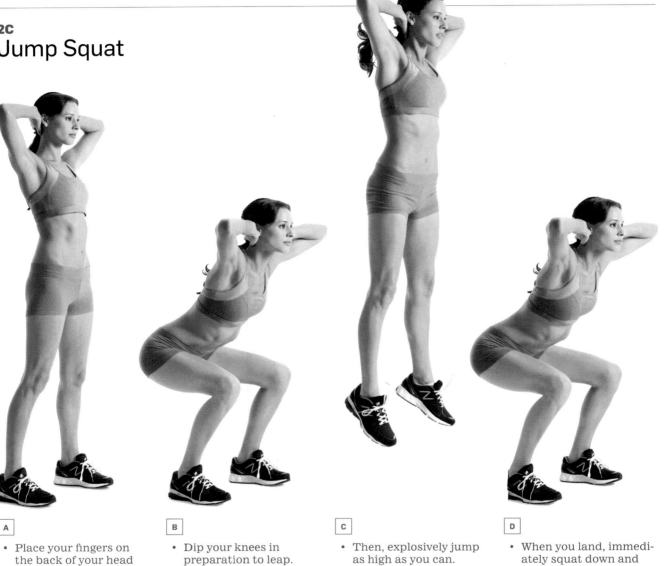

A
- Place your fingers on the back of your head and pull your elbows back so that they're in line with your body.

B
- Dip your knees in preparation to leap.

C
- Then, explosively jump as high as you can.

D
- When you land, immediately squat down and jump again.

REPS As many as possible in 30 seconds **SETS** 4

2D

Rolling Side Plank

A B

- Get into a plank position, but then immediately roll onto your right elbow so that you're performing a side plank. Hold for 1 to 2 seconds.

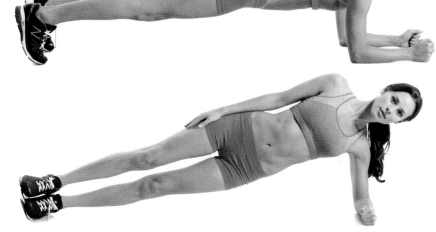

C

- Roll your body over onto both elbows—into a plank—and hold for a second.

D

- Next, roll all the way up onto your left elbow so that you're performing a side plank facing the opposite direction. Hold for another 1 to 2 seconds.
- Continue repeating until time is up.

REPS As many as possible in 45 seconds **SETS** 4

The Abs Workout B

Perform 3A to 3C sequentially, resting 45 seconds between exercises and 90 seconds after you finish all exercises in the group. Complete all the exercises in this group a total of three times. After your last circuit, rest 90 seconds and proceed to Group 4.

3A

Dumbbell Chest Press on Swiss Ball

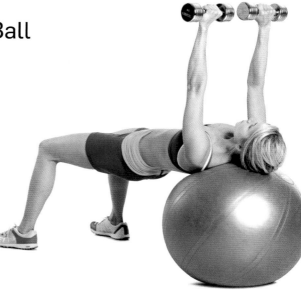

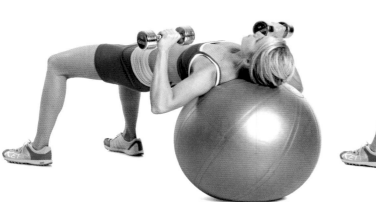

A

- Grab a pair of dumbbells and lie on your back on a Swiss ball.
- Raise your hips so that your body forms a straight line from your knees to your shoulders. Your arms should be straight up and your palms facing out but turned slightly inward.

B

- Without changing the angle of your hands, lower the dumbbells to the sides of your chest.
- Pause, then press the weights back up to the starting position as quickly as you can.

REPS 10–12 **SETS** 3

3B
Stepup and Single-Arm Press

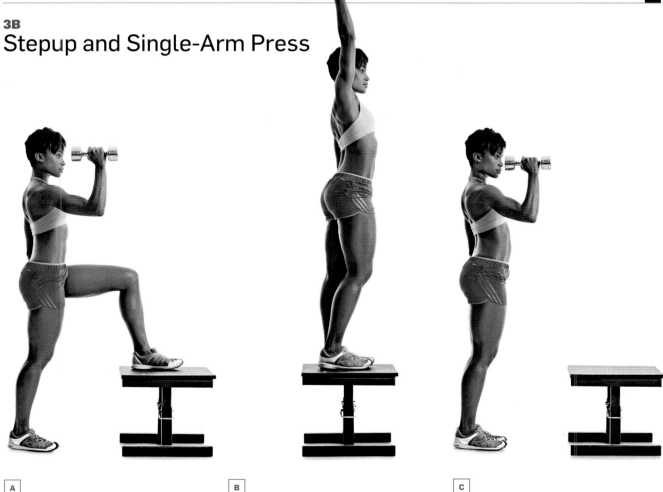

- Grab a dumbbell and hold it in your right hand, with your arm bent 90 degrees, so that the dumbbell is just above your shoulder. Your palm should be in line with your shoulder. Place your left foot on a box or step that's about knee height.

REPS 15/side **SETS** 3

B

- Push down with your left heel, and step up onto the box as you push the dumbbell straight above your right shoulder.

C

- Lower your arm and return to the starting position.
- Do all of the prescribed repetitions with your left foot on the box and the weight in your right hand.
- Switch arms and legs, and repeat.

The Abs Workout B

3C
Single-Arm Reverse Lunge and Press

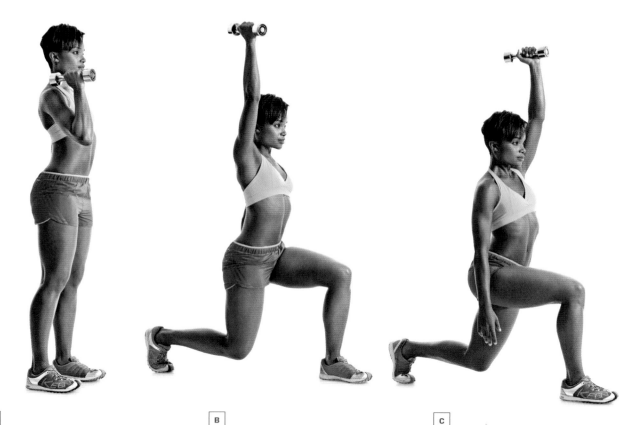

A
- Stand with your feet slightly closer than shoulder-width apart. Grab a dumbbell with your right hand and hold it next to your right shoulder, your palm facing in.

B
- Step backward with your right leg and lower your body into a reverse lunge as you simultaneously press the dumbbell straight above your shoulder.
- To return to the starting position, lower the dumbbell as you push yourself back up. That's 1 rep.

C
- Complete all your reps, then switch arms and legs and repeat.

REPS 8/side **SETS** 3

HOW TO DO IT

Perform the one exercise in Group 4 for a total of 4 sets, resting 30 to 60 seconds between them.

4
DB Lunge to Curl to Press

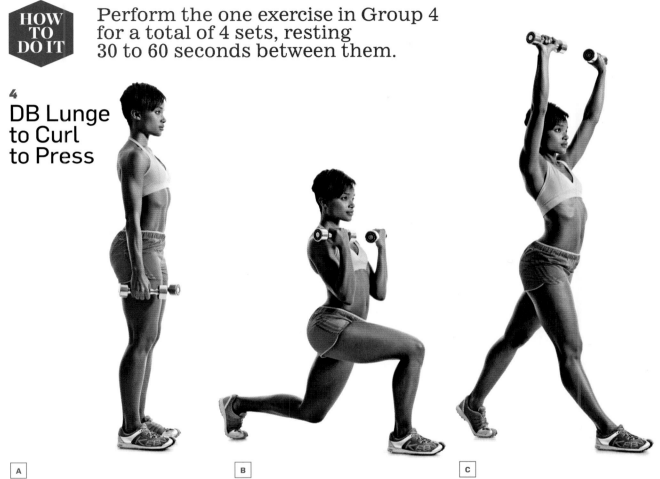

A
- Hold a pair of dumbbells at arm's length at your sides.

B
- Step forward with your right leg and lower your body until your front knee is bent at least 90 degrees.
- Curl the dumbbells to your chest as you sink down, and as you rise, rotate your wrists so that your palms face forward.

C
- Press the dumbbells overhead when you are in the standing position.
- Return your arms to the starting position.
- Repeat, this time stepping forward with your left leg.

REPS 6 lunges/leg (12 total curls and presses) **SETS** 4

The Best Abs Exercises Ever Created

THESE CUTTING-EDGE MOVES
WILL WORK EVERY MUSCLE IN YOUR BODY AND HELP YOU
GET BACK IN SHAPE FASTER THAN EVER.

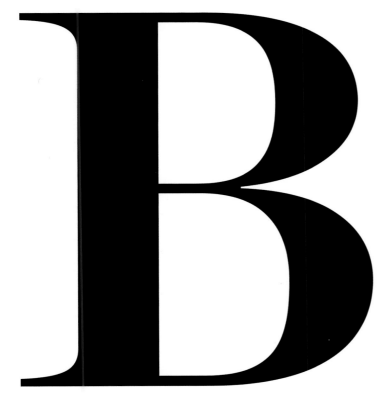

ack when you first

started exercising, you probably had a workout that seemed like it provided all the right ingredients you needed to lose weight, fit into your skinny jeans, and have more energy. A few reps here, a couple sets there, and you were done. But while your muscles felt like they were working, and sweat dripped from your brow and covered your shirt, the movements you did rarely took off the pounds or came close to creating a slimmer new you.

So what did you do wrong? Technically, nothing. You did the exercises and worked hard. That should be enough to lose weight—but it's not. The secret to a lean bod isn't wrapped in just any random mix of exercise. You need variety, but that doesn't mean simply trying every machine in

The Best Abs Exercises Ever Created

the gym. If you want to see your abs, the movements you perform must challenge your entire body and not individual muscles like your arms and shoulders. When that's achieved, you activate more muscle fibers, burn more calories, and—poof!—start to see your abs.

In order to put an end to your frustrating workouts, we had some of the best fitness minds handpick their favorite exercises. Some exercises may look familiar, like pushups, squats, and lunges. These are part of any great routine. But where most workouts stop is where these workouts actually begin. Our experts created a list of hundreds of moves that will work every muscle in your body, including your abs. We call these the best abs exercises ever created because they work you harder and faster for guaranteed results.

As you look through these exercises, it's important that you keep an open mind. You see, some exercises might seem easy and others bizarre. But we promise that these moves will bring out the best in your body and work your body in the ways it needs. Just don't be surprised if you don't see familiar machine-related exercises to tone your legs. Or a healthy diet of curls and pressdowns to sculpt your arms. If you do what you've always done, you'll get the same results you've always received. And that's the last thing that we—or our expert fitness advisors—want you to experience.

Not only will these exercises keep you from straying from your workout, they'll actually have you looking forward to your next gym day. And while a great workout doesn't require much equipment, these exercises will provide enough variety that you can do them in your own home or with the expensive machines you'll find at your local training facility. The big difference: These moves are so original that you'll be excited by the challenge of something new. And they'll work all of the regions that make up your core: upper abs, lower abs, obliques, transverse abdominis, and lower back muscles. Even if you've never lifted a weight before, you'll find that these exercises are more fun than you'd have imagined. But even better—they'll do more than make you sweat. They'll actually produce changes you can see and appreciate.

The best part? These exercises will literally reinvent how you view your abs. You see, there's more than 100 abs exercises in this program that don't include even the slightest crunching movement—and yet these moves work the muscles in your midsection harder than ever before. What's more, because these exercises simulate real-life movements, you'll build a body that won't experience as many aches and pains. Therein is the beauty of these moves: You'll be working every muscle in your body, sweating, melting calories and transforming your body into a new slim and trim version without even realizing it. And in no time, you'll have reshaped your abs, butt, thighs and arms and traded in the older version of you for the gorgeous body you've always wanted.

CHAPTER 7

Tone Every Inch

The Abs Exercise Rating System makes it easy to figure out which exercises are right for you on any given day. Just look for the key:

EASY   **MODERATE**   **HARD CORE**

So, if you're looking to upgrade your workout, or want to create your own, use our guide to find the right level of difficulty for your expertise.

The Abs Advantage

Creating your own flat belly plan requires a healthy dose of core exercises. But the best workouts include exercises that challenge every muscle in your abs without you even knowing it. We've included dozens of these exercises for you to use in your workouts. Just look for the exercises highlighted in yellow. They have been specially designed to work more muscles, shrink your belly, and leave you with a toned, tight body in a fraction of the time.

■

Upper Body Exercise: Chest

Sculpt and tone your upper body
and fight off fat.

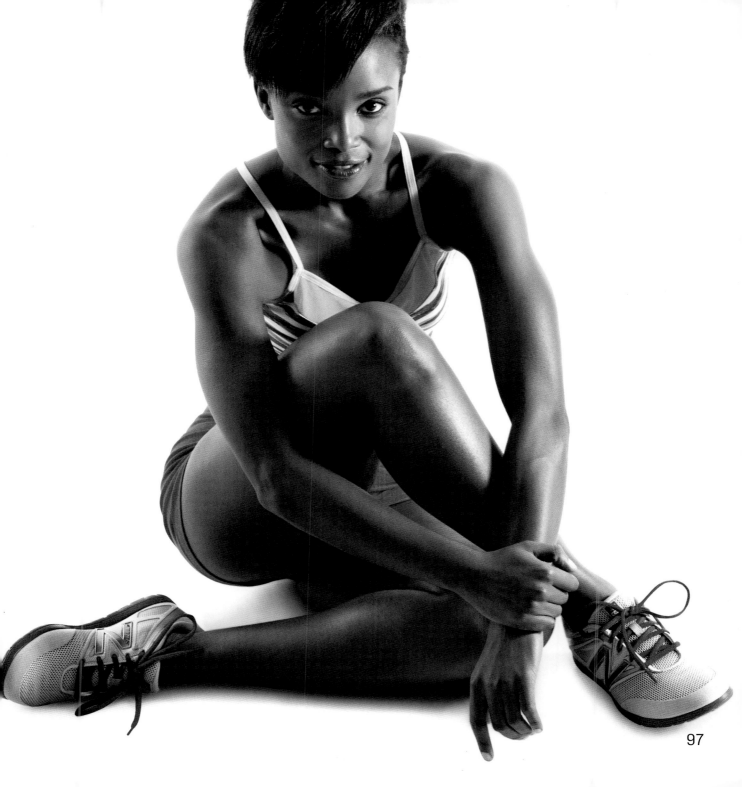

97

Upper Body Exercises: Chest

Pushups ●

A
- Get on all fours, and place your hands on the floor slightly wider than and in line with your shoulders. Your body should form a straight line from your ankles to your shoulders.
- Squeeze your abs as tight as possible and keep them contracted for the entire exercise.

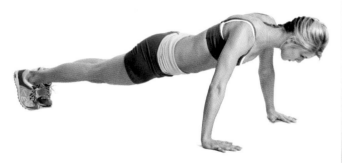

B
- Lower your body until your chest nearly touches the floor, making sure that you tuck your elbows close to the sides of your torso.
- Pause, then push yourself back to the starting position.

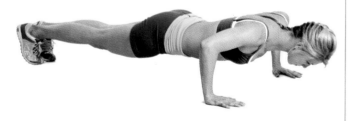

> ● **PUSHUPS—SIMPLIFIED!** *If you struggle with normal pushups, bend your knees and cross your ankles behind you. Your body should still form a straight line from your ankles to your shoulders. Then, lower your body until your chest nearly touches the floor and press back up to the starting position.*

Incline Dumbbell Press ●

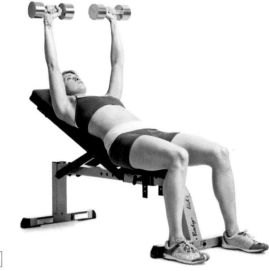

A
- Set an adjustable bench to an incline of 30 to 45 degrees.
- Grab a pair of dumbbells and lie faceup on the bench.
- Hold the dumbbells directly above your shoulders with your arms straight.

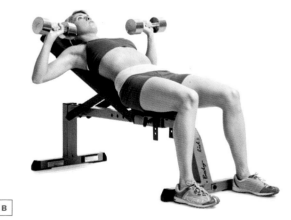

B
- Lower the dumbbells to the sides of your chest, pause, and then press the weights back above your chest.

Pushup Plus ●

A

- Get on all fours and place your hands on the floor slightly wider than and in line with your shoulders. Your body should form a straight line from your ankles to your shoulders.
- Squeeze your abs as tight as possible and keep them contracted for the entire exercise.

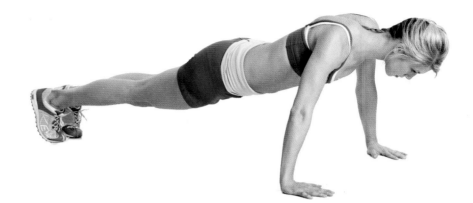

B

- Lower your body until your chest nearly touches the floor.
- Pause, then push yourself back to the starting position.

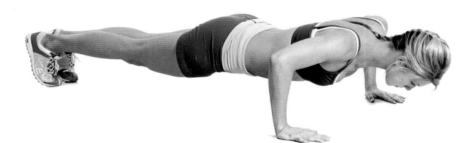

C

- Once your arms are straight, push your upper back toward the ceiling. It's a subtle move, but it should feel like your shoulder blades are flaring out.
- Pause, then repeat the entire movement.

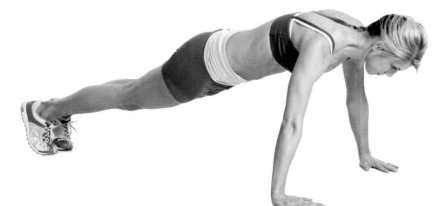

Upper Body Exercises: Chest

Pike Pushups ●

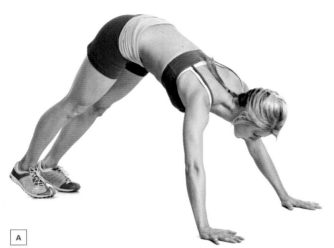

A

- Start in a traditional pushup position, but walk your feet toward your hands and raise your hips into the air. Your body should look like an inverted V.

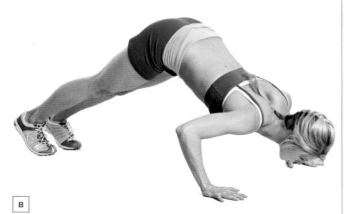

B

- Keeping your hips raised, lower your body until your chin nearly touches the floor.
- Pause, then press back up to the starting position.

Dumbbell Chest Press ●

A

- Grab a pair of dumbbells and lie faceup on a flat bench.
- Hold the dumbbells above your chest with your arms straight. The dumbbells should be nearly touching, and your palms should be facing your feet.

B

- Keeping your elbows tucked close to your body, lower the weights to the sides of your chest.
- Pause, then press the dumbbells back above your chest.

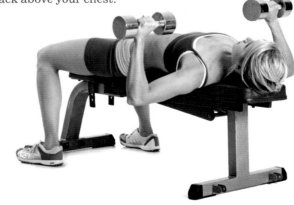

Dumbbell T-Pushup ●

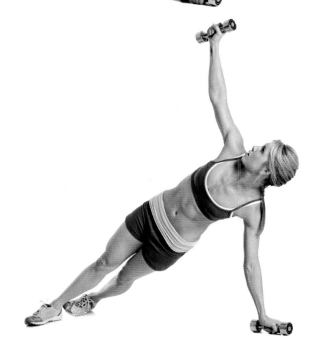

A

- Place a pair of dumbbells (preferably hex dumbbells) on the floor about shoulder-width apart.
- Start in a pushup position and grab the dumbbells.

B

- Perform a pushup while holding the dumbbells.

C

- As you press back up, rotate your body to the right and pull the dumbbell in your right hand up and above your shoulder. In the top position, your right arm should be straight and your body turned to the side so that you form the letter T.
- Lower the dumbbell back to the starting position, perform another pushup, and repeat—this time turning to the left.

● **T-PUSHUPS—SIMPLIFIED!** *If the Dumbbell T-Pushup is too difficult, simply perform the exercise without the dumbbells. The movement will be identical, but you won't have the added resistance.*

Upper Body Exercises: Chest

Pushup and Step Out ●

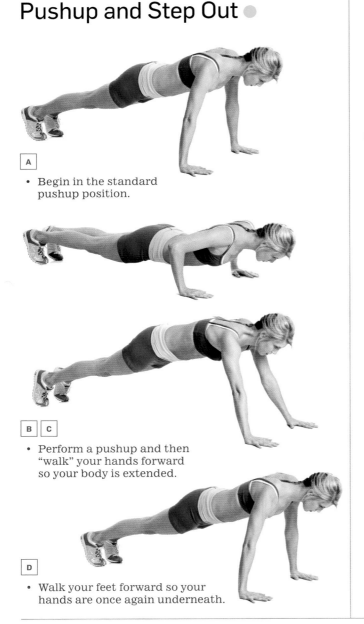

A

- Begin in the standard pushup position.

B C

- Perform a pushup and then "walk" your hands forward so your body is extended.

D

- Walk your feet forward so your hands are once again underneath.

Single-Leg Pushups ●

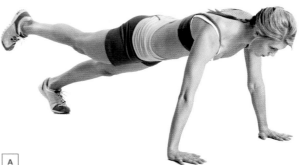

A

- Begin in the standard pushup position with your body forming a straight line from your ankles to your shoulders.
- Raise one foot off the floor.

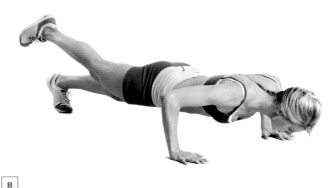

B

- Lower your body toward the floor and then press back up, all the while keeping your leg off the floor.
- Try to perform all reps without lowering your leg.

Pushup Jacks

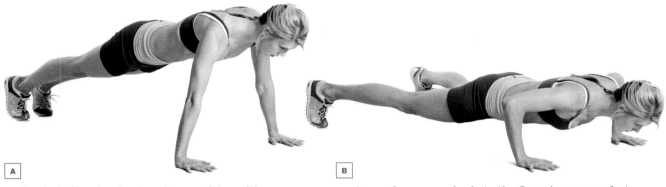

A
- Begin in the standard pushup position with your body forming a straight line from your ankles to your shoulders.

B
- As you lower your body to the floor, jump your feet outward so that your feet end up shoulder-width apart at the bottom of the movement.
- As you press your body back up, jump your legs back together and return to the starting position.

Grasshopper Pushup

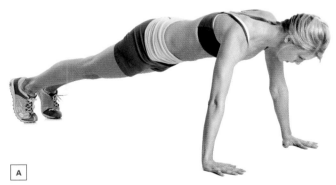
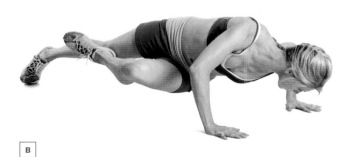

A
- Begin in the standard pushup position with your body forming a straight line from your ankles to your shoulders.
- Bend your right knee and slide your leg underneath your body.

B
- Perform a pushup, trying to prevent your right leg from touching the floor.
- Press back up, return your right leg to the starting position, and then repeat with your left leg.

Upper Body Exercises: Chest

Incline Pushup on Bench ●

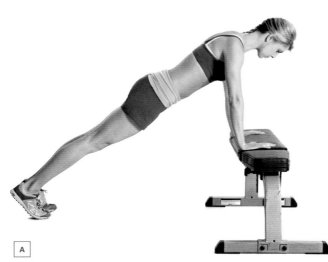

A

- Begin in the standard pushup position, but place your hands on a bench (or a box) instead of the floor. Your body should still form a straight line from your shoulders to your ankles.

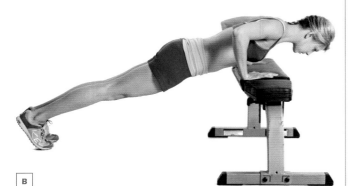

B

- Lower your chest to the bench, pause, and then press back up to the starting position.

Alternating Cable Press ●

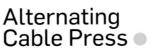

A

- Attach a D-handle to a cable station and adjust the pulley so the handle is at chest height.
- With your right hand, grab the high pulley handle and face away from the weight stack.
- Stagger your feet and make sure the handle is positioned in front of your shoulder. Your arm should be parallel to the floor.

B

- Push the handle forward and straighten your arm in front of you.
- Pause and return to the starting position.
- Perform all reps on one side, then switch hands and repeat.

Pushup with Hand Raise ●

A

- Begin in the standard pushup position with your body forming a straight line from your ankles to your shoulders.
- Lower your body to the floor and then press back up.

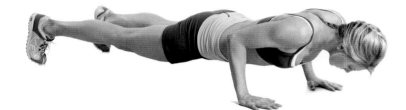

B

- As you return to the starting position, raise your right hand so it's in line with your body.
- Hold for 2 seconds, and then return your hand to the starting position.

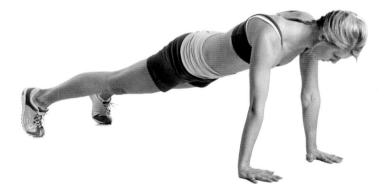

C

- Do another pushup and then repeat, this time raising your left hand.

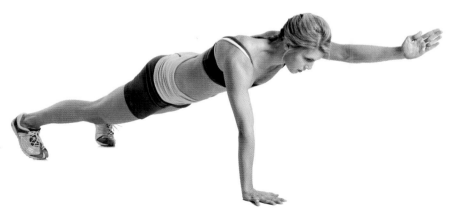

Upper Body Exercises: Chest

Single-Leg Pushup with Shoulder Touch ●

A

- Begin in the standard pushup position with your body forming a straight line from your ankles to your shoulders.

B

- Raise one foot off the floor and perform a pushup. As you press back up, take your left hand and touch your right shoulder.

C

- Return your hand to the starting position and perform another pushup. This time, take your right hand and touch your left shoulder.
- Continue alternating legs and arms on each rep.

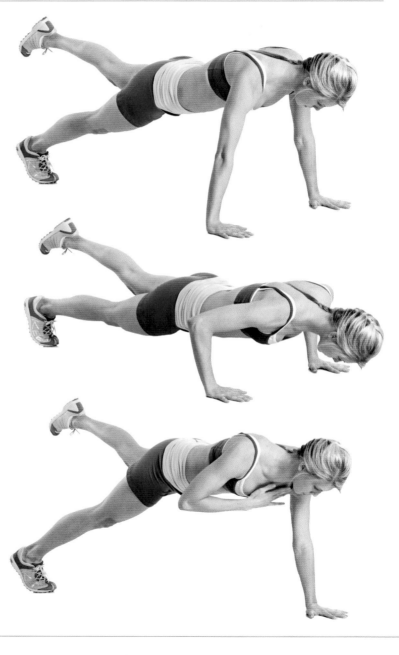

Resistance Band Forward Punches

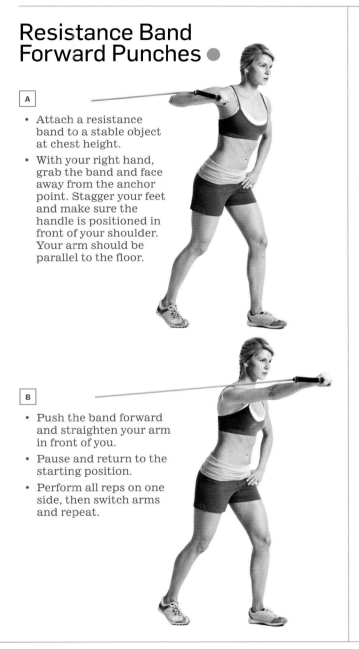

A

- Attach a resistance band to a stable object at chest height.
- With your right hand, grab the band and face away from the anchor point. Stagger your feet and make sure the handle is positioned in front of your shoulder. Your arm should be parallel to the floor.

B

- Push the band forward and straighten your arm in front of you.
- Pause and return to the starting position.
- Perform all reps on one side, then switch arms and repeat.

Spider-WOMAN Pushups

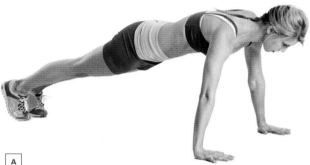

A

- Begin in the standard pushup position with your body forming a straight line from your ankles to your shoulders.

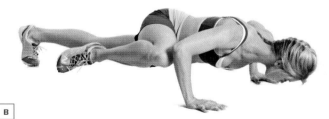

B

- As you lower your body toward the floor, lift your right foot off the floor. Bring your right leg out to the side and try to touch your knee to your right elbow.
- Reverse the movement, then push your body back up to the starting position.
- Perform another pushup, but try to touch your left knee to your left elbow.
- Alternate sides on each repetition.

107

Upper Body Exercises: Chest

Dumbbell Pushup Row ●

A

- Place a pair of dumbbells about shoulder-width apart on the floor. Grab the dumbbell handles and position yourself in a pushup position.

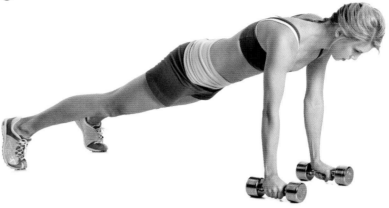

B

- Lower your body to the floor and then press back up.

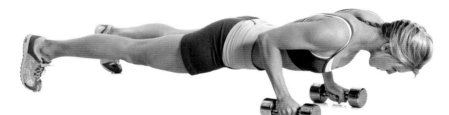

C

- Once you're back in the starting position, pull the dumbbell in your right hand up toward the side of your chest.
- Pause, then return the dumbbell back to the floor and repeat with your left hand. That's 1 rep. Try to prevent your torso from rotating each time you row the weight.

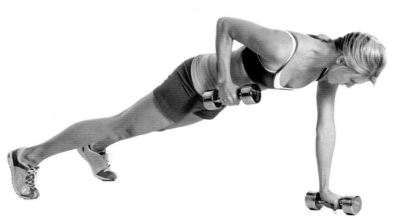

TRX Atomic Pushups ●

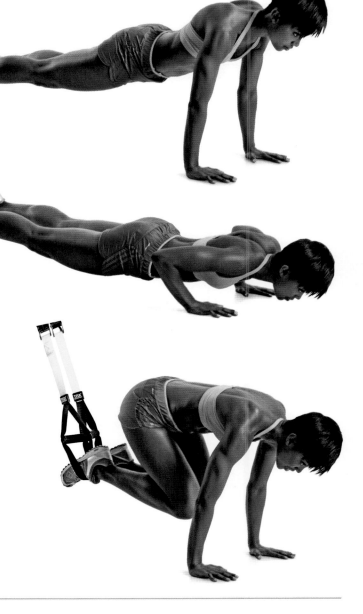

A

- Place both feet in the foot cradles of a TRX.
- Get into pushup position with your body forming a straight line from your shoulders to your ankles.

B

- Perform a pushup by lowering your body until your chest is just above the floor and then pressing back up.

C

- Bring your knees toward your elbows in a crunching movement.
- Pause and return to the starting position.

Upper Body Exercise: Back

Look stunning in any backless dress and balance your body.

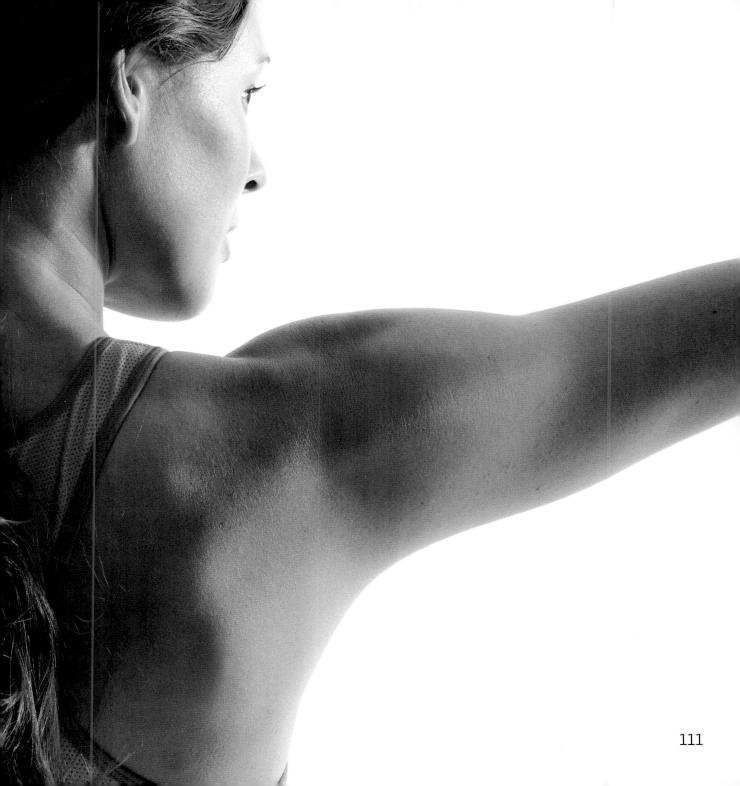

Upper Body Exercises: Back

Barbell Bent-Over Row ●

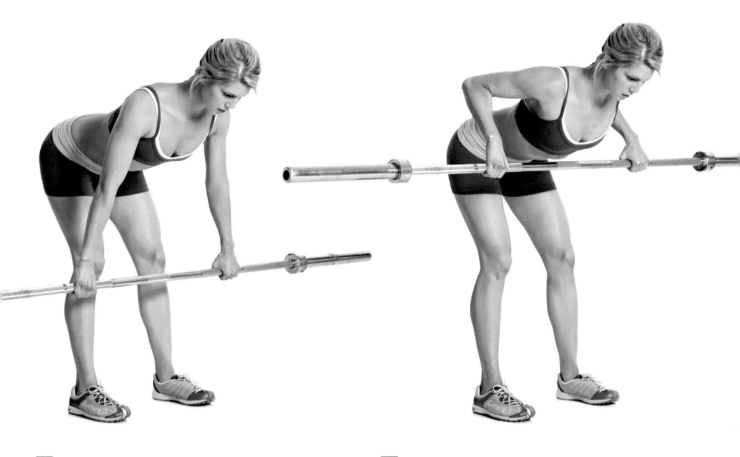

A

- Grab a barbell with an overhand grip with your hands about shoulder-width apart.
- Hold the bar at arm's length, and then bend at your hips and lower your torso until it's almost parallel to the floor. Your knees should be slightly bent and your lower back naturally arched.

B

- Squeeze your shoulder blades together and pull the bar up to your upper abs.
- Pause, then return the bar back to the starting position.

Inverted Row ●

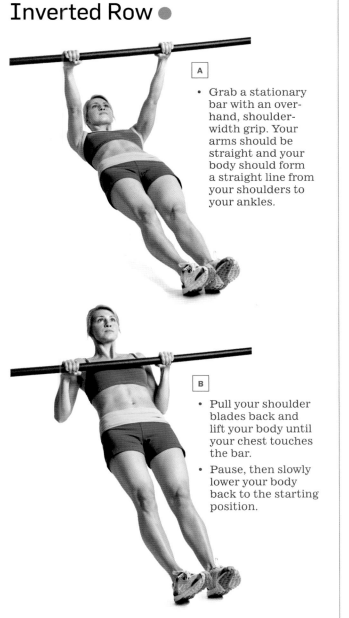

A

- Grab a stationary bar with an overhand, shoulder-width grip. Your arms should be straight and your body should form a straight line from your shoulders to your ankles.

B

- Pull your shoulder blades back and lift your body until your chest touches the bar.
- Pause, then slowly lower your body back to the starting position.

Dumbbell Bent-Over Row ●

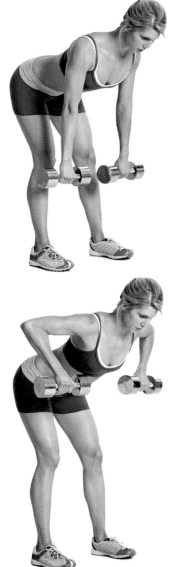

A

- Grab a pair of dumbbells with an overhand grip with your hands about shoulder-width apart.
- Hold the dumbbells at arm's length, and then bend at your hips and lower your torso until it's almost parallel to the floor. Your knees should be slightly bent and your lower back naturally arched.

B

- Squeeze your shoulder blades together and pull the dumbbells up to the sides of your torso.
- Pause, then return to the starting position.

Upper Body Exercises: Back

Band Pull-Apart ●

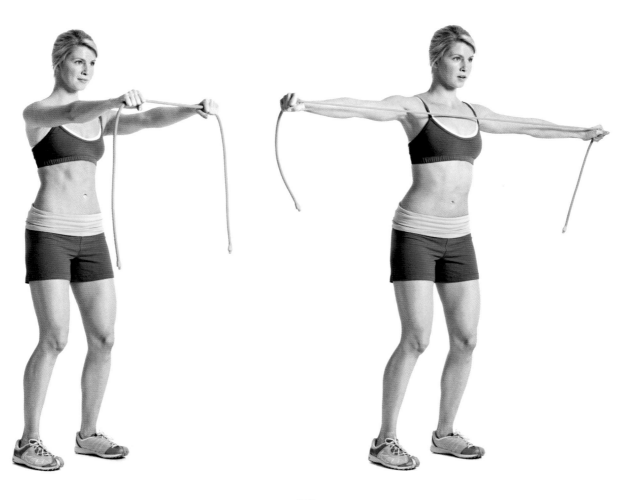

A

- Grab a resistance band in both hands and hold the ends a little more than shoulder-width apart.
- Raise your arms so that the band is at arm's length in front of your chest.

B

- Pull each end of the band and squeeze your shoulder blades together. (Try to snap the band in half.)
- Pause, then return your hands to the starting position.

Assisted Chinups ●

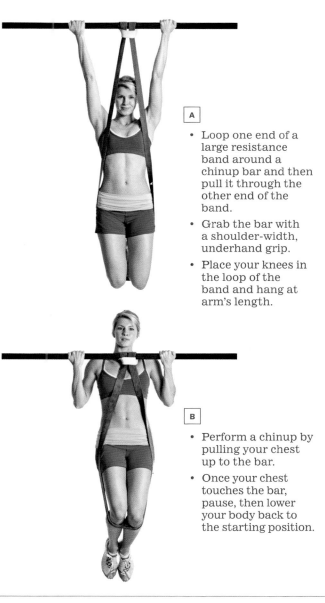

A

- Loop one end of a large resistance band around a chinup bar and then pull it through the other end of the band.
- Grab the bar with a shoulder-width, underhand grip.
- Place your knees in the loop of the band and hang at arm's length.

B

- Perform a chinup by pulling your chest up to the bar.
- Once your chest touches the bar, pause, then lower your body back to the starting position.

Split Stance Single-Arm Cable Row ●

A

- Attach a D-handle to the pulley on a cable station and set the cable to about chest height.
- Grab the handle in your right hand, step away from the cable tower, and stand in a staggered stance.

B

- Pull the handle toward your right side by squeezing your shoulder blade back.
- Pause, then return to the starting position.
- Perform all reps, switch hands, and repeat.

115

Upper Body Exercises: Back

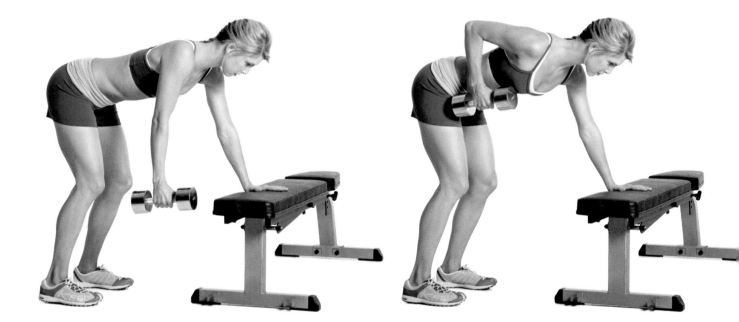

3-Point Dumbbell Row ●

A

- Grab a dumbbell in your right hand.
- Push your hips back and bend over until your torso is almost parallel to the floor. Place your left hand on a bench in front of your body. Your right arm should hang at arm's length with your palm facing your other arm.

B

- Keeping your elbow close to your body, pull the dumbbell up to your chest by squeezing your shoulder blade back.
- Pause, then lower back to the starting position.
- Complete all prescribed reps, then switch arms and repeat.

Seated Lat Pulldown ●

A

- Sit at a lat pulldown station and grab the bar with an overhand grip that's just beyond shoulder width. Your arms should be completely straight and your torso upright.

B

- Pull your shoulder blades down and back, and bring the bar to your chest.
- Pause, then return to the starting position.

Dumbbell Row with Rotation ●

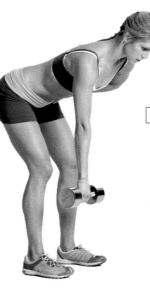

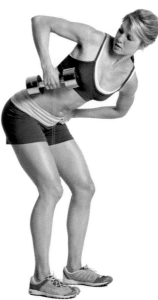

A

- Grab a dumbbell with an overhand grip in your right hand.
- Hold the dumbbell at arm's length, and then bend at your hips and lower your torso until it's almost parallel to the floor. Your knees should be slightly bent, your lower back naturally arched, and your other hand on your hip.

B

- Squeeze your shoulder blades back and then pull the dumbbell up to the sides of your torso and rotate your torso upward.
- Pause, then return to the starting position.
- Complete all prescribed reps, switch arms, and repeat.

Upper Body Exercises: Back

Kneeling Mixed Grip Pulldown ●

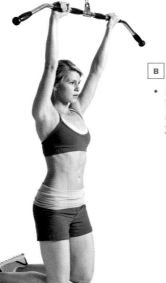

A

- Attach a bar to a lat pulldown station and grab the bar with a mixed grip—one hand over, the other under.
- Kneel on the floor so that your body forms a straight line from your shoulders to your knees.

B

- Squeeze your shoulder blades down and back, and then bring the bar to your chest.

45-Degree Cable Row ●

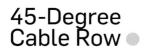

A

- Attach a D-handle to the pulley on a cable station and set the cable to the highest setting.
- Grab the handle in your right hand, step away from the cable tower, and stand in a staggered stance.

B

- Pull the handle down and toward your right side by squeezing your shoulder blade back.
- Pause, then return to the starting position.
- Perform all reps, switch hands, and repeat.

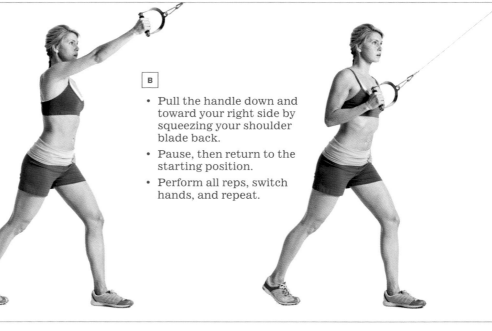

Resistance Band Bent-Over Row ●

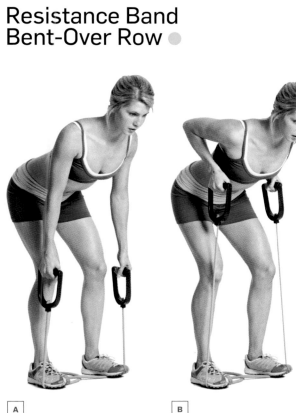

A

- Grab a resistance band and step on it with one foot (use both feet for more resistance).
- Hold the band in each hand at arm's length, about shoulder-width apart, and then bend at your hips and lower your torso until it's almost parallel to the floor. Your knees should be slightly bent and your lower back naturally arched.

B

- Squeeze your shoulder blades together and pull the band up to your upper abs.
- Pause, then return the bar back to the starting position.

Resistance Band Pulldown ●

A

- Loop one end of a large resistance band around a chinup bar and then pull it through the other end of the band.
- Grab the band with both hands about shoulder-width apart and your arms straight.

B

- Squeeze your shoulder blades down and back, and pull each hand to the side of your chest.
- Pause, then return to the starting position.

Upper Body Exercise: Arms

Fight off arm flab and build lean, sexy biceps and triceps.

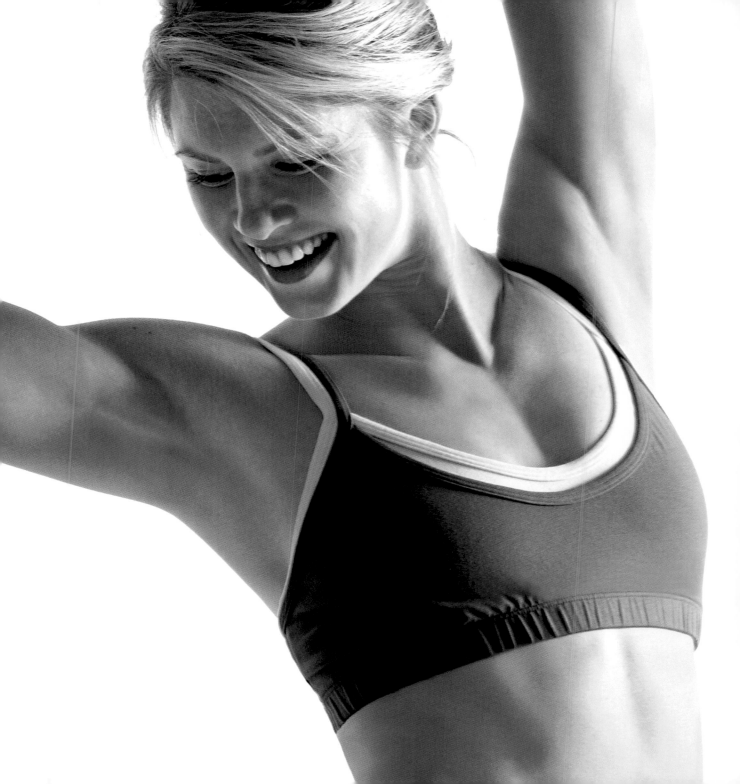

Upper Body Exercises: Arms

Triceps Rope Extensions ●

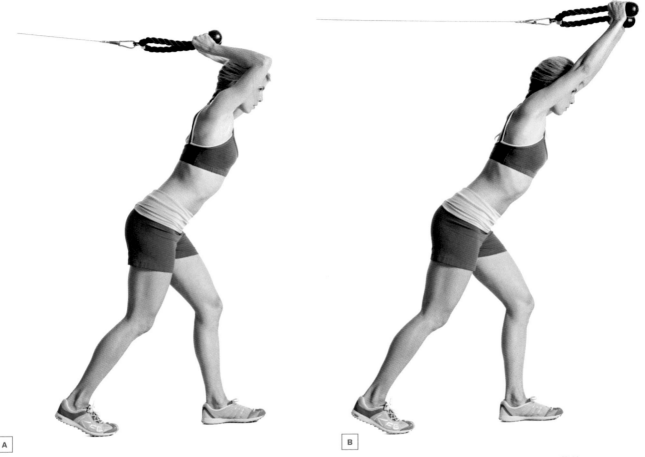

A

- Attach a rope attachment to a cable station and set it at a height above your head.
- Grab the rope with each hand and stand with your back to the cable station.
- Stand in a staggered stance, bend at your torso, and hold the rope behind your head with your elbows bent 90 degrees.

B

- Without moving your upper arms, pull the rope forward until your arms are straight.
- Pause, then return to the starting position.

Dumbbell Biceps Curl ●

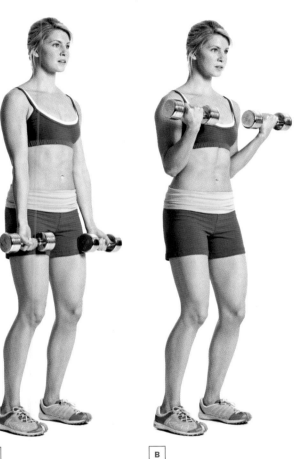

A

B

- Grab a pair of dumbbells and let them hang at arm's length next to your sides with your palms facing forward.

- Without moving your upper arms, bend your elbows and curl the dumbbells as close to your shoulders as you can.

- Pause, then lower the weights back to the starting position.

Resistance Band Biceps Curl ●

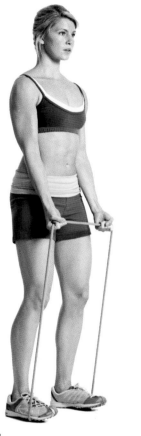
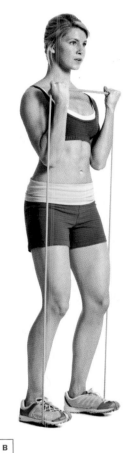

A

B

- Stand on one end of a resistance band with both feet about shoulder-width apart.

- Grab the other end of the band with your hands about shoulder-width apart and your arms at your sides.

- Without moving your upper arms, bend your arms and pull the band as close to your shoulders as you can.

- Pause, then lower the band to the starting position.

Upper Body Exercises: Arms

Resistance Band Overhead Triceps Press ●

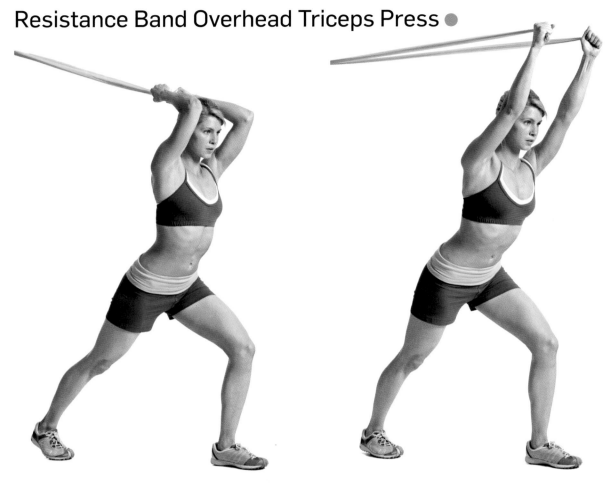

A

- Loop one end of a large resistance band around a chinup bar (or a secure object) and then pull it through the other end of the band.

- Grab the band with each hand and your back to the anchor point. Stand in a staggered stance, one foot in front of the other.

- Hold the band behind your head, your elbows pointing forward and bent 90 degrees.

B

- Without moving your upper arms, push your forearms forward until your arms are straight.

- Pause, then return to the starting position.

Dips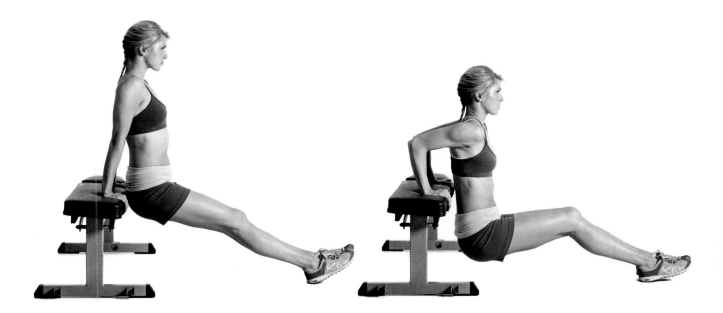

A

- Hoist yourself up on a bench with your torso perpendicular to the floor. You'll maintain this posture throughout the exercise.
- Bend your knees and cross your ankles.

B

- Slowly lower your body until your shoulder joints are below your elbows.
- Push back up until your elbows are nearly straight but not locked.

Upper Body Exercise: Shoulders

Look great in any tank top by targeting these muscles.

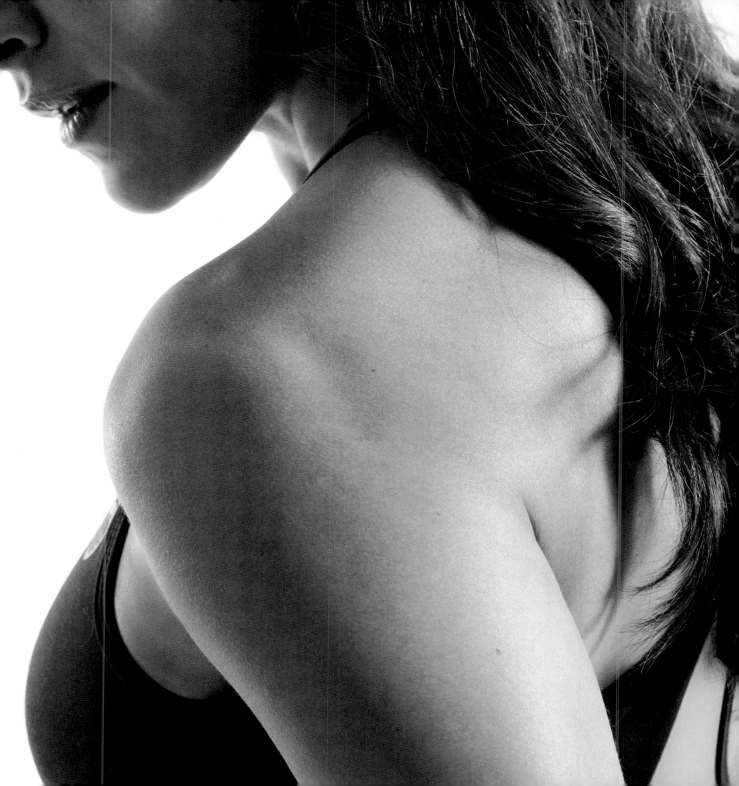

Upper Body Exercises: Shoulders

Barbell Shoulder Press ●

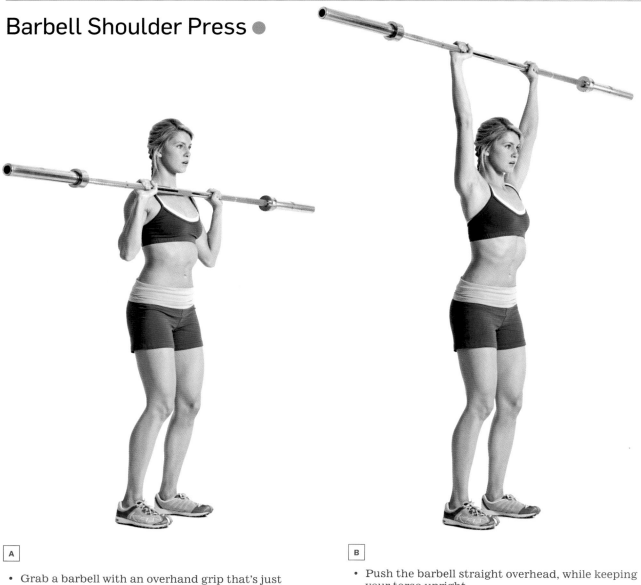

A

- Grab a barbell with an overhand grip that's just beyond shoulder width and hold it at shoulder level in front of your body. Stand with your feet shoulder-width apart and your knees slightly bent.

B

- Push the barbell straight overhead, while keeping your torso upright.
- Pause, then lower the bar back to the starting position.

Dumbbell Lateral Shoulder Raises ●

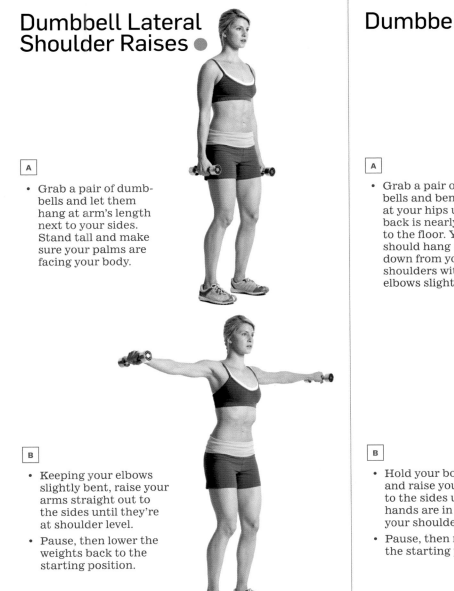

A

- Grab a pair of dumbbells and let them hang at arm's length next to your sides. Stand tall and make sure your palms are facing your body.

B

- Keeping your elbows slightly bent, raise your arms straight out to the sides until they're at shoulder level.
- Pause, then lower the weights back to the starting position.

Dumbbell Rear Lateral Raise ●

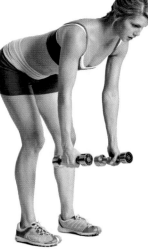

A

- Grab a pair of dumbbells and bend forward at your hips until your back is nearly parallel to the floor. Your arms should hang straight down from your shoulders with your elbows slightly bent.

B

- Hold your body still and raise your arms out to the sides until your hands are in line with your shoulders.
- Pause, then return to the starting position.

Upper Body Exercises: Shoulders

T Raise ●

A

- Lie chest down on an adjustable bench set to a low incline. Your arms should hang straight down from your shoulders, and your palms should be facing each other.

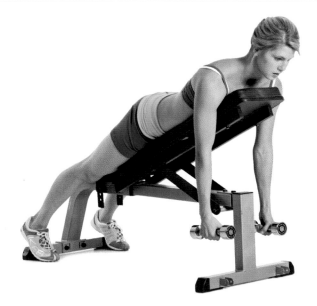

B

- Raise your arms straight out to your sides until they're in line with your body.
- At the top of the movement, your arms and torso should form a T.
- Pause, then lower your arms back to the starting position.

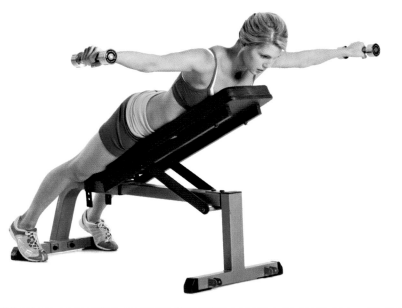

Y Raise

A

- Lie chest down on an adjustable bench set to a low incline. Your arms should hang straight down from your shoulders, and your palms should be facing each other.

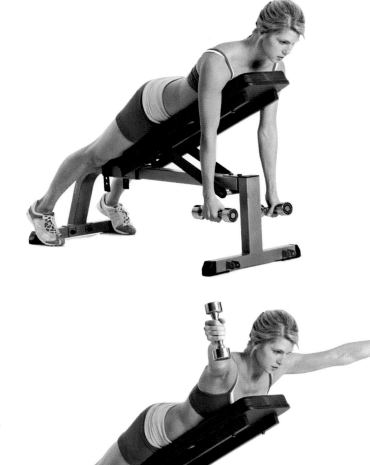

B

- Raise your arms at a 30-degree angle to your body until they are in line with your body.
- At the top of the movement, your arms and torso should form a Y.
- Pause, then lower back to the starting position.

Upper Body Exercises: Shoulders

I Raise ●

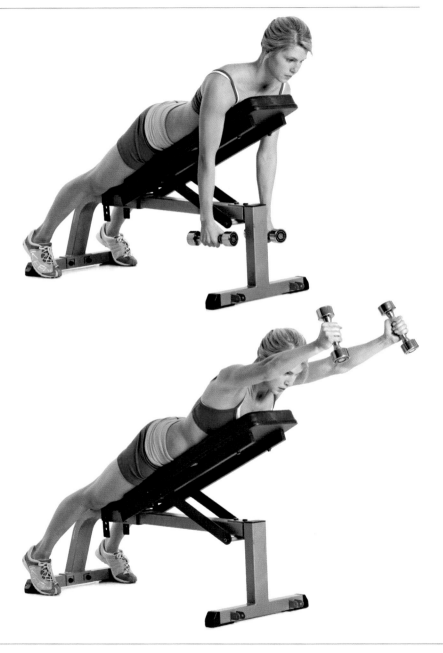

A

- Lie chest down on an adjustable bench set to a low incline.
- Your arms should hang straight down from your shoulders, and your palms should be facing each other.

B

- Raise your arms straight up until they're in line with your body.
- Your arms and torso should form the letter I.
- Pause, then lower back to the starting position.

Dumbbell Overhead Press ●

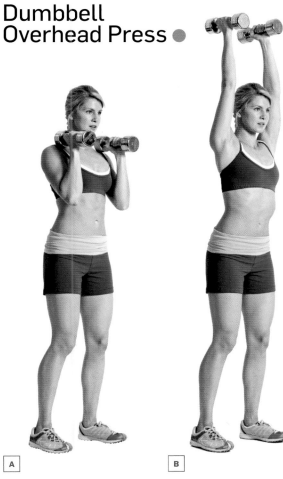

A

- Grab a pair of dumbbells and hold them just outside your shoulders with your palms facing each other.

B

- Press the weight overhead until your arms are completely straight.
- Pause, then slowly lower the dumbbells back to the starting position.

One-Arm Overhead Press ●

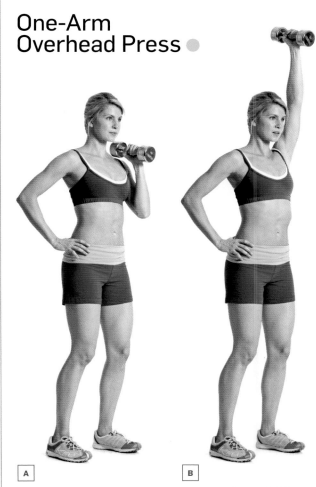

A

- Grab one dumbbell with one hand and hold it just outside your shoulder with your palm facing your head.

B

- Press the weight overhead until your arm is completely straight.
- Pause, then slowly lower the dumbbell back to the starting position.
- Complete all reps, then grab the dumbbell with your other hand and repeat.

Upper Body Exercises

DB Alternating Shoulder Press with Twist ●

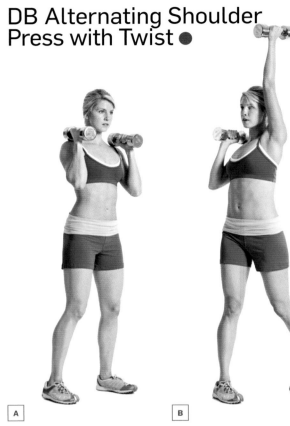

A

- Grab a pair of dumb-bells and hold them just outside your shoulders with your palms facing each other.

B

- Rotate your torso to the right, pivot your left foot, and press the dumbbell in your left hand overhead.
- Reverse the movement and return to the starting position.
- Rotate to the left and press the dumbbell in your right hand overhead.
- Continue alternating back and forth.

Wall Slide ●

A

- Lean your head, upper back, and butt against the wall.
- Place your hands and arms against the wall in the "high-five" position, your elbows bent 90 degrees and your upper arms at shoulder height. Hold for 1 second.
- Don't allow your head, upper back, or butt to lose contact with the wall.

B

- Keeping your elbows, wrists, and hands pressed into the wall, slide your elbows down toward your sides as far as you can.
- Squeeze your shoulder blades together.
- Slide your arms back up the wall as high as you can while keeping your hands in contact with the wall.
- Lower and repeat.

TRX Rows

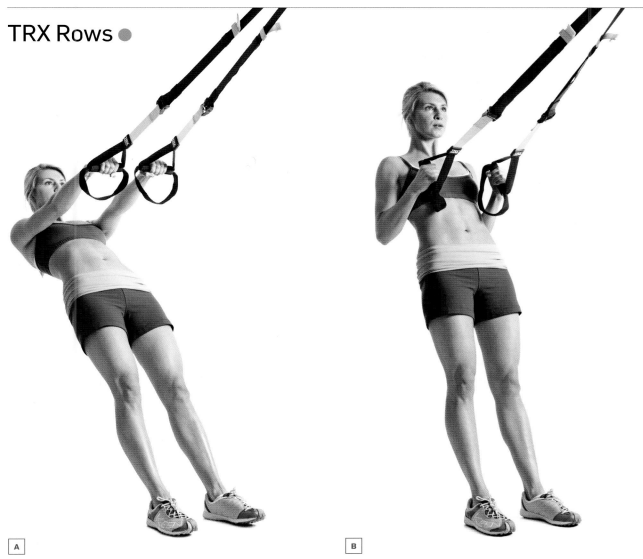

A

- Hold on to the TRX and back away until you feel tension in the straps.
- Your body should form a 45- to 60-degree angle to the floor, and your arms should be close to parallel to the floor, palms facing down.

B

- Pull your body toward the anchor point by bringing the handles toward the sides of your chest as you rotate your palms inward.
- Your elbows should be at 45 degrees.
- Pause and return to the starting position.

Total Body Exercises

The Best Way to Blast Fat?
With moves that work all of your muscles.

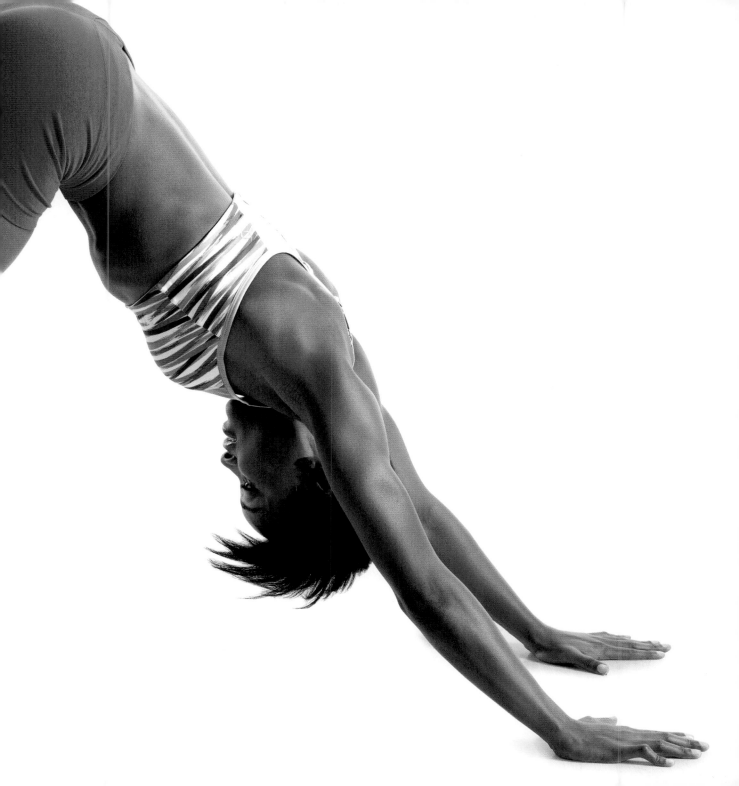

Total Body Exercises

Jumping Jack ●

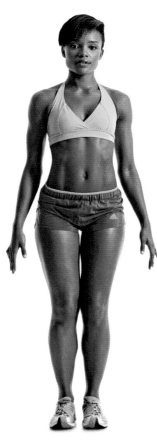

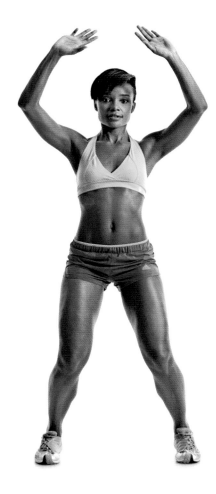

A

- Stand with your feet together and your hands at your sides.

B

- Simultaneously raise your arms above your head and jump your feet out to the sides.
- Immediately, reverse the movement and jump back to the starting position.
- Repeat for all reps.

Band Curl to Squat to Press ●

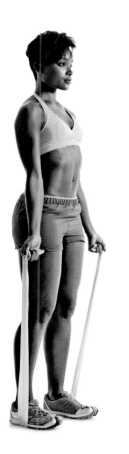 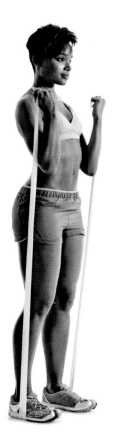 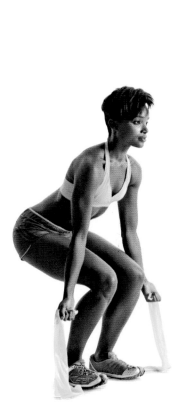 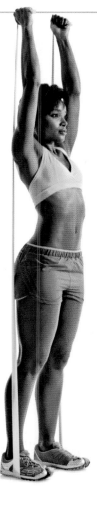

A

- Stand on a resistance band with your feet shoulder-width apart.
- Grab the ends of the band with your hands about shoulder-width apart and your arms at your sides.

B

- Without moving your upper arms, bend your arms and pull the band as close to your shoulders as you can.
- Pause, then lower the band to the starting position.

C

- Push your hips back and squat down until your upper thighs are at least parallel to the floor.

C

- Immediately, explode upward, stand up, and press the band overhead. That's 1 rep.

Total Body Exercises

Squat Thrust ●

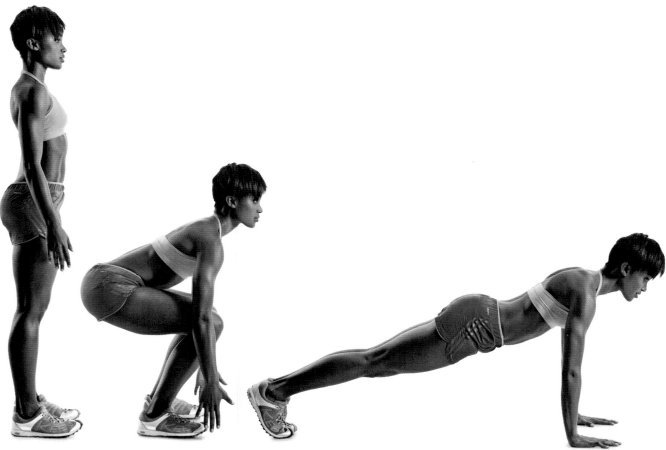

A
- Stand with your feet shoulder-width apart and your arms at your sides.

B
- Push your hips back, bend your knees, and lower your body as deep as you can into a squat.

C
- Place your hands on the floor, and kick your legs backward into a pushup position.
- Kick your legs back to the squat position. Stand up and jump. That's 1 rep.

Squat to Stand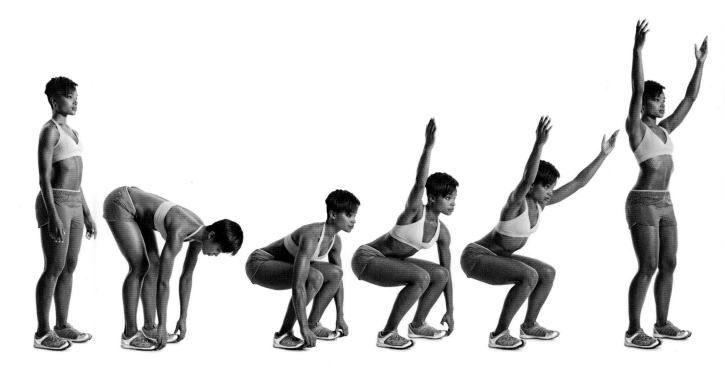

A
- Stand tall with your legs straight and your feet shoulder-width apart.

B
- Keeping your legs straight, bend over and grab your toes. (If you need to bend your knees, you can, but bend them only as much as necessary.)

C
- Without letting go of your toes, lower your body into a squat as you raise your chest and shoulders up.

D
- Staying in the squat position, raise your right arm up high and wide.

B
- Then raise your left arm.

B
- Now stand up.

Total Body Exercises

Goblet Squat to Press ●

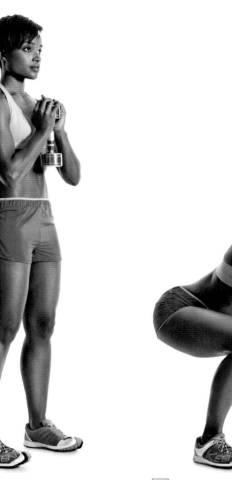

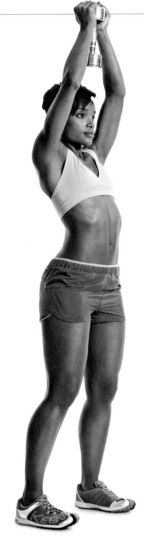

- Hold a dumbbell vertically next to your chest, with both hands cupping the dumbbell head.

- Push your hips back and lower your body into a squat until your upper thighs are at least parallel to the floor. Your elbows should brush the insides of your knees in the bottom position.

- Pause, then press your body back up and press the dumbbell overhead.
- Lower the dumbbell back to the starting position.

Dumbbell Squat Thrust

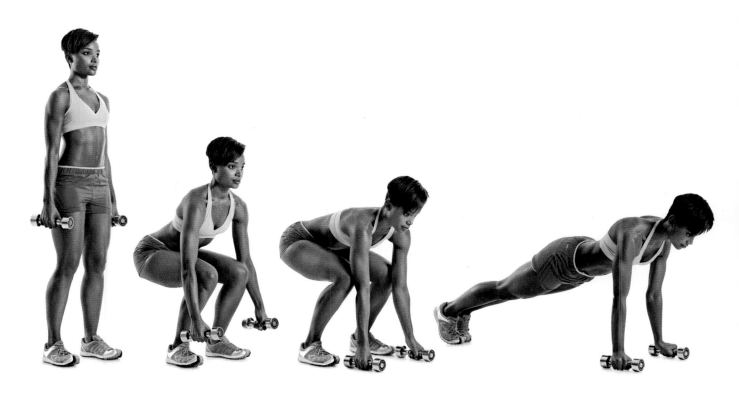

A
- Stand with your feet shoulder-width apart and your arms at your sides holding a pair of dumbbells.

B
- Push your hips back, bend your knees, and lower your body as deep as you can into a squat.

C
- Place the dumbbells on the floor, then kick your legs backward into a pushup position.

D
- Kick your legs back to the squat position.
- Stand up and jump. That's 1 rep.

Total Body Exercises

Dumbbell Push Press ●

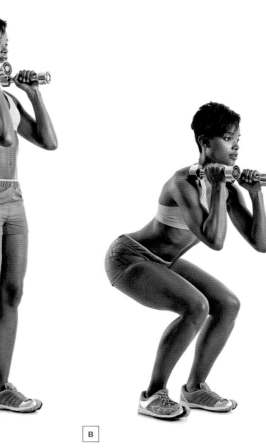

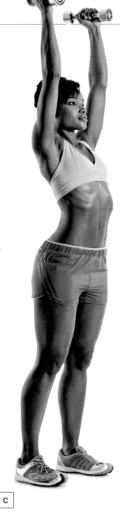

A

- Grab a pair of dumbbells and hold them just outside your shoulders with your palms facing each other.

B

- Bend your knees and lower your body into a half squat.

C

- Press the weight overhead as you stand up tall and explode upward, pressing through your heels.
- Pause, then slowly lower the dumbbells back to the starting position.

Dumbbell Snatch ●

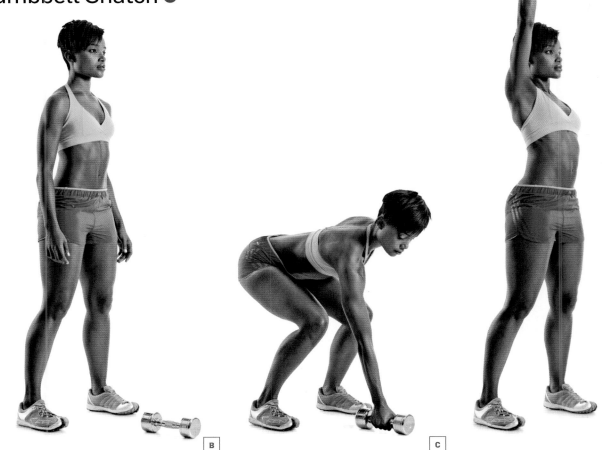

A

- Place a dumbbell on the floor and stand over it with your feet wider than shoulder-width apart.

B

- Bend at your hips and knees, and squat down until you can grab the dumbbell with one hand, without rounding your upper back.

C

- Keeping the dumbbell close to your body, pull the dumbbell upward and try to throw it at the ceiling without letting go.
- As you raise the dumbbell, your forearm should rotate up and back, until your arm is straight and your palm is facing forward.
- Pause and then lower the weight back to the starting position.

Total Body Exercises

Dumbbell Swing ●

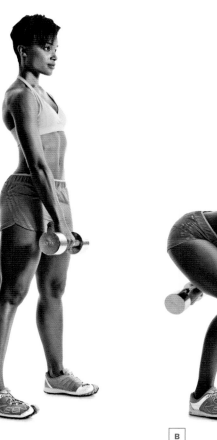

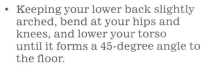

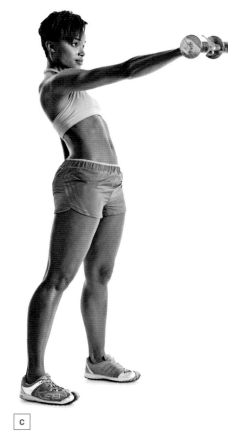

A

- Grab a dumbbell (or kettlebell) with an overhand grip and hold it with one hand in front of your waist at arm's length.
- Set your feet slightly wider than shoulder-width apart.

B

- Keeping your lower back slightly arched, bend at your hips and knees, and lower your torso until it forms a 45-degree angle to the floor.
- Now swing the dumbbell between your legs.

C

- Keeping your arm straight, thrust your hips forward, straighten your knees, and swing the dumbbell up to chest level as you rise to standing position.
- Reverse the movement and swing the dumbbell back between your legs again. That's 1 rep.
- Do all reps, then switch arms and repeat.

Dumbbell Curl to Squat to Press ●

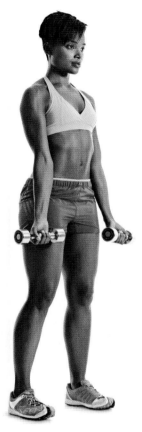
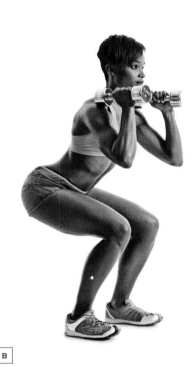
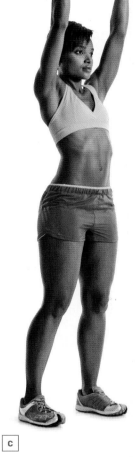

A

- Grab a pair of dumbbells and let them hang at arm's length next to your sides with your palms facing forward.

B

- Without moving your upper arms, bend your elbows and curl the dumbbells as close to your shoulders as you can.
- Immediately push your hips back and lower your body into a squat, until your thighs are at least parallel to the floor.

C

- Stand up and press the dumbbells over your head. That's 1 rep.
- Return to the starting position and repeat.

Total Body Exercises

Dumbbell Clean ●

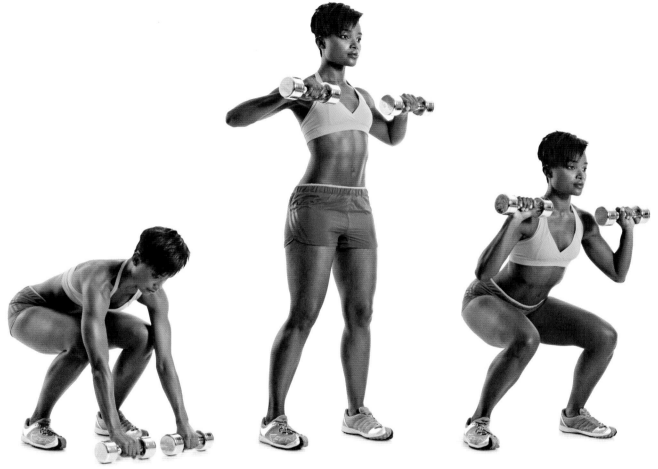

A
- Squat over a pair of dumbbells and grab them with an overhand grip.

B
- Stand and lift both weights up to chest height.

C
- Quickly drop underneath the weights and "catch" them on your shoulders, with your elbows high.
- Drop your elbows, keeping the dumbbells at shoulder level.

Dumbbell High Pull

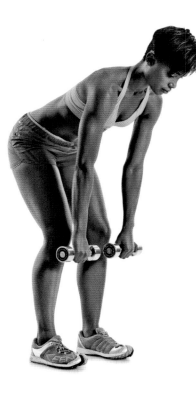

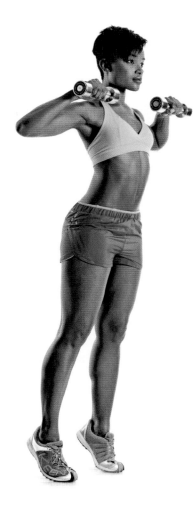

A

- Grab a pair of dumbbells with an overhand grip and hold them just below knee height.

B

- Explosively pull the dumbbells upward, rise onto your toes, and bend your elbows as you bring the weights up to shoulder height. Return to the starting position.

Total Body Exercises

Reverse Lunge and SA Cable Row

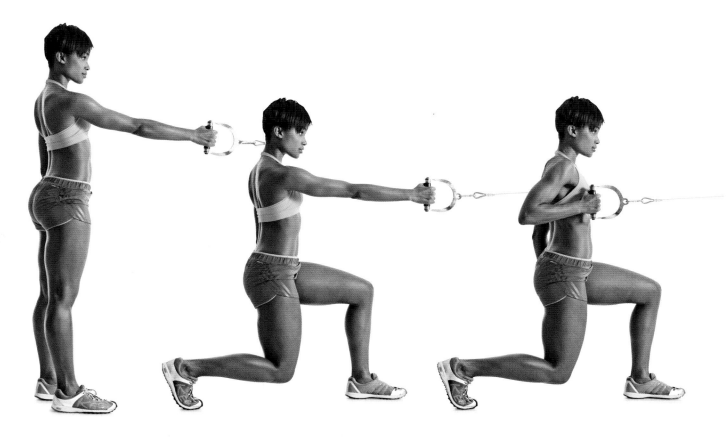

A
- Attach a D-handle at hip height to a cable station.
- Grab the handle and step away from the tower until your arm is extended in front of your body.

B
- Step backward into a lunge and lower your body until your front knee is bent 90 degrees.

C
- Pause, row the cable to the side of your chest, and then return to the starting position.
- Perform all reps, and then switch arms and repeat the process, stepping back with your other leg.

Dumbbell Hang Jump Shrugs ●

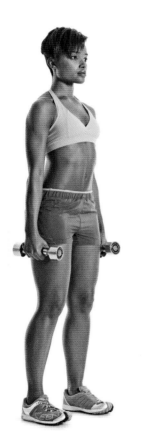

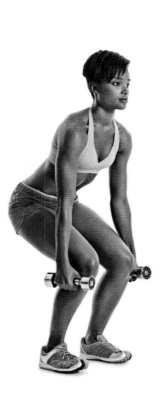

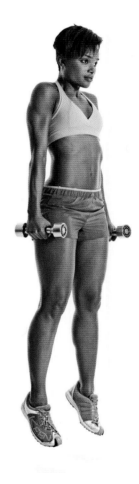

A

- Grab a pair of dumbbells and let them hang at arm's length with your palms facing each other.

B

- Push your hips back, slightly bend your knees, and lower the dumbbells until they are just below your knees.

C

- In one movement, explode upward and shrug your shoulders as high as you can, while keeping your arms straight.
- Land softly on the floor, dip your knees, and repeat.

151

Total Body Exercises

Lunge with Biceps Curl ●

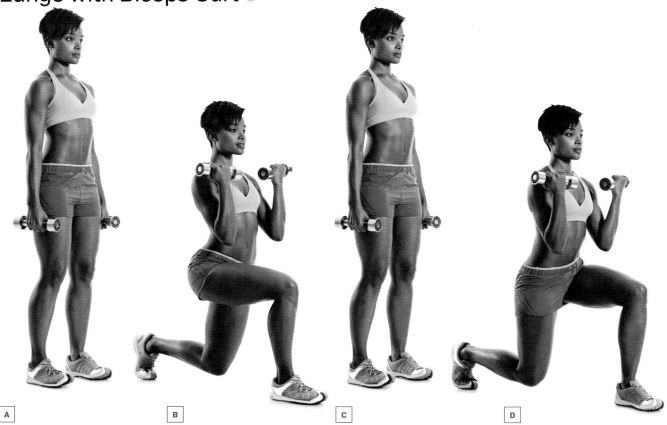

A
- Grab a pair of dumbbells and hold them at arm's length next to your sides, your palms facing each other.
- Stand tall with your feet hip-width apart.

B
- Step forward with your right leg and lower your body until your front knee is bent 90 degrees.
- At the same time as you lunge, curl both dumbbells up to your shoulders.

C
- Lower the dumbbells, and then return to the starting position.

D
- Step forward with the other leg and repeat.
- Continue alternating legs.

Lunge and Reach ●

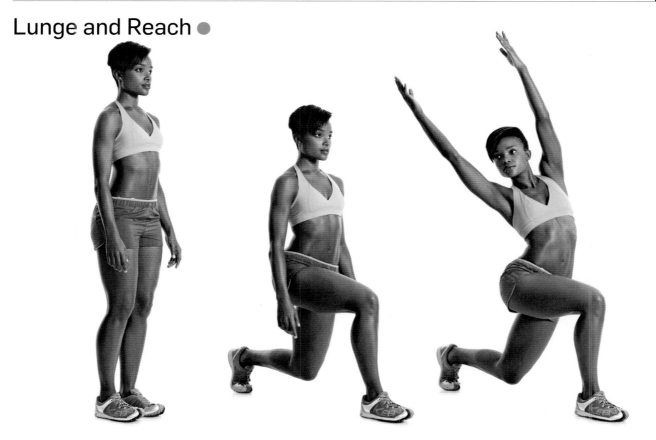

A

- Stand tall with your arms hanging at your sides.

- Brace your core and hold it that way.

B

- Lunge back with your right leg, lowering your body until your left knee is bent at least 90 degrees.

C

- As you lunge, reach back with both hands over your shoulders and to the left.

- Reverse the movement back to the starting position.

- Complete the prescribed number of repetitions with your left leg, then step back with your left leg and reach over your right shoulder for the same number of reps.

- Keep your torso upright for the entire movement.

Total Body Exercises

Side Lunge with Biceps Curl ●

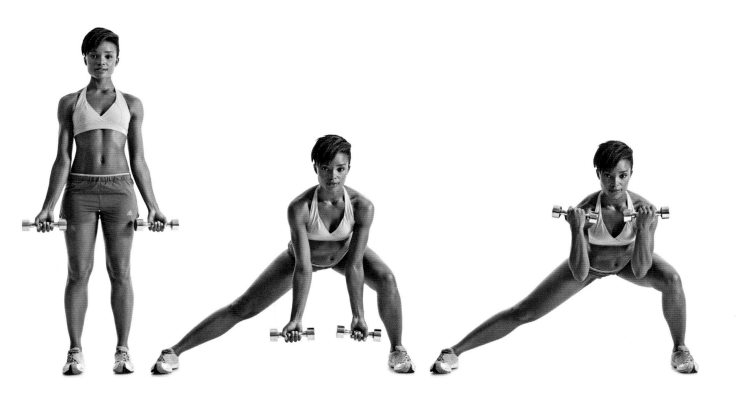

A

- Hold a pair of dumbbells at arm's length with your palms facing forward and your feet shoulder-width apart.

B

- Lift your left foot and take a step to the left as you push your hips backward and lower your body by dropping your hips and bending your left knee.
- Your right leg should remain straight in the "bottom" position of the lunge.

C

- Curl both arms up.
- Lower the weight and return to the starting position.
- Repeat the entire process, this time stepping to the right.

Dumbbell Renegade Crawl ●

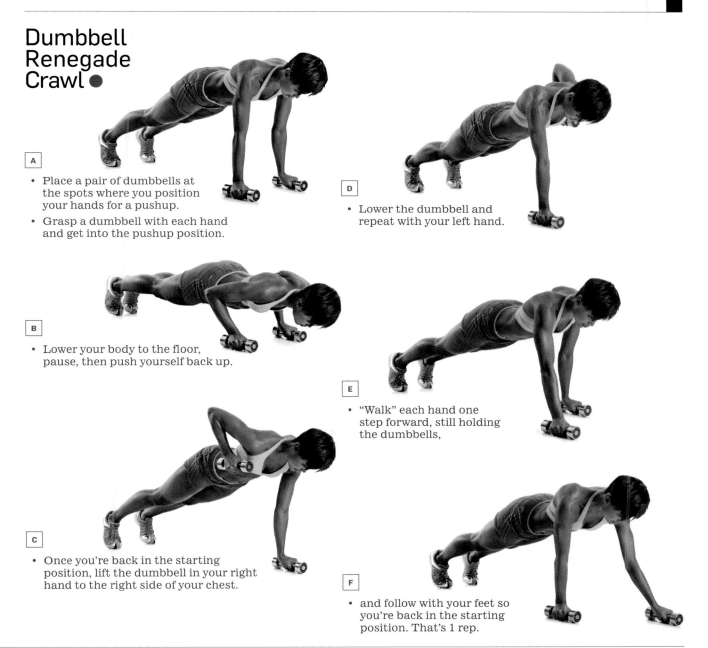

A
- Place a pair of dumbbells at the spots where you position your hands for a pushup.
- Grasp a dumbbell with each hand and get into the pushup position.

B
- Lower your body to the floor, pause, then push yourself back up.

C
- Once you're back in the starting position, lift the dumbbell in your right hand to the right side of your chest.

D
- Lower the dumbbell and repeat with your left hand.

E
- "Walk" each hand one step forward, still holding the dumbbells,

F
- and follow with your feet so you're back in the starting position. That's 1 rep.

Total Body Exercises

Squat and Cable Row ●

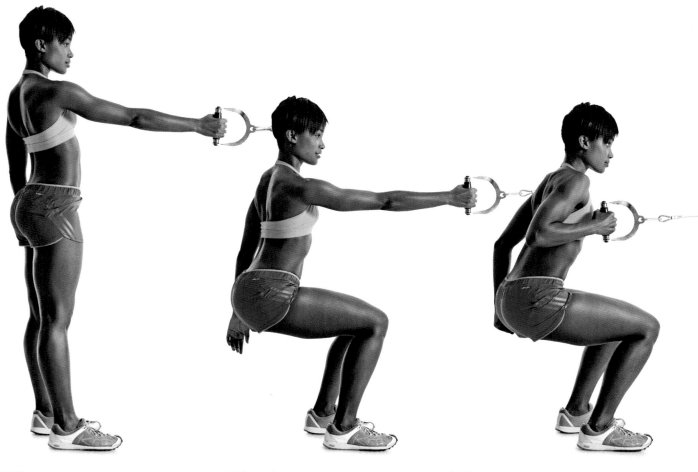

A
- Attach a D-handle at hip height to a cable station.
- Grab the handle with one hand and step away from the tower until your arm is extended in front of your body.

B
- Push your hips back and lower your body into a squat until your thighs are at least parallel to the floor.

C
- Pause, row the cable to the side of your chest, and then return to the starting position.
- Perform all reps, then switch arms and repeat the process.

Split Squat and Overhead Press ●

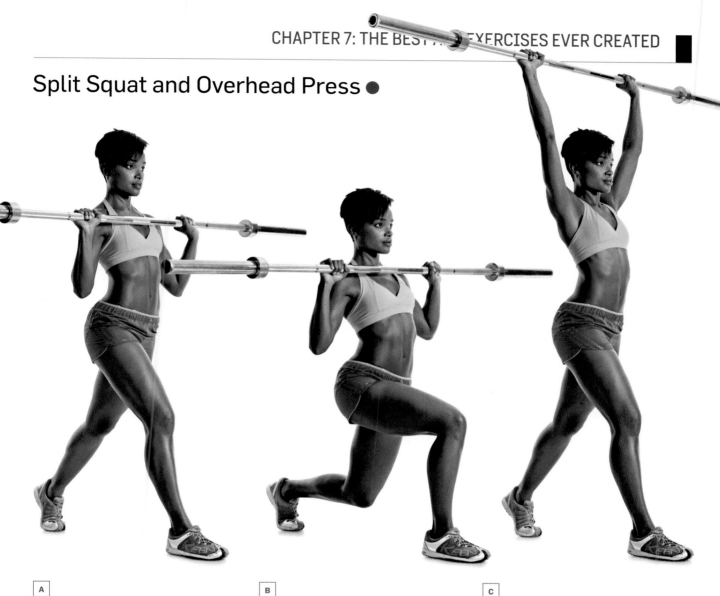

A

- Grab a bar with an overhand grip around shoulder-width apart and hold it at shoulder height.
- Stand in a staggered stance with your right foot in front of your left and your front knee slightly bent.

B

- Lower your body as far as you can, or until your back knee nearly touches the floor.

C

- Push yourself back up to the starting position. As you stand up, press the bar overhead.
- Return to the starting position and repeat.

Total Body Exercises

Squat to Overhead Press ●

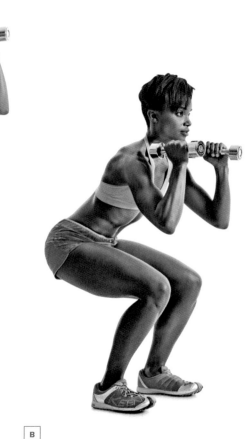
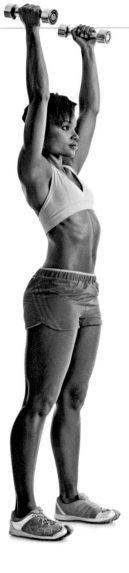

A

- Grab a pair of dumbbells and hold them next to your shoulders, your palms facing each other.
- Stand tall with your feet shoulder-width apart.

B

- Lower your body until the tops of your thighs are at least parallel to the floor.

C

- Push your body back to standing position as you press the dumbbell directly over your shoulders.
- Lower the dumbbells back to the starting position.

Squat with Alternating Shoulder Press ●

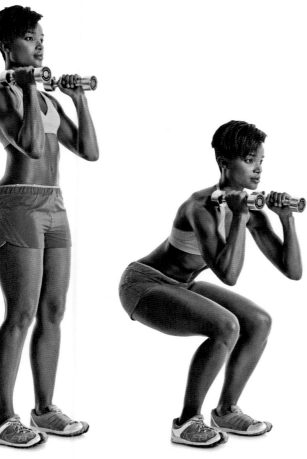

A
- Grab a pair of dumbbells and hold them next to your shoulders, your palms facing each other. Stand tall with your feet shoulder-width apart.

B
- Lower your body until the tops of your thighs are at least parallel to the floor.

C
- Push your body back to a standing position as you press one dumbbell directly over your shoulder.

D
- Lower the dumbbell back down, squat again, and then press the other dumbbell overhead. That's 1 rep.

Total Body Exercises

Inchworm ●

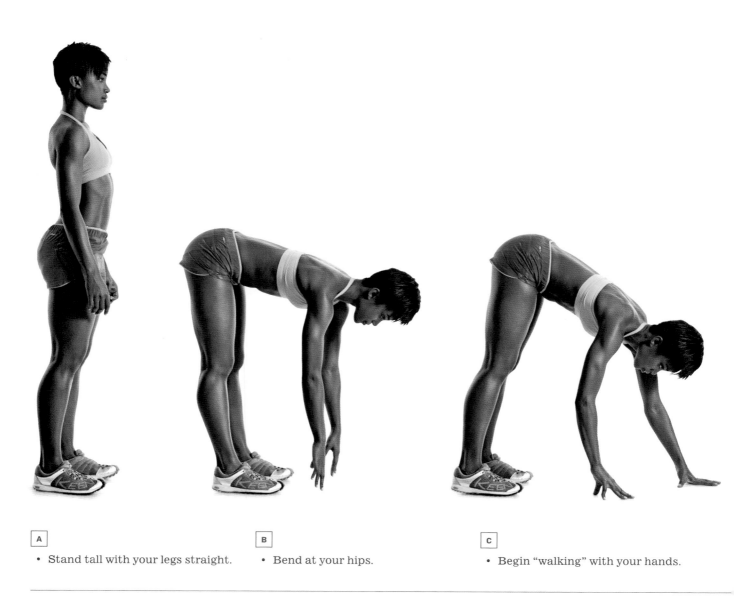

A
- Stand tall with your legs straight.

B
- Bend at your hips.

C
- Begin "walking" with your hands.

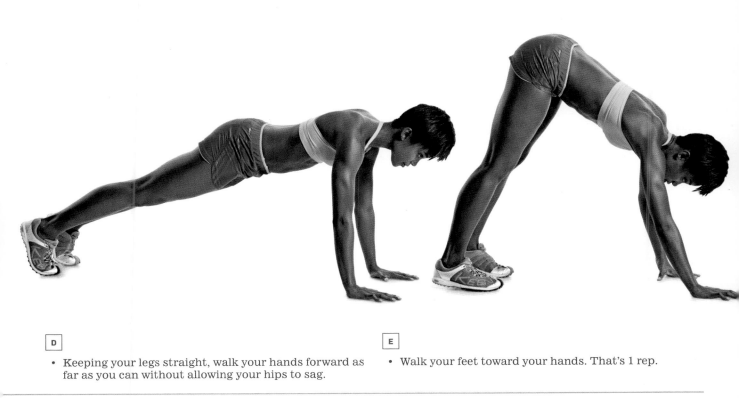

D

- Keeping your legs straight, walk your hands forward as far as you can without allowing your hips to sag.

E

- Walk your feet toward your hands. That's 1 rep.

Total Body Exercises

Kettlebell Windmill ●

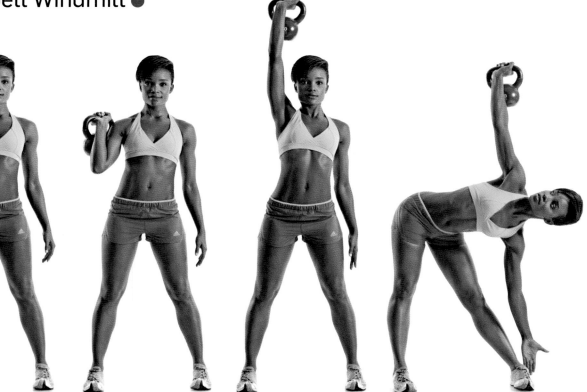

A
- Stand with your feet wider than hip-width apart, and hold the kettlebell in your left hand.

B
- Raise it next to your left shoulder,

C
- then press it overhead.

D
- Rotate your chest to the left and look up at the kettlebell as you try to touch your right hand to your right foot.
- Pause, then return to the starting position, keeping your left arm extended.
- Do the prescribed number of reps before lowering the weight, then repeat on the other side.

Resistance Band Squat and Row ●

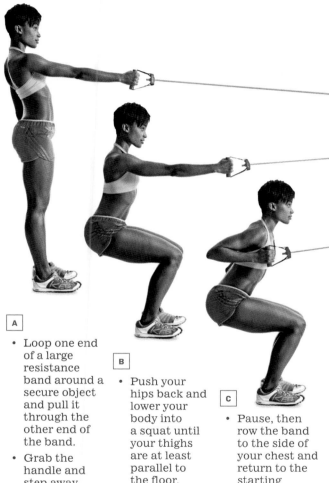

A

- Loop one end of a large resistance band around a secure object and pull it through the other end of the band.
- Grab the handle and step away from the anchor point until your arm is extended in front of your body.

B

- Push your hips back and lower your body into a squat until your thighs are at least parallel to the floor.

C

- Pause, then row the band to the side of your chest and return to the starting position.
- Perform all reps, then switch arms and repeat the process.

One-Arm Overhead Farmer's Carry ●

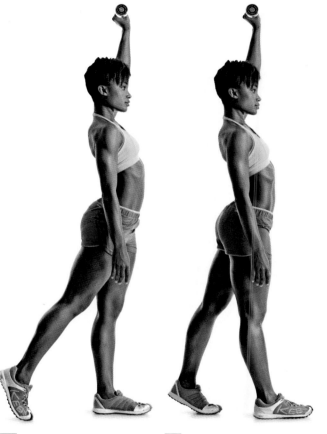

A

- Hold a dumbbell in your right hand straight above your shoulder with your arm completely straight and your palm facing out.

B

- Keeping your arm locked in this position, walk forward the prescribed number of steps while maintaining your upright posture.
- Complete all reps, switch arms, and repeat.

Total Body Exercises

Resistance Band Squat and Overhead Press

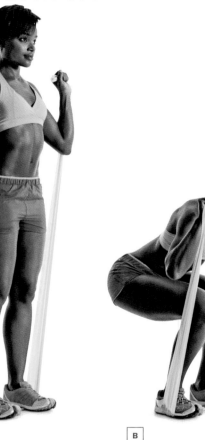

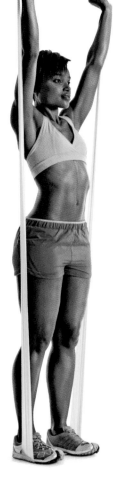

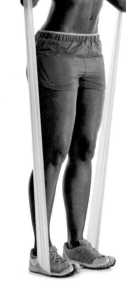

A

- Grab the ends of a resistance band in each hand and stand on the middle with your feet shoulder-width apart.
- Hold the ends at shoulder height with your palms facing away from your body.

B

- Push your hips back, bend your knees, and lower your body into a squat until your upper thighs are at least parallel to the floor.

C

- Press back up to the starting position, pressing your arms overhead until your arms are straight.

D

- Lower your arms. That's 1 rep.

Resistance Band Squat and Press ●

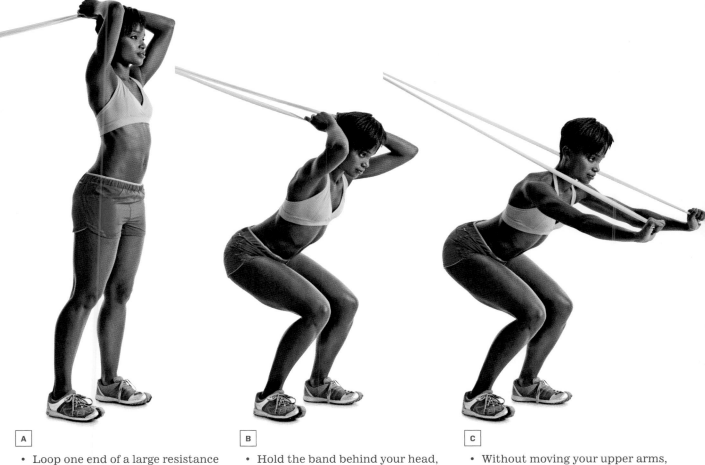

A

- Loop one end of a large resistance band around a secure object and then pull it through the other end of the band.
- Grab the band with each hand and your back to the anchor point. Stand in a staggered stance, one foot in front of the other.

B

- Hold the band behind your head, your elbows pointing forward and bent 90 degrees.

C

- Without moving your upper arms, push your forearms forward until your arms are straight.
- Pause, then return to the starting position.

Lower Body Exercises

Blast away cellulite, tighten your tush, and fit into your skinny jeans.

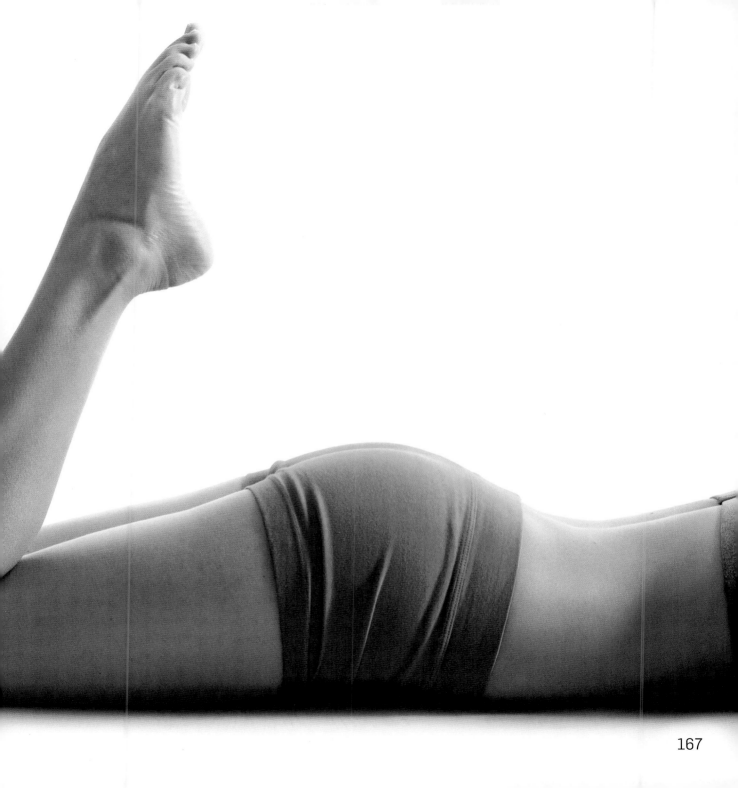

Lower Body Exercises

Barbell Squat ●

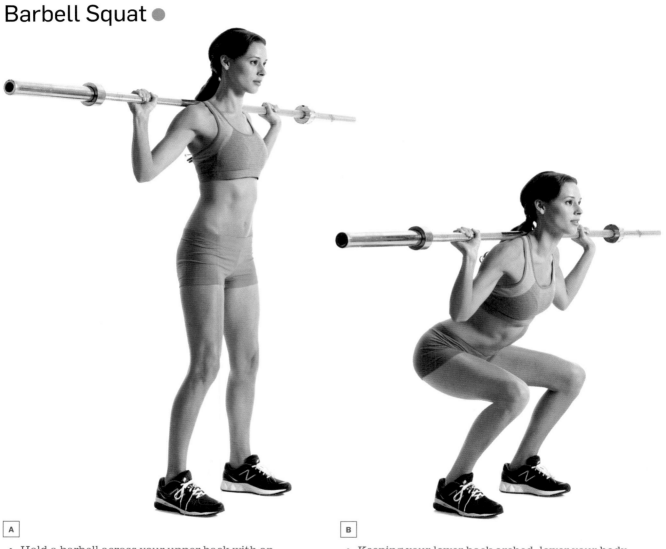

A

- Hold a barbell across your upper back with an overhand grip and your feet shoulder-width apart.

B

- Keeping your lower back arched, lower your body as deep as you can by pushing your hips back and bending your knees.
- Pause, then reverse the movement back to the starting position.

Bodyweight Squat ●

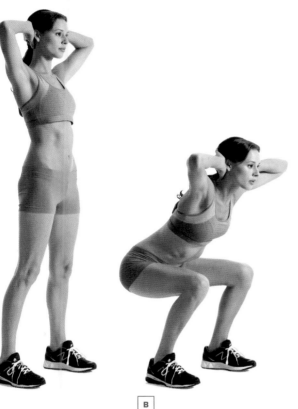

A
- Stand tall with your feet shoulder-width apart and place your fingers on the back of your head.

B
- Pull your shoulders and elbows back, and lower your body as far as you can by pushing your hips back and bending your knees.
- Pause, then push yourself back to the starting position.

Dumbbell Front Squat ●

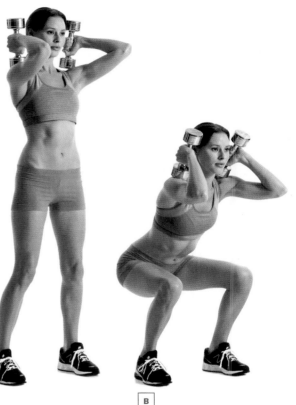

A
- Stand with your feet shoulder-width apart. Hold a pair of dumbbells so that your palms are facing each other, and rest one of the dumbbell heads on the meatiest part of each shoulder.
- Keep your body as upright as you can at all times, as your upper arms remain parallel to the floor.

B
- Brace your abs and lower your body as far as you can by pushing your hips back and bending your knees.
- Pause, then push yourself back to the starting position.

Lower Body Exercises

Skater Jumps ●

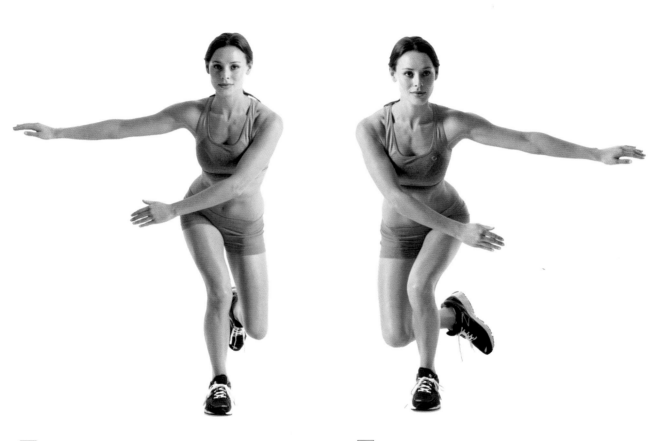

A

- Stand on your right foot with your right knee slightly bent, and place your left foot just behind your right ankle.
- Bend your right knee and lower your body into a partial squat.
- Bound to the left by jumping off your right foot.

B

- Land on your left foot and bring your right foot behind your left as you reach toward the floor with your right hand.
- Repeat the move back toward the right, landing on your right foot and reaching with your left hand.

Squat Jumps ●

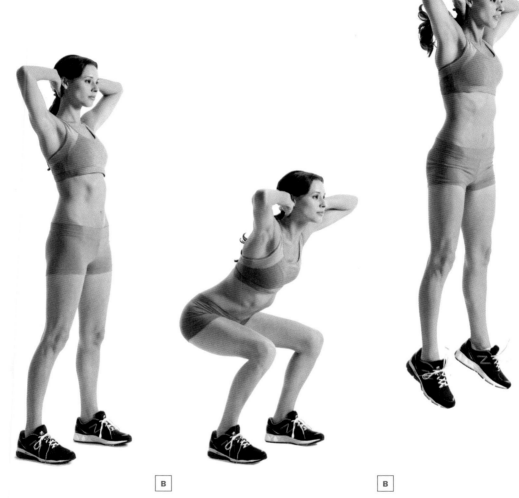

A
- Place your fingers on the back of your head and pull your elbows back so that they're in line with your body.

B
- Dip your knees in preparation to leap.

B
- Explosively jump as high as you can, raising your arms up in the air as you jump.
- When you land, immediately squat down and jump again.

Lower Body Exercises

Dumbbell Split Squat ●

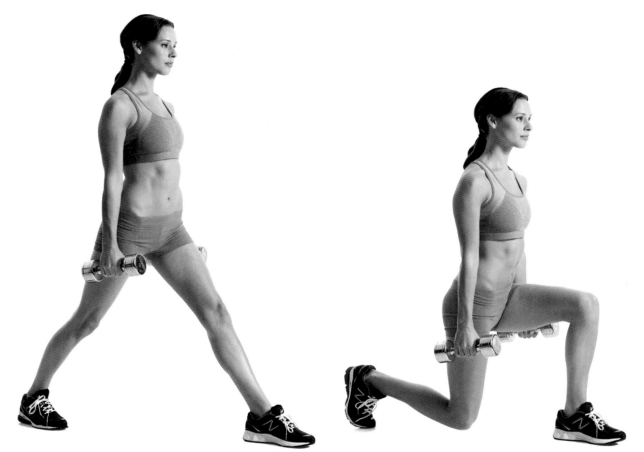

A

- Hold a pair of dumbbells at arm's length next to your sides, your palms facing each other. Stand in a staggered stance, your left foot in front of your right.

B

- Slowly lower your body as far as you can. Your rear knee should nearly touch the floor.
- Pause, then push yourself back up to the starting position.
- Complete the prescribed number of reps, then do the same number of reps with your right foot in front of your left.

Dumbbell Squat ●

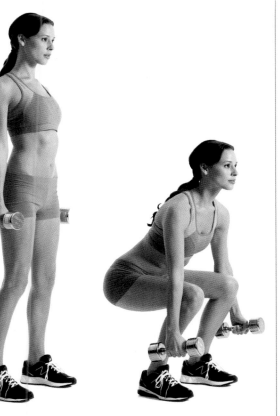

A

- Hold a pair of dumb-bells at arm's length next to your sides, your palms facing each other.

B

- Brace your abs, and lower your body as far as you can by pushing your hips back and bending your knees.
- Pause, then push back up to the starting position.

Single-Arm Dumbbell Squat ●

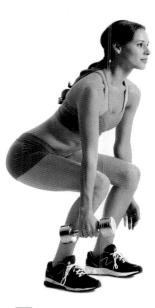
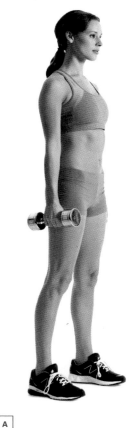

A

- Hold one dumbbell at arm's length next to your side, your palm facing your torso.

B

- Brace your abs, and lower your body as far as you can by pushing your hips back and bending your knees.
- Pause, then push back up to the starting position.
- Do all reps, switch the dumbbell to your other hand, and repeat.

173

Lower Body Exercises

Single-Arm Dumbbell Front Squat ●

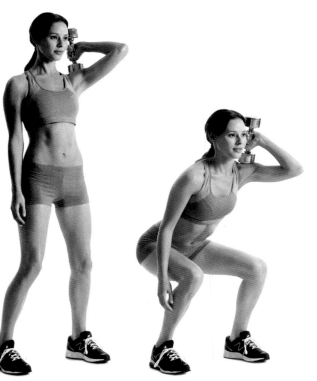

A

- Hold a dumbbell in your left hand and let your other arm rest at your side. Rest one of the dumbbell heads on the meatiest part of your right shoulder.
- Keep your body as upright as you can at all times as your left upper arm remains parallel to the floor.

B

- Brace your abs and lower your body as far as you can by pushing your hips back and bending your knees.
- Pause, then push yourself back to the starting position.
- Do all reps, switch the dumbbell to the other hand, and repeat.

Goblet Squat ●

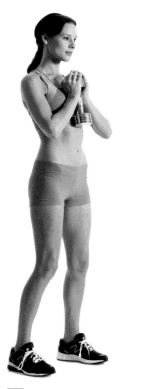

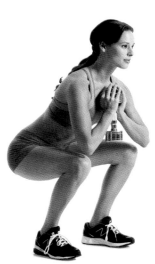

A

- Hold a dumbbell vertically next to your chest, with both hands cupping the dumbbell head.

B

- Push your hips back and lower your body into a squat until your upper thighs are at least parallel to the floor. Your elbows should brush the insides of your knees in the bottom position.
- Pause, then press your body back up to the starting position.

Box Jumps

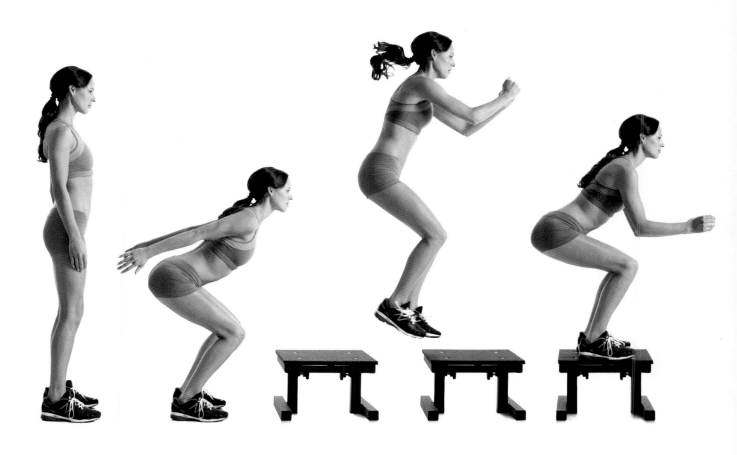

A

- Stand in front of a sturdy, secure box that's high enough so that you have to jump with great effort in order to land on top of it. Your feet should be shoulder-width apart.

B **C** **D**

- Dip your knees, and then explosively jump into the air and land on the top of the box with a "soft" landing.
- Step down and return to the starting position.

Lower Body Exercises

Dumbbell Squat Jumps ●

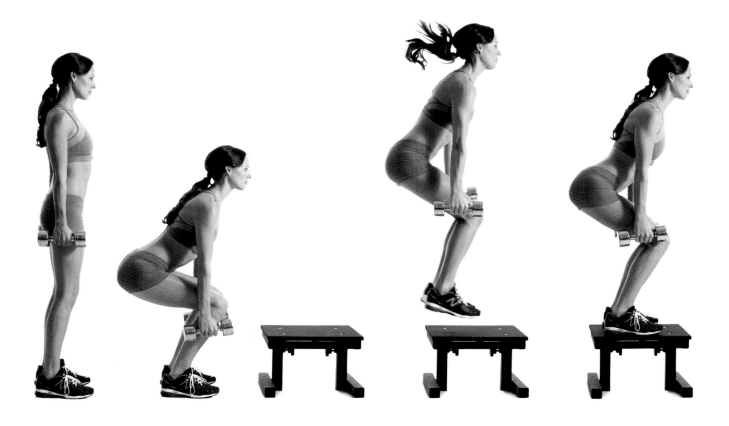

A

- Grab a pair of dumbbells and hold them at your sides. Stand in front of a sturdy, secure box that's high enough so that you have to jump with great effort in order to land on top of it. Your feet should be shoulder-width apart.

B **C** **D**

- Dip your knees, and then explosively jump into the air and land on the top of the box with a "soft" landing.
- Step down and return to the starting position.

One-Arm Dumbbell Sumo Front Squat ●

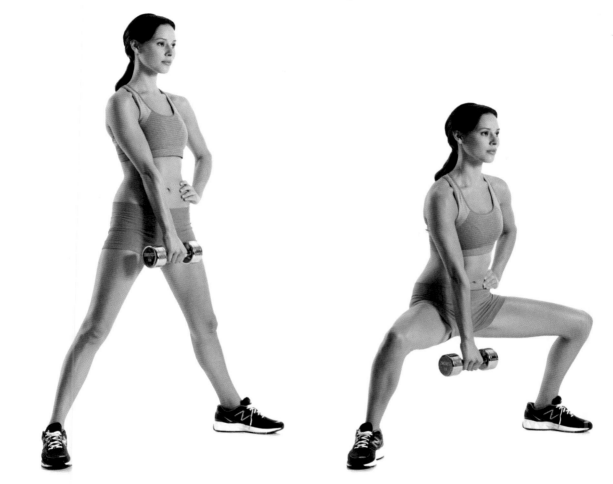

A

- Grab a dumbbell in one hand and hold it at arm's length in front of your waist.
- Set your feet about twice shoulder-width with your toes turned slightly outward.

B

- Push your hips back and lower your body into a squat until your upper thighs are at least parallel to the floor.
- Pause, then press your body back up to the starting position.

Lower Body Exercises

Band Lateral Squats ●

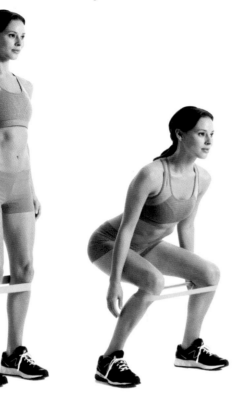

A
- Place both legs between a mini resistance band and position the band just below your knees.

B
- Take a side step to the right and push your hips back and bend your knees so you lower your body into a squat.
- Stand back up. That's 1 rep.
- Complete the prescribed number of reps, then sidestep to your left for the same number of reps. That's 1 set.

Calf Raise ●

A
- Grab a dumbbell in your right hand and stand on a step or weight plate.
- Cross your left foot behind your right ankle, and balance your body on the ball of your right foot, with your right heel on the floor or hanging off the step.

B
- Lift your right heel as high as you can.
- Pause, then lower and repeat.
- Complete the prescribed number of reps with your right leg, then do the same number with your left leg while holding the dumbbell in your left hand.

Overhead Split Squat ●

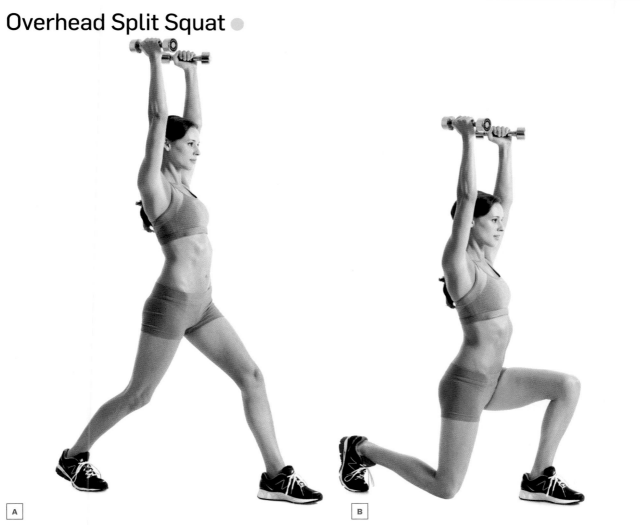

A

- Hold a pair of dumbbells directly over your shoulders, with your arms completely straight. Squeeze your abs tight for the entire exercise. Stand in a staggered stance, your left foot in front of your right foot.

B

- Push your hips back and bend your knees so you lower your body into a squat.
- Pause, then push yourself back up to the starting position.
- Perform the prescribed number of reps, and then do the same number of reps with your right foot in front of your left.

Lower Body Exercises

Split Jumps ●

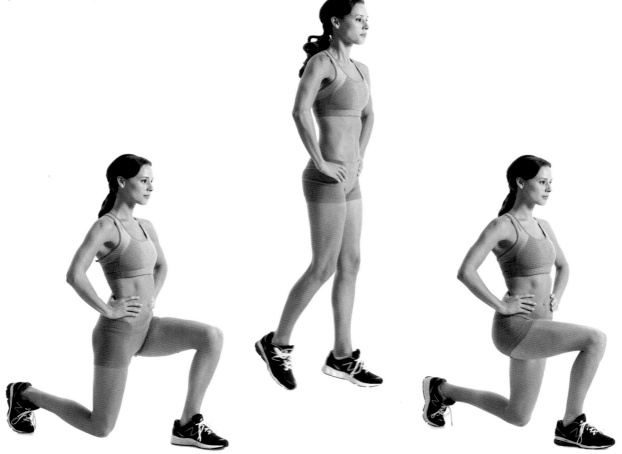

A

- Stand in a staggered stance, your left foot in front of your right foot.
- Lower your body as far as you can.

B

- Quickly jump into the air with enough force that you can switch the direction of your feet in the air.

C

- Land with your right foot in front of your left.
- Continue alternating back and forth with each repetition.

Dumbbell Split Jumps

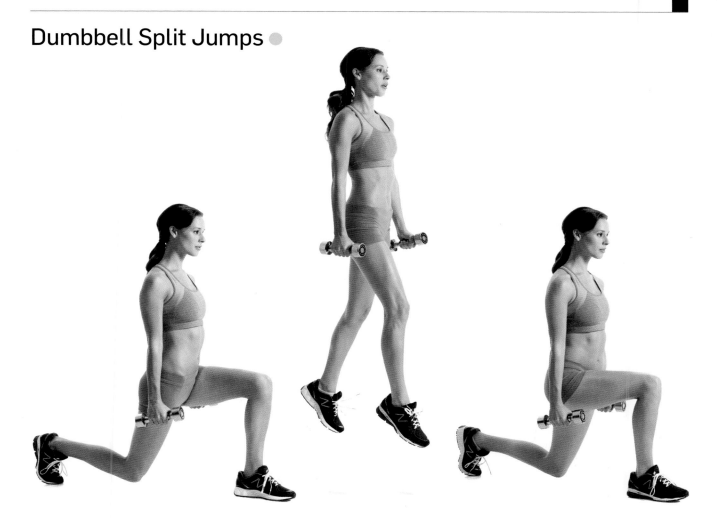

A

- Hold a pair of dumbbells at arm's length next to your sides, your palms facing each other. Stand in a staggered stance, your left foot in front of your right foot.
- Lower your body as far as you can.

B

- Quickly jump into the air with enough force that you can switch the direction of your feet in the air.

C

- Land with your right foot in front of your left.
- Continue alternating back and forth with each repetition.

Lower Body Exercises

Dumbbell Walking Lunges ●

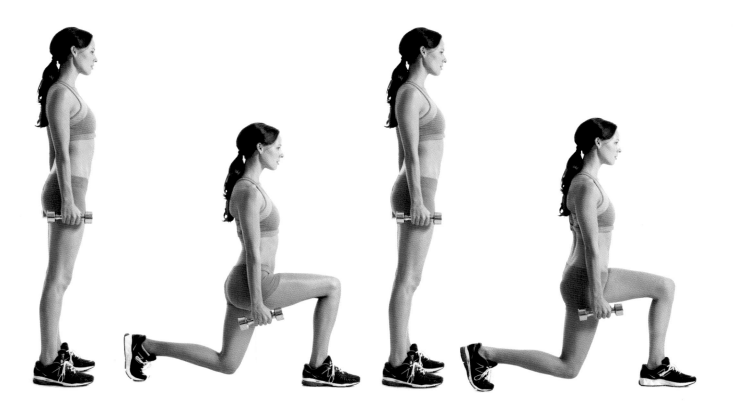

A

- Grab a pair of dumb-
  bells and hold them at
  arm's length at your
  sides, your palms facing
  each other.

B

- Step forward with your
  right leg and slowly
  lower your body until
  your front knee is bent
  at least 90 degrees.

C

- Pause, then push
  yourself to the starting
  position as quickly as
  you can.

D

- Complete the pre-
  scribed number of reps
  with your right leg, then
  do the same number
  with your left leg.

Bodyweight Lunges ●

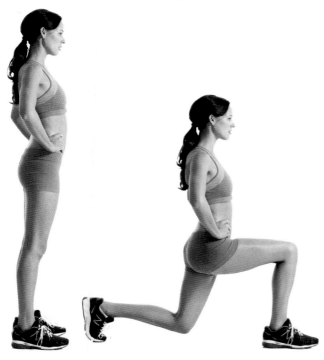

A

- Place your hands on your hips, pull your shoulders back, and stand as tall as you can.

B

- Step forward with your right leg and slowly lower your body until your front knee is bent at least 90 degrees.
- Pause, then push yourself to the starting position as quickly as you can.
- Complete the prescribed number of reps with your right leg, then do the same number with your left leg.

Dumbbell Lateral Lunge ●

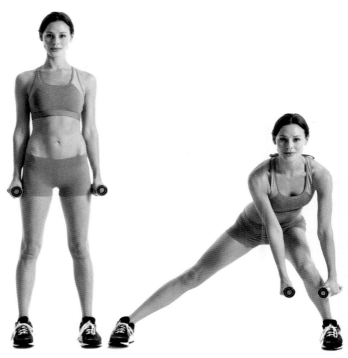

A

- Hold a pair of dumbbells at arm's length next to your sides, your palms facing each other.

B

- Lift your left foot and take a big step to your left as you push your hips backward and lower your body by dropping your hips and bending your left knee.
- Pause, then quickly push yourself back to the starting position.

Lower Body Exercises

Bodyweight Lateral Lunge ●

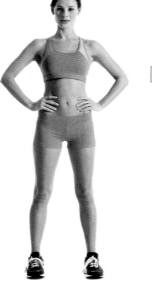

A

- Place your hands on your hips, pull your shoulders back, and stand as tall as you can.

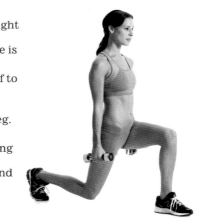

B

- Lift your left foot and take a big step to your left as you push your hips backward and lower your body by dropping your hips and bending your left knee.
- Pause, then quickly push yourself back to the starting position.

One Dumbbell Lunge ●

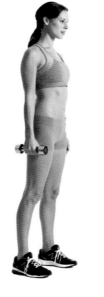

A

- Grab a dumbbell in one hand and hold it at arm's length at your side, your palm facing your body.

B

- Step forward with your right leg and slowly lower your body until your front knee is bent at least 90 degrees.
- Pause, then push yourself to the starting position as quickly as you can.
- Repeat with your other leg.
- Complete the prescribed number of reps, alternating legs, then switch the dumbbell to the other hand and repeat.

Cross-Behind Lunges

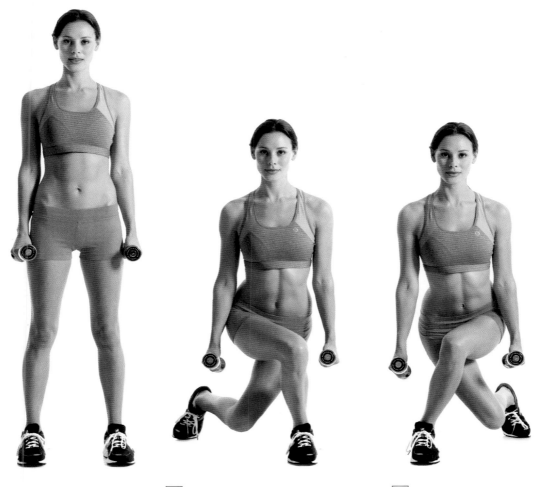

A

- Grab a pair of dumbbells and hold them at arm's length at your sides, your palms facing each other.

B

- Step forward and to the side so that your lead foot ends up in front of your back foot (like a curtsy).
- Lower your body until your front knee is bent at least 90 degrees.

C

- Pause, then return to the starting position and repeat with your other leg.

Lower Body Exercises

Goblet Reverse Lunge ○

A

- Hold a dumbbell vertically next to your chest, with both hands cupping the dumbbell head.

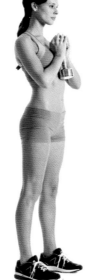

B

- Step backward with your left leg.
- Lower your body into a lunge until your front leg is bent 90 degrees. Pause, then return to the starting position.
- Do all your reps and then repeat with your other leg.

Dumbbell Reverse Lunge ●

A

- Grab a pair of dumbbells and hold them at arm's length next to your sides, your palms facing each other.

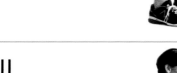
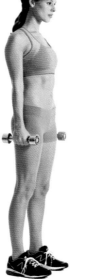

B

- Step backward with your left leg.
- Lower your body into a lunge until your front leg is bent 90 degrees. Pause, then return to the starting position.
- Do all your reps and then repeat with your other leg.

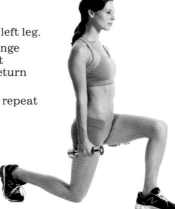

Reverse Lunge and Rotate

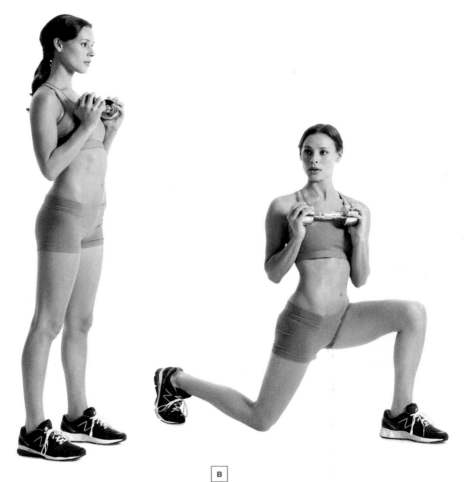

A

- Grab a dumbbell and hold it by the ends, just below your chin. Stand tall with your feet less than shoulder-width apart.

B

- Step backward with your left leg and lower your body into a lunge until your front leg is bent 90 degrees. As you lunge, rotate your upper body toward the same side as the leg you're using to step backward.
- Pause, then return to the starting position.
- Repeat on your other leg and continue alternating back and forth.

Lower Body Exercises

Lateral Bound with Pause ●

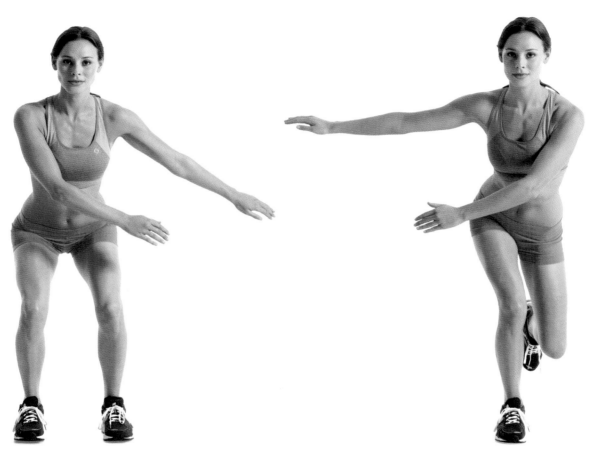

A

- Stand with your hips pushed back and knees slightly bent.
- Dip your knees slightly, and then explosively hop off your right leg, swinging your arms and moving to your left.

B

- Land on your left foot and pause until you remove all momentum.
- Then reverse the movement to the right. That's 1 rep.

Rear-Foot Elevated Split Squat

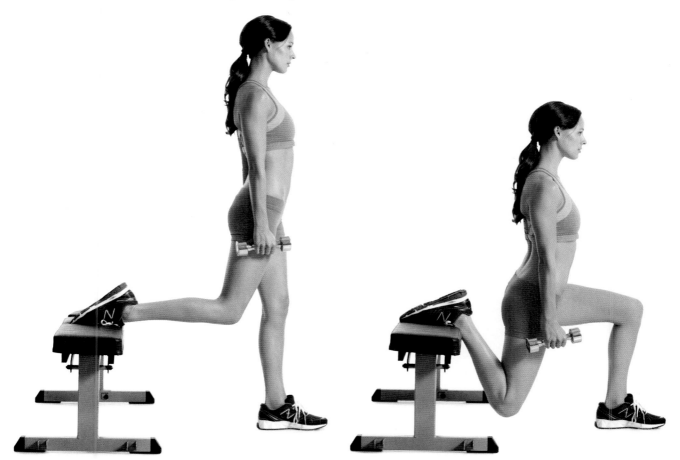

A

- Hold a pair of dumbbells at arm's length next to your sides, your palms facing each other.
- Stand in a staggered stance with your left foot in front of your right, and place the instep of your back foot on a bench.

B

- Lower your body as far as you can, pause, then push your body back up to the starting position.
- Do all reps with your left foot forward, then do the same number with your right foot in front of your left.

Lower Body Exercises

Dumbbell Deadlift ●

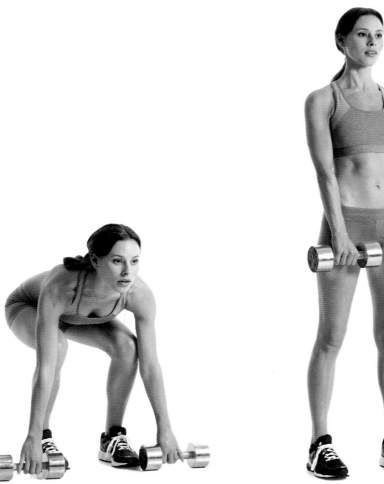

A

- Set a pair of dumbbells on the floor in front of you.
- Bend at your hips and knees, and grab the dumbbells with an overhand grip.

B

- Without allowing your lower back to round, stand up with the dumbbells and thrust your hips forward.
- Lower your body back to the starting position.

Snatch Grip Deadlift ●

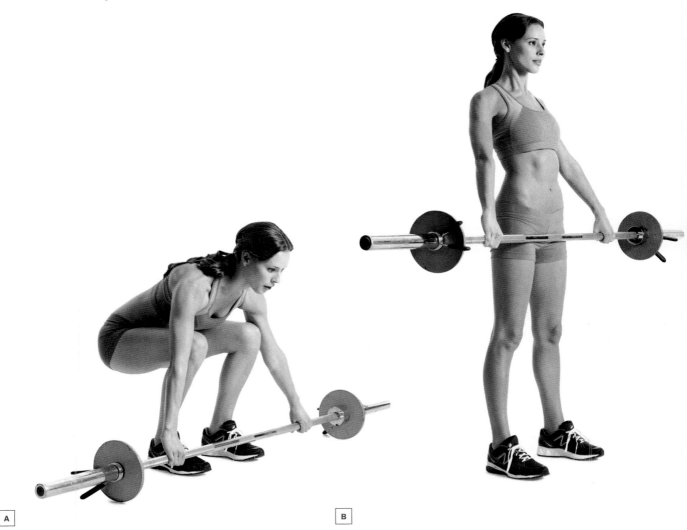

A

- Load a barbell and roll it up against your shins.
- Bend at your hips and knees, and grab the bar with an overhand grip that's about twice shoulder-width.

B

- Without allowing your lower back to round, stand up, thrust your hips forward, and squeeze your glutes.
- Pause, then lower the bar back to the floor while keeping it as close to your body as possible.

Lower Body Exercises

Barbell Romanian Deadlift ●

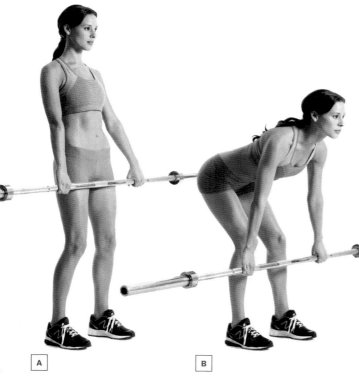

A

- Grab a barbell with an overhand grip that's just beyond shoulder-width and hold it at arm's length in front of your hips. Your knees should be slightly bent and chest pushed out. This is the starting position.

B

- Without changing the bend in your knees, bend at your hips and lower your torso until it's almost parallel to the floor.
- Pause, then raise your torso back to the starting position.

One Dumbbell Single-Leg Romanian Deadlift ●

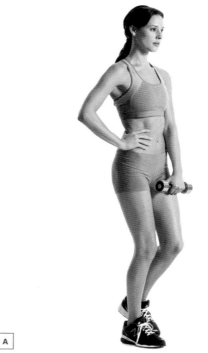

A

- Grab a dumbbell in your left hand, and hold it at arm's length in front of your thighs. Stand with your feet hip-width apart and your knees slightly bent. Balance on your right leg.
- Without changing the bend in your knee, bend at your hips and lower your torso until it's almost parallel to the floor.
- Pause, then raise your torso back to the starting position.
- As you push your hips back, your leg should raise off the floor and stay in line with your body.
- Make sure your back stays naturally arched through-out the entire movement as you keep the dumbbell as close to your body as possible.
- Perform all reps, then hold the dumbbell in your right hand and balance on your left leg and repeat.

Single-Leg Romanian Deadlift ●

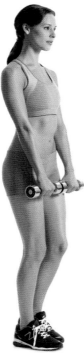

A

- Grab a pair of dumbbells with an overhand grip, and hold them at arm's length in front of your thighs. Stand with your feet hip-width apart and your knees slightly bent. Balance on one leg.
- Without changing the bend in your knee, bend at your hips and lower your torso until it's almost parallel to the floor.
- Pause, then raise your torso back to the starting position.
- As you push your hips back, your leg should raise off the floor and stay in line with your body.
- Make sure your back stays naturally arched throughout the entire movement as you keep the dumbbell as close to your body as possible.
- Perform all reps, then balance on your other leg and repeat.

Dumbbell Romanian Deadlift ●

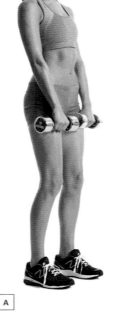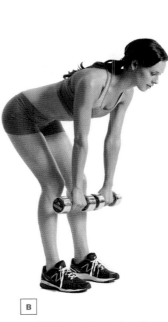

A

- Grab a pair of dumbbells with an overhand grip, and hold them at arm's length in front of your thighs. Stand with your feet hip-width apart and your knees slightly bent.

B

- Without changing the bend in your knees, bend at your hips and lower your torso until it's almost parallel to the floor.
- Pause, then raise your torso back to the starting position.

Lower Body Exercises

Sumo Deadlift ●

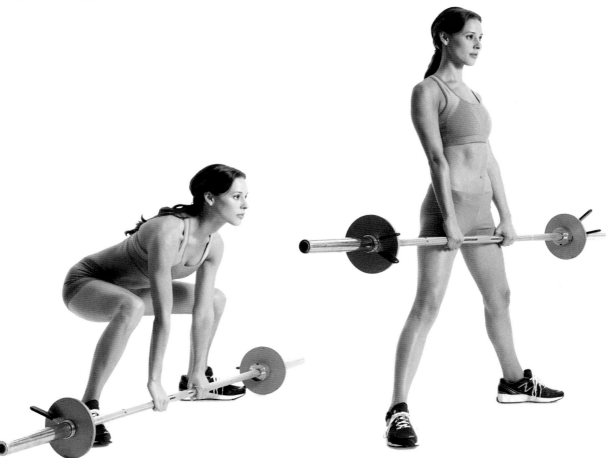

A

- Load a barbell and roll it up against your shins. Set your feet about twice shoulder-width apart with your toes pointed out an angle.
- Bend at your hips and knees, and grab the center of the bar with an overhand grip and your hands about 12 inches apart.

B

- Without allowing your lower back to round, stand up, thrust your hips forward, and squeeze your glutes.
- Pause, then lower the bar back to the floor while keeping it as close to your body as possible.

Barbell Hip Raise ●

A

- Sit on the floor with your upper back against a stable bench, your knees bent and feet flat on the floor.
- Put a padded barbell across your hips and grab the barbell with an overhand grip, about shoulder-width apart.

B

- Keeping your back against the bench and the barbell just below your pelvis, raise your hips—while squeezing your glutes—until your hips are in line with your body.
- Return to the starting position, and repeat.

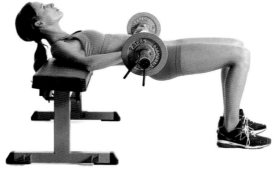

Single-Leg Hip Raise ●

A

- Lie faceup on the floor with your right knee bent and your left leg straight.
- Raise your left leg until it's in line with your right thigh, and place your arms out to the sides.

B

- Push your hips upward, keeping your left leg elevated.
- Pause, then slowly lower your body and leg back to the starting position.
- Complete the prescribed number of reps with your left leg, then switch legs and do the same number with your right leg.

Lower Body Exercises

Hip Raise ●

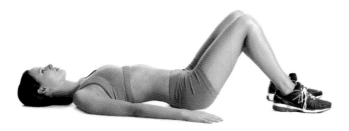

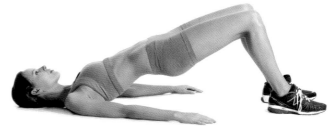

A

- Lie faceup on the floor with your knees bent and your feet flat on the floor.

B

- Raise your hips so your body forms a straight line from your shoulders to your knees.
- Pause in the up position, then lower your body back to the starting position.

Resistance Band Hip Raise ●

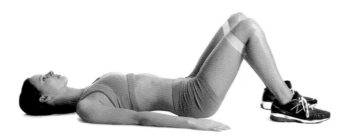

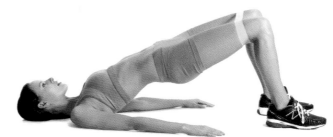

A

- Place a mini resistance band just above your knees, and lie faceup on the floor with your knees bent and your feet flat on the floor.

B

- Press your knees outward against the band and raise your hips so your body forms a straight line from your shoulders to your knees.
- Pause in the up position, then lower your body back to the starting position.

Swiss Ball Hip Raise and Leg Curl ●

A

- Lie faceup on the floor, and place your lower legs and heels on a Swiss ball.

B

- Push your hips up so that your body forms a straight line from your shoulders to your knees.

C

- Pull your heels toward your body and roll the ball as close as possible to your butt.
- Pause, then reverse the motion and roll the ball back until your body is in a straight line.
- Lower your hips to the floor and repeat.

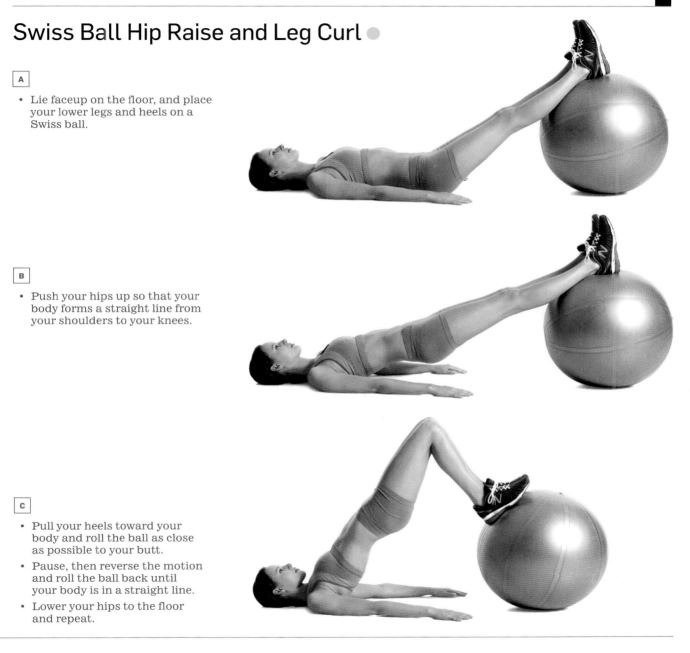

Lower Body Exercises

Stepups ●

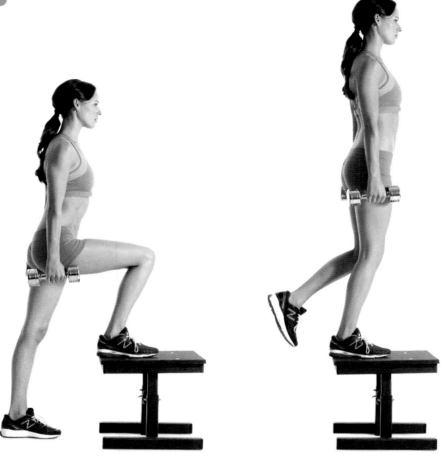

A

- Grab a pair of dumbbells and hold them at arm's length at your sides.
- Stand in front of a step or bench and place your left foot firmly on the step. The step should be high enough that your knee is bent 90 degrees.

B

- Press your left heel into the step, and push your body up until your left leg is straight and you're standing on one leg on the step, keeping your right foot elevated.
- Lower your body back down until your right foot touches the floor. That's 1 rep.
- Complete the prescribed number of reps with your left leg, then do the same number with your right.

Crossover Stepups ●

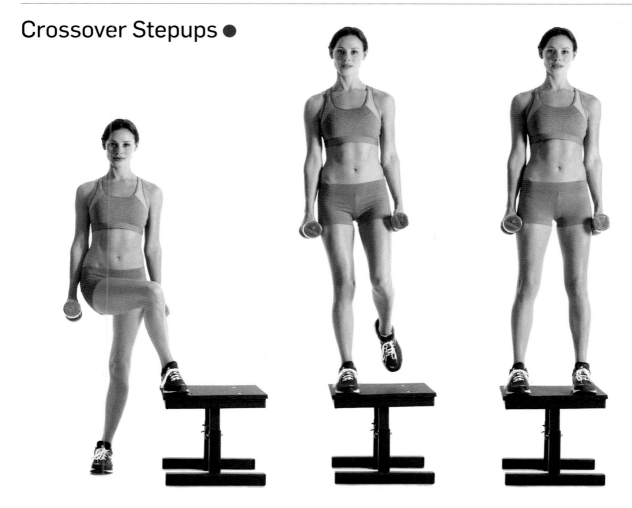

A

- Grab a pair of dumbbells and stand with your left side next to a step that's at knee height.
- Place your right foot on the step.

B **C**

- Press through your right heel and push your body up onto the step until both legs are straight.
- Lower your body back to the starting position.
- Perform the prescribed number of reps with your right leg, then switch to your left leg and repeat.

Lower Body Exercises

Lateral Band Walks ●

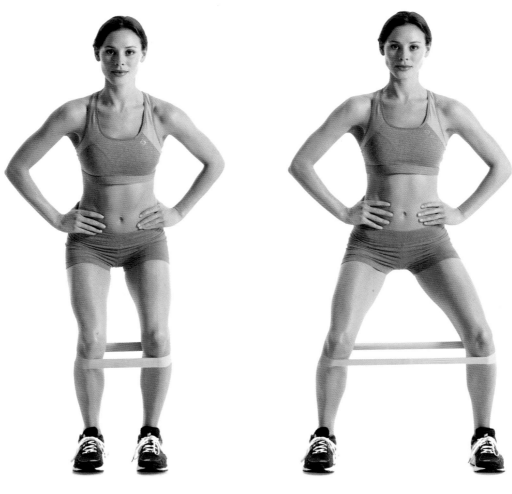

A

- Place both legs between a mini resistance band, and position the band just below your knees.

B

- Take small steps to your right for the prescribed number of reps.
- Sidestep back to your left for the same number of reps. That's 1 set.

Side Lying Clam ●

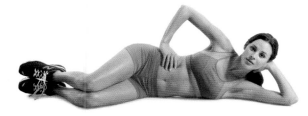

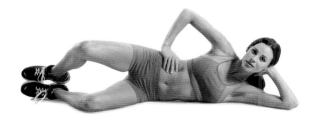

A

- Lie on the floor on your left side, with your hips and knees bent 45 degrees. Your right leg should be on top of your left leg, your heels together.

B

- Keeping your feet in contact with each other and your left leg on the floor, raise your right knee as high as you can without moving your pelvis.
- Pause, then return to the starting position.
- Do all reps, then roll to your other side and repeat.

Side Lying Hip Abduction ●

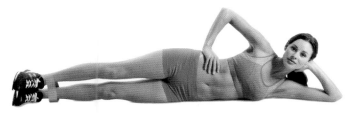

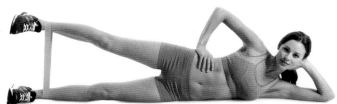

A

- Lie on the floor on your left side and loop a mini resistance band around your ankles.

B

- Without moving any other part of your body, raise your right leg as high as you can. Your legs should remain straight the entire time.
- Pause, then return to the starting position.
- Do all reps, roll to your other side, and repeat.

Lower Body Exercises

Bird Dog ●

A

- Get down on your hands and knees with your palms flat on the floor and shoulder-width apart. Your thighs should be perpendicular to the floor.

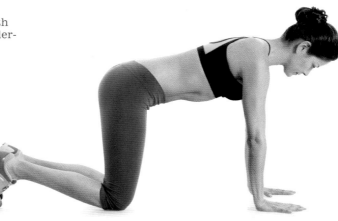

B

- Without allowing your lower back to rise or round, squeeze your abs, and raise your right arm and left leg until they're in line with your body.
- Hold for 5 seconds, then return to the starting position.
- Repeat with your left arm and right leg. Continue alternating back and forth.

Valslide Reverse Lunge ●

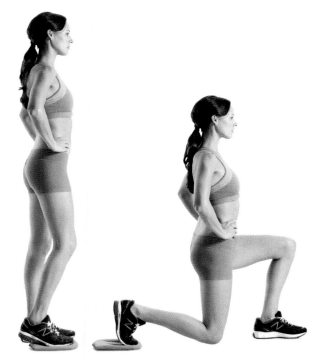

Valslide Side Lunge ●

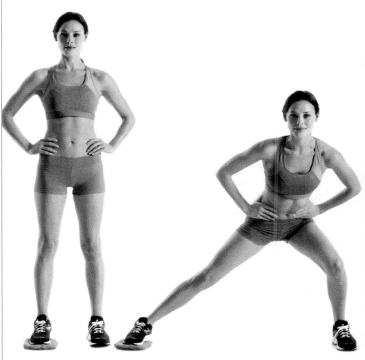

A

- Stand upright and place the ball of your right foot on the middle of the Valslide.

B

- Slide your right foot back until your left knee is bent 90 degrees, and then return to the starting position.
- As you stand, press through your left heel, making sure your left leg does all the work bringing your body back to the standing position.
- Do all reps, stand on the Valslide with your left foot, and repeat.

A

- Stand upright and place your right foot on the Valslide.

B

- Slide your right foot to the side as you push your hips back, bend your left leg, and lower into a squat. Make sure that your toes remain pointing forward and your right leg remains straight.
- Slide your right leg back and return to the starting position.
- Perform all reps and repeat on your other leg.

Lower Body Exercises

TRX Leg Curl ●

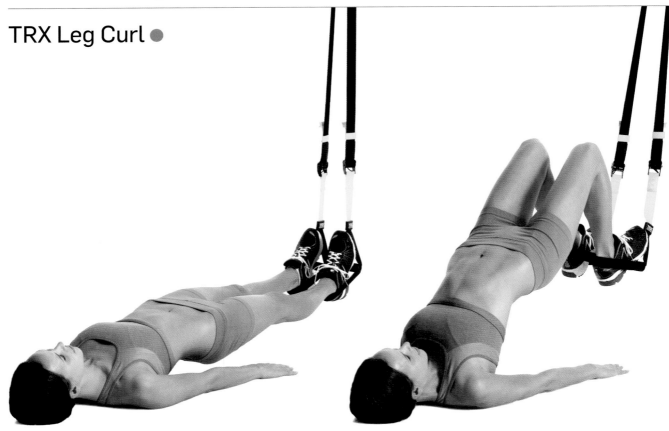

A

- Lie faceup on the floor and place both of your feet in the foot cradles of the TRX.

B

- Push your hips up so that your body forms a straight line from your shoulders to your knees.
- Pull your heels toward your body so your feet are as close as possible to your butt.
- Pause, then reverse the motion until your body is in a straight line.
- Lower your hips to the floor and then repeat.

TRX Squat Jumps

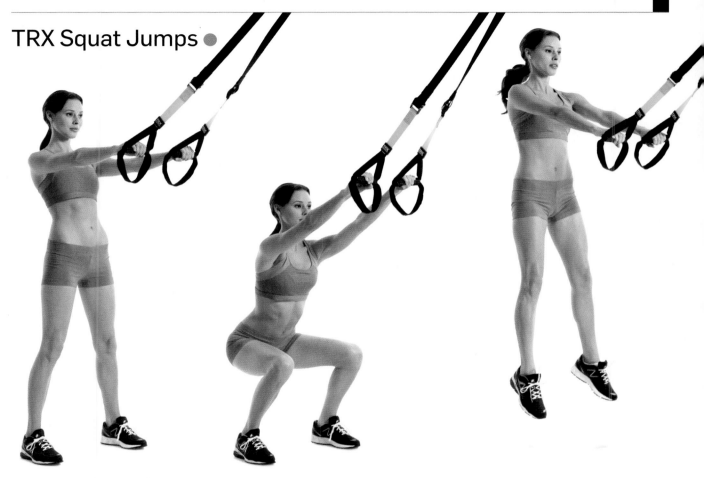

A

- Hold on to the TRX and back away until you feel tension in the straps. Your body should be almost perpendicular to the floor, and your arms should be parallel to the floor, palms facing down.

B

- Push your hips back, bend your knees, and lower your body into a squat until your upper thighs are at least parallel to the floor.

C

- Immediately jump up as high as you can while holding on to the handles.
- Land back in the starting position, lower your body again, and repeat.

Abs

Unlock the potential of your body
and achieve your flat-belly dreams.

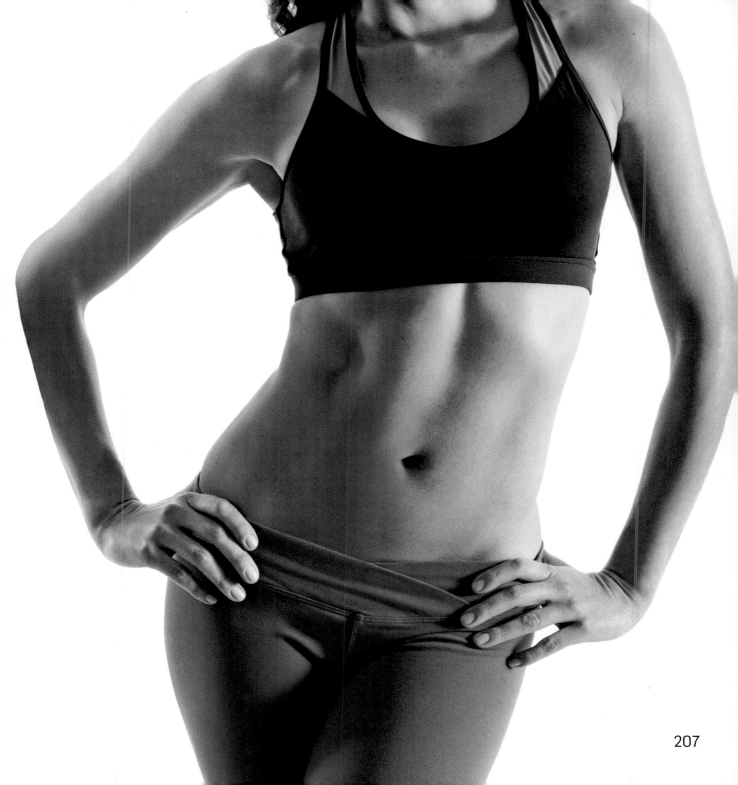

Abs Exercises

Situps ●

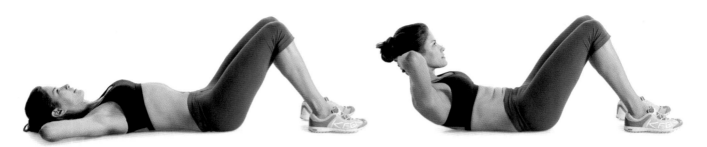

A

- Lie on your back with your your knees bent and your feet flat on the floor.
- Place your fingertips behind your ears and pull your shoulder blades back so your elbows are out to the sides.

B

- Contract your abs and then raise your body up toward your knees.
- Pause, then slowly roll back down to the starting position.

Plank ●

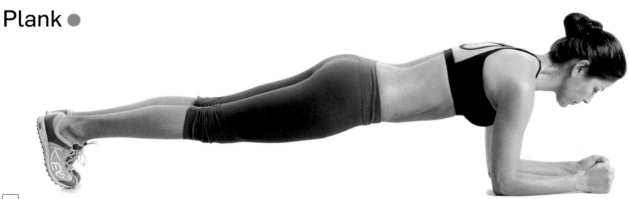

A

- Start to get in a pushup position, but bend your elbows and rest your weight on your forearms instead of on your hands. Your body should form a straight line from your shoulders to your ankles.
- Brace your core by contracting your abs as if you were about to be punched in the gut.
- Hold this position as directed.

Plank to Pushup

A

- Start to get in a pushup position, but bend your elbows and rest your weight on your forearms instead of on your hands. Your body should form a straight line from your shoulders to your ankles.
- Brace your core by contracting your abs as if you were about to be punched in the gut.

B **C**

- Press your body up into the top position of a pushup by extending your arms one at a time.
- Pause, then reverse the movement and return to your elbows. That's 1 rep.

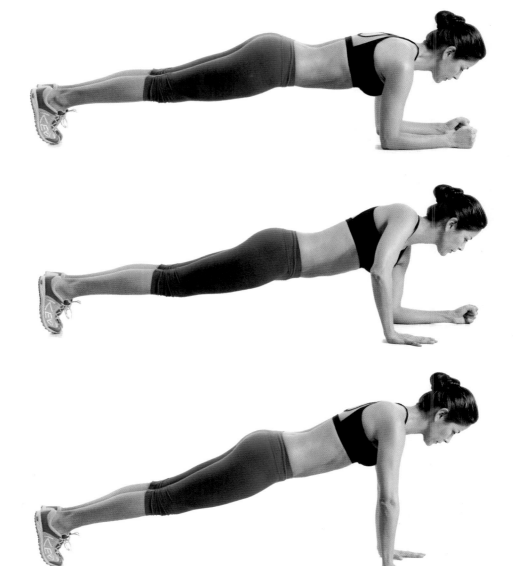

Abs Exercises

Front Plank
with Weight Transfer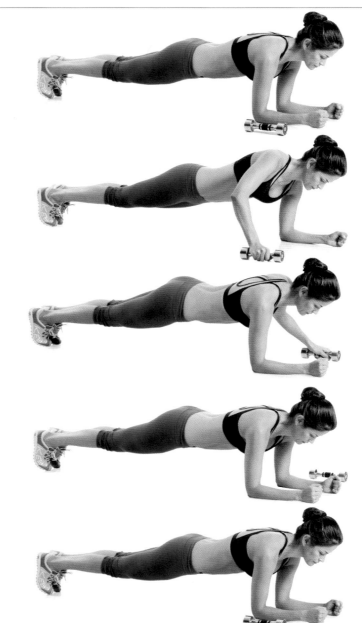

A

- Assume the plank position with a light weight to the outside of your right elbow.

B　**C**

- Pick up the weight with your right hand and pass it to your left hand.

D

- Place the weight to your left.

E

- Move the weight back to the other side. That's 1 rep.
- Make sure you brace your abs to keep your torso from rotating as you lift the weight.

Side Plank ●

A

- Lie on your left side with your knees straight.
- Prop your upper body up on your left elbow and forearm.
- Brace your core by contracting your abs forcefully as if you were about to be punched in the gut.
- Raise your hips until your body forms a straight line from your ankles to your shoulders.
- Hold as directed, then switch sides and repeat.

Hands-Free Side Plank ●

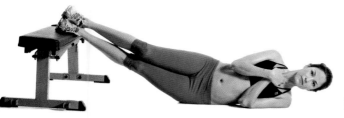

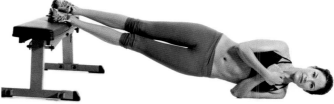

A

- Lie on your left side with your knees straight.
- Place both of your feet on a bench and cross both of your arms across your chest, so your left shoulder is on the floor.
- Squeeze your glutes and prop your upper body up on your left shoulder. Brace your core by contracting your abs forcefully as if you were about to be punched in the gut.

B

- Raise your hips until your body forms a straight line from your ankles to your shoulders. Hold for the required duration, then switch sides and repeat.

Abs Exercises

Mountain Climbers ●

A

- Assume a pushup position with your arms completely straight.
- Your body should form a straight line from your shoulders to your ankles.

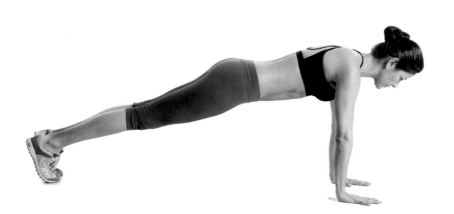

B

- Lift your right foot off the floor and slowly raise your knee as close to your chest as you can.

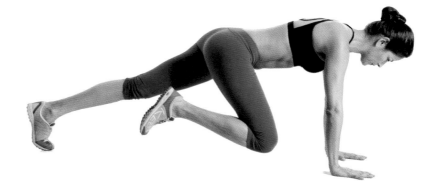

C

- Return to the starting position and repeat with your left leg.
- Continue alternating for the prescribed number of reps or time.

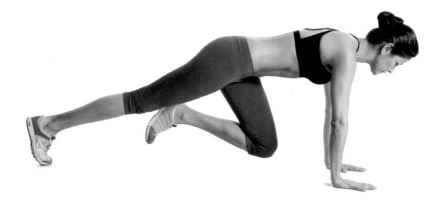

Side Plank and Rotate

A

- Lift your body into a side plank, and start with your right arm raised straight above you so that it's perpendicular to the floor.

B

- Reach under and behind your torso with your right hand, keeping your abs braced.
- Lift your arm back up to the starting position. That's 1 rep.
- Do all reps, roll onto your other side, and repeat.

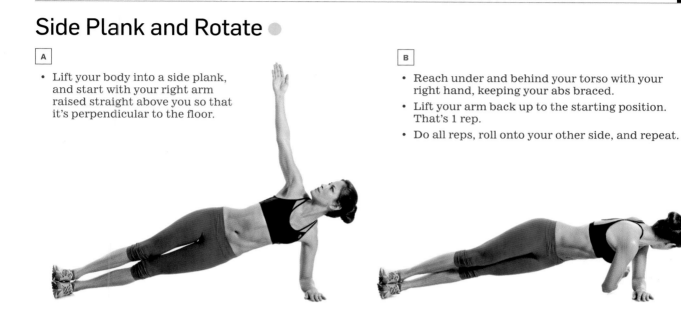

Plank Jumping Jacks

A

- Start to get in a pushup position, but bend your elbows and rest your weight on your forearms instead of on your hands. Your body should form a straight line from your shoulders to your ankles.
- Brace your core by contracting your abs as if you were about to be punched in the gut.

B

- Jump your feet out to the sides as if you were performing a jumping jack, making sure that your upper body doesn't rotate.
- Quickly return your feet to the starting position. That's 1 rep.

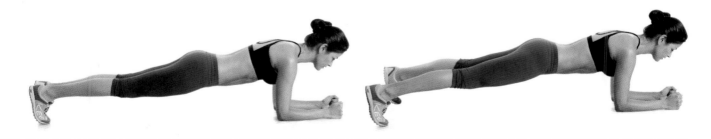

Abs Exercises

Plank with Arm Extension

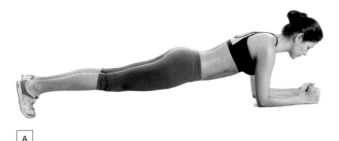

A

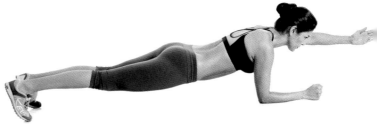

B

- Start to get in a pushup position, but bend your elbows and rest your weight on your forearms instead of on your hands. Your body should form a straight line from your shoulders to your ankles.
- Brace your core by contracting your abs as if you were about to be punched in the gut.

- Raise and straighten your right arm, and hold it so that it's parallel to the rest of your body.
- Hold as directed, lower to the starting position, then raise your other arm and repeat.

Lateral Plank Walks ●

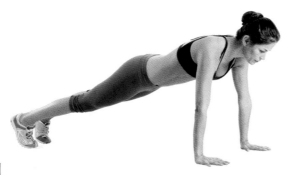

A

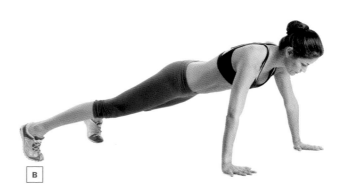

B

- Lower onto all fours and place your weight on your hands so you're in the start position of a pushup.

- "Walk" your right hand and right foot to the right, followed by your left hand and foot.
- Continue this process for 10 steps. Make sure you keep your abs tight and don't allow your body to rotate.
- Reverse the direction and walk your way back to the starting position.

Alternating Superman Plank and Reach ●

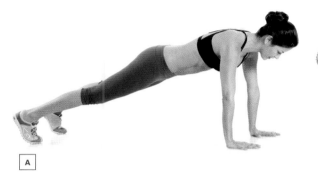

A

- Lower onto all fours and place your weight on your hands so you're in the start position of a pushup. Move your feet so that they're about shoulder-width apart. Your body should form a straight line from your shoulders to your ankles.

B

- Raise your left foot and right arm off the floor and hold.
- Return to the floor and repeat with your right foot and left arm. That's 1 rep.
- Make sure that when you raise your arm and leg, your body doesn't rotate and your hips don't raise.

Planking Frog Tucks ●

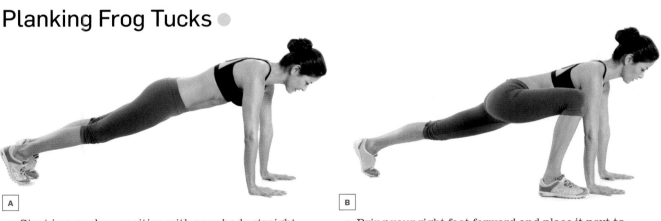

A

- Start in a pushup position with your body straight from your shoulders to your ankles.

B

- Bring your right foot forward and place it next to your right hand (or as close as you can). Try to prevent your hips from sagging or rising.
- Return your leg to the starting position and repeat with your left leg. That's 1 rep.

Abs Exercises

Cross-Body Mountain Climbers ●

A

- Assume a pushup position with your arms completely straight. Your body should form a straight line from your shoulders to your ankles.

B

- Lift your right knee toward your left elbow, lower, then raise your left knee toward your right elbow. That's 1 rep.

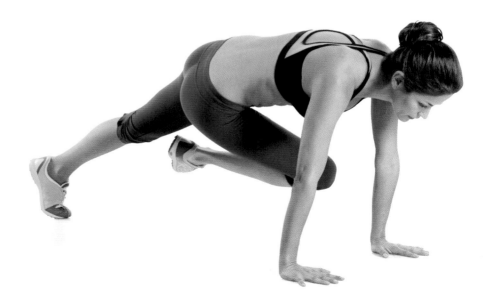

One-Leg Plank ●

A

- Start to get in a pushup position, but bend your elbows and rest your weight on your forearms instead of on your hands. Your body should form a straight line from your shoulders to your ankles.
- Brace your core by contracting your abs as if you were about to be punched in the gut.

B

- Raise one foot a few inches off the floor and hold.
- Lower your foot and repeat with your other foot. That's 1 set.

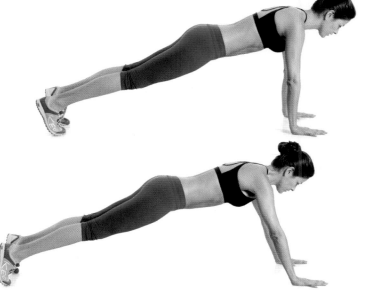

Extended Plank ●

A

- Lower onto all fours and place your weight on your hands so you're in the start position of a pushup.
- Your body should form a straight line from your shoulders to your ankles.

B

- Squeeze your abs as if you're about to be punched in the stomach, and hold for the prescribed time.

Abs Exercises

Side Plank with Row ●

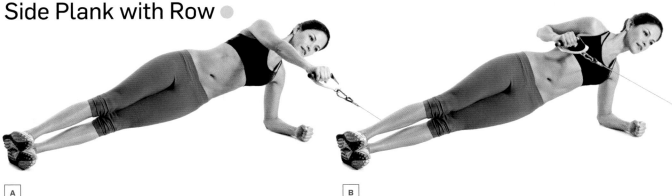

A

- Attach a handle to the low pulley of a cable machine and grab it with your right hand.
- Brace your core and raise your body into a side plank on your left side.

B

- Bend your elbow and pull the handle to your rib cage, keeping your hips pushed up and forward.
- Slowly straighten your arm back in front of you.
- Complete all reps on your left side, then switch to your right side, grab the handle with your left hand, and repeat.

Front Plank with Pulldown ●

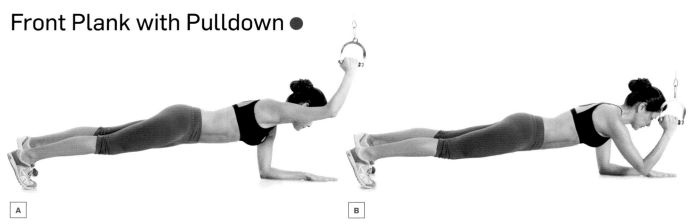

A

- Attach a handle to the high pulley of a cable machine and grab it in your right hand.
- Start to get in a pushup position, but bend your elbows and rest your weight on your left forearm and feet. Your body should form a straight line from your shoulders to your ankles.

B

- With your palm facing your body, bend your right elbow and pull the cable down toward the floor, and then return to the starting position.
- Complete all reps, switch arms, and repeat.

Rolling Plank ●

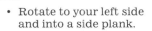

- Begin in a plank position with your body forming a straight line from your shoulders to your ankles.

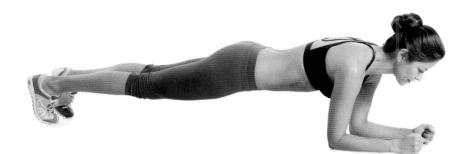

B

- Rotate to your left side and into a side plank.

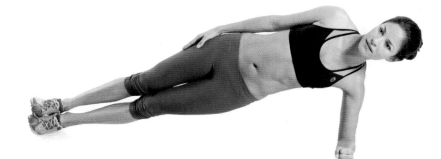

C

- Hold for 10 seconds, then rotate into a right side plank and hold for another 10 seconds. That's 1 rep.
- Return to a plank position and repeat.

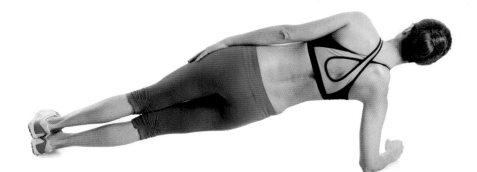

Abs Exercises

Swiss Ball Mountain Climber ●

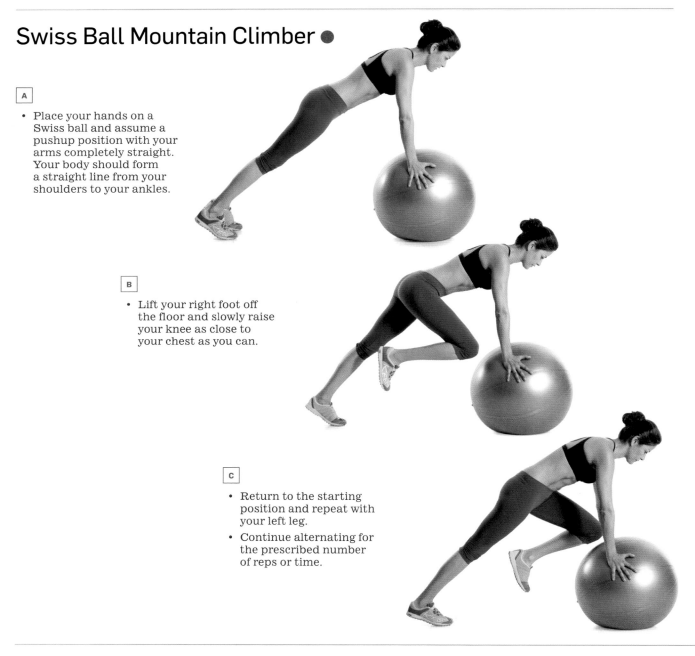

A
- Place your hands on a Swiss ball and assume a pushup position with your arms completely straight. Your body should form a straight line from your shoulders to your ankles.

B
- Lift your right foot off the floor and slowly raise your knee as close to your chest as you can.

C
- Return to the starting position and repeat with your left leg.
- Continue alternating for the prescribed number of reps or time.

Swiss Ball Jackknife

A

- Assume a pushup position with your arms completely straight.
- Rest your shins on a Swiss ball so that your body forms a straight line from your shoulders to your ankles.

B

- Without changing your lower back posture, roll the Swiss ball toward your chest by pulling it forward with your feet.
- Pause, then return the ball to the starting position by lowering your hips and rolling the ball backward.

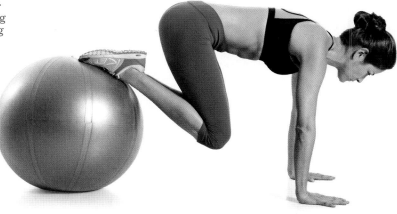

Abs Exercises

Stability Ball Reverse Leg Lifts ●

A

- Lie on a Swiss ball with your legs bent.
- Hold on to a sturdy object for support.
- Your lower back should be in the middle of the ball and your knees slightly bent.

B **C**

- Lift your hips up and bring your knees toward your chest until your legs are perpendicular to the floor.
- Pause, then lower your legs back to the starting position.

Stability Ball Side Crunches

A

- Lie sideways on a Swiss ball and brace your right foot against a wall or a heavy object. Place your fingers behind your ears.

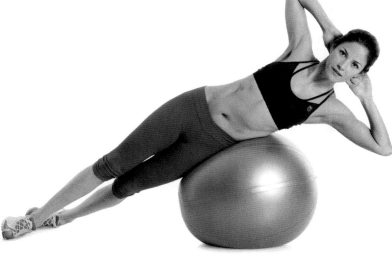

B

- Lift your shoulders and crunch sideways toward your hip.
- Pause, then return to the starting position.
- Complete the prescribed number of reps on that side, then do the same number on your other side.

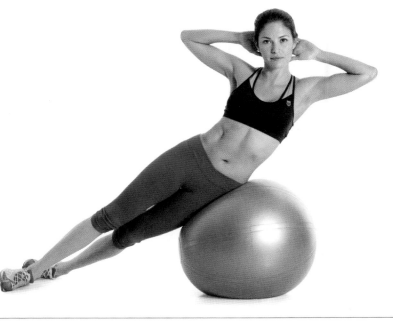

Abs Exercises

Stability Ball Reaching Crunches ●

A

- Lie with your hips, lower back, and shoulders in contact with a Swiss ball and hold a weight plate across your chest.

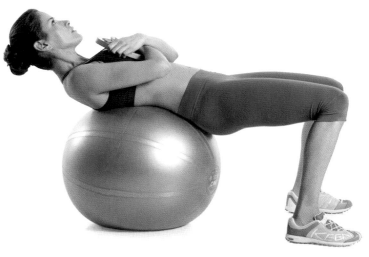

B

- Raise your head and shoulders and crunch your rib cage toward your pelvis.
- Pause, then return to the starting position.

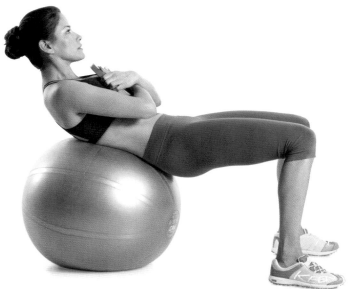

Dumbbell Side Bend ●

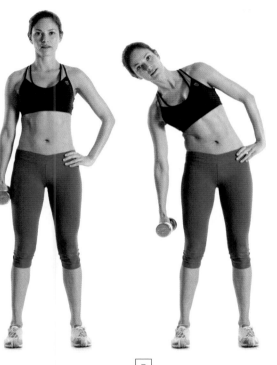

A

- Stand with your feet shoulder-width apart.
- Hold a dumbbell in your right hand at your side with your arms straight.

B

- Squeeze your abs tight and, without twisting your upper body, slowly bend to the right as far as you can, lowering the weight toward your right knee.
- Pause, then slowly return to an upright position.
- Complete all reps to the right, hold the dumbbell in your left hand, and repeat on your other side.

Low Cable Chops ●

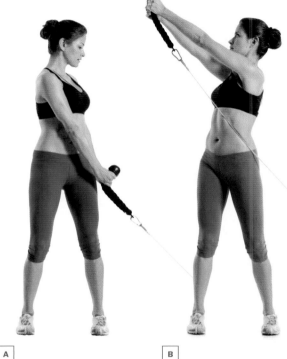

A

- Attach a rope handle to the low pulley of a cable station. Stand tall with your feet shoulder-width apart, your knees slightly bent, and grab the rope with both hands at arm's length in front of your right hip.

B

- Brace your core, and in one movement pull the rope past your left shoulder as you simultaneously rotate your torso to the left.
- Reverse the movement to return to the starting position.
- Complete the prescribed number of reps to your left side, then do the same number rotating to your right.

Abs Exercises

Dumbbell Reverse Chops (Low to High) ●

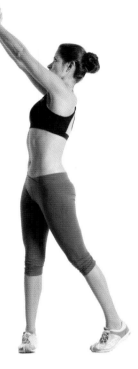

A

- Stand with your feet shoulder-width apart. Grab a dumbbell and hold it with both hands just outside your right ankle.

B

- Brace your core, and in one movement pull the dumbbell up past your left shoulder as you simultaneously rotate your torso to the left.
- Reverse the movement to return to the starting position.
- Complete the prescribed number of reps to your left side, then do the same number starting with the dumbbell just outside your left ankle, rotating to your right.

Resistance Band Chops ●

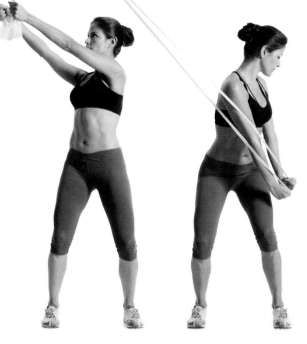

A

- Loop one end of a large resistance band around a chinup bar and then pull it through the other end of the band.
- Clasp both hands around the band and step away so that your right side faces the anchor point. Your shoulders should be turned toward the band.

B

- In one movement, while keeping your arms straight, rotate your torso down and across your body so your hands end up outside your left hip.
- Pause, then return to the starting position.
- Do all reps to your left side, then repeat with your left side facing the anchor point.

Resistance Band High Low Chop ●

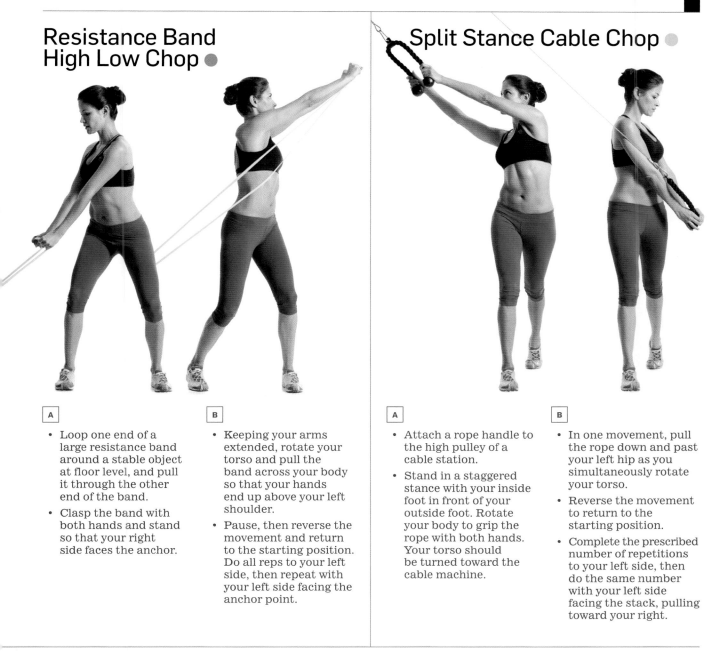

A

- Loop one end of a large resistance band around a stable object at floor level, and pull it through the other end of the band.
- Clasp the band with both hands and stand so that your right side faces the anchor.

B

- Keeping your arms extended, rotate your torso and pull the band across your body so that your hands end up above your left shoulder.
- Pause, then reverse the movement and return to the starting position. Do all reps to your left side, then repeat with your left side facing the anchor point.

Split Stance Cable Chop ●

A

- Attach a rope handle to the high pulley of a cable station.
- Stand in a staggered stance with your inside foot in front of your outside foot. Rotate your body to grip the rope with both hands. Your torso should be turned toward the cable machine.

B

- In one movement, pull the rope down and past your left hip as you simultaneously rotate your torso.
- Reverse the movement to return to the starting position.
- Complete the prescribed number of repetitions to your left side, then do the same number with your left side facing the stack, pulling toward your right.

Abs Exercises

Band Tight Rotation ●

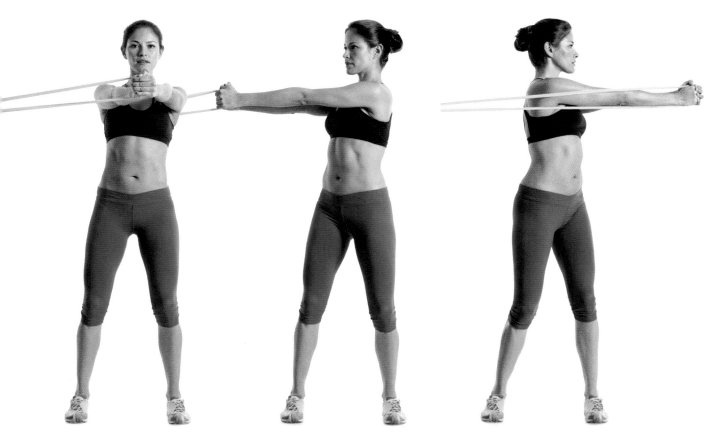

A

- Attach a resistance band to a stable object at waist height.
- Clasp the band with both hands and stand so that your right side faces the anchor, holding the band in front of your chest.
- Step away until you feel light tension.

B

- Keeping your hips square and your core engaged, rotate your upper body to the right so your arms are in line with your right shoulder. That's 1 rep.

C

- Quickly reverse, twisting all the way to the left so your arms are in line with your left shoulder.
- Continue alternating as fast as you can for the prescribed number of reps.
- On the next set, stand with your right side facing the anchor.

Tight Rotations ●

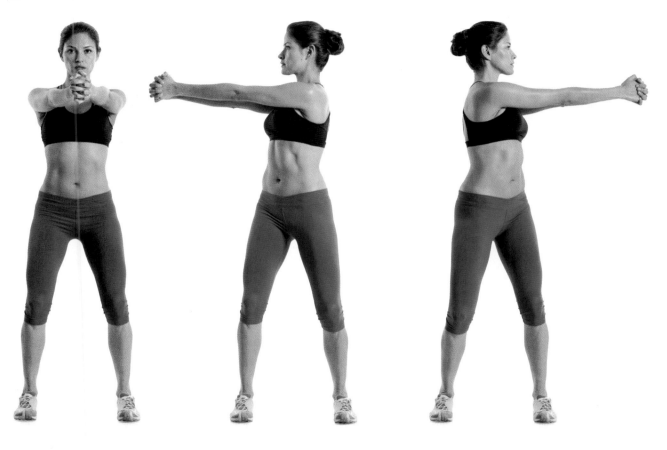

- Stand with your feet more than hip-width apart and your arms extended in front of you, palms together.

B

- Keeping your hips square and your core engaged, rotate your upper body to the right so your arms are in line with your right shoulder. That's 1 rep.

C

- Quickly reverse, twisting all the way to the left so your arms are in line with your left shoulder.

- Continue alternating as fast as you can for the prescribed number of reps.

Abs Exercises

Dumbbell Seated Core Stabilization ●

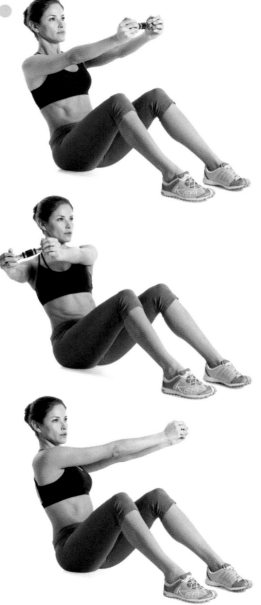

A

- Sit on the floor with your knees bent.
- Hold a dumbbell straight out in front of your chest.
- Lean back so your torso is at a 45-degree angle to the floor, and brace your core.

B

- Without moving your torso, slowly (take 2 seconds) rotate your arms to the right as far as you can.
- Pause for 3 seconds.

C

- Slowly rotate your arms to the left as far as you can.
- Pause again, then continue to alternate back and forth for the allotted time.

Side Pillar Jacks

A

- Lie on your left side with your knees straight.
- Prop your upper body up on your left elbow and forearm.
- Raise your hips until your body forms a straight line from your shoulders to your ankles.

B

- Raise your top leg as high as you can and hold it that way for 2 seconds.
- Lower it back to the starting position. That's 1 rep.
- Perform the prescribed number of reps, then turn around so that you're lying on your right side and repeat.

Abs Exercises

Seated Twist ●

A

- Sit on the floor with your knees bent and your feet flat.
- Hold your arms straight out in front of your chest with your palms together.

B

- Lean back so your torso is at a 45-degree angle to the floor.
- Brace your core and rotate to the right as far as you can.

C

- Pause, then reverse your movement and twist all the way back to the left as far as you can.

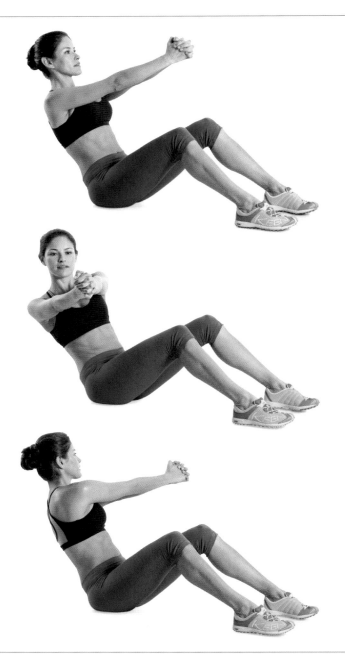

Swiss Ball Rollout

A

- Sit on your knees in front of a Swiss ball, and place your forearms and fist on the ball. Your elbows should be bent about 90 degrees.

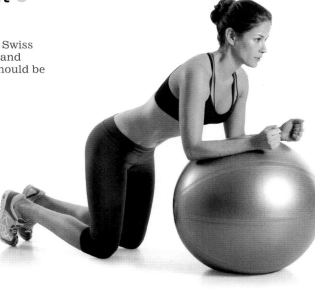

B

- Keeping your core braced, slowly roll the ball forward, straightening your arms and extending your body as far as you can without allowing your lower back to collapse.
- Use your abs to pull the ball back to your knees.

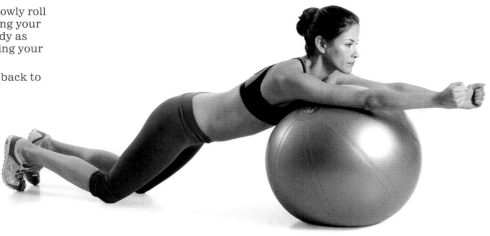

Abs Exercises

Swiss Ball Stir the Pot ●

- Assume a plank position with your forearms on a Swiss ball. Your body should form a straight line from your shoulders to your ankles.
- Squeeze your abs and glutes as hard as you can.

B C

- Use your forearms to move the ball in small circles while keeping the rest of your body in the original position.
- Make one circle moving to the right and then one to the left. That's 1 rep.

Swiss Ball Pike

A

- Assume a pushup position with your arms completely straight. Position your hands slightly wider than and in line with your shoulders.
- Rest your shins on a Swiss ball. Your body should form a straight line from your shoulders to your ankles.

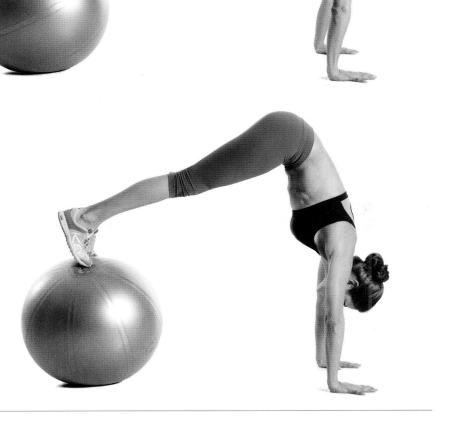

B

- Without bending your knees, roll the Swiss ball toward your body by raising your hips as high as you can.
- Pause, then return the ball to the starting position by lowering your hips and rolling the ball backward.

Abs Exercises

One-Arm Dumbbell Carry ●

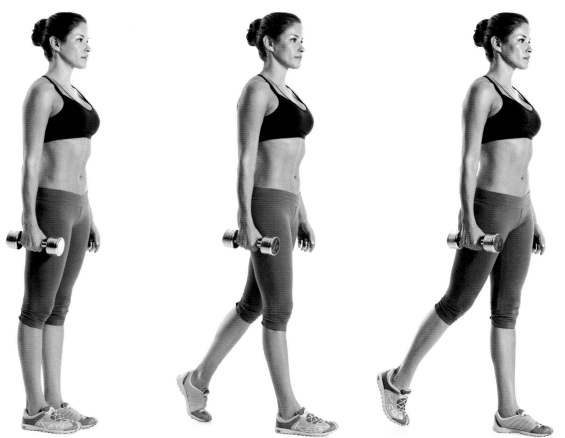

A

- Grab a dumbbell and hold it like a suitcase, keeping your shoulders square and upright.

B **C**

- Maintain that posture as you walk with the dumbbell at your side for the prescribed number of reps or steps.
- Put the dumbbell down, pick it up with your other hand, and walk back.
- Make sure that you squeeze your abs tight the entire time and don't lean your body to the left or right as you walk.

Cable Core Press ●

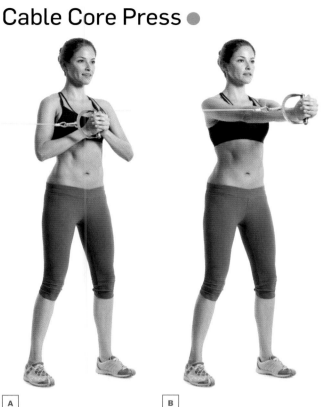

A

- Attach a handle to a cable machine at chest height.
- Grab the handle with your hands clasped and stand with your right side facing the weight stack. Spread your feet about shoulder-width apart.

B

- Step away from the stack until you feel tension in the cable.
- Hold the handle against your chest and slowly press your arms in front of you until they're completely straight.
- Hold for 2 seconds, then return your hands to the starting position.
- Do all your reps, then turn around and repeat with your left side facing the weight stack.

Slide Out ●

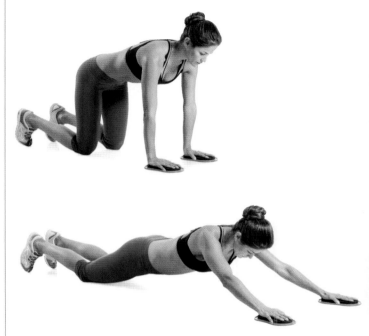

A

- Kneel on the floor and place both hands on a Valslide. Your hands should be under your shoulder.

B

- Slowly push the Valslide forward, extending your body as far as you can without allowing your hips to sag.
- Use your abs to pull your hands back to below your shoulders.

Abs Exercises

Reverse Crunch •

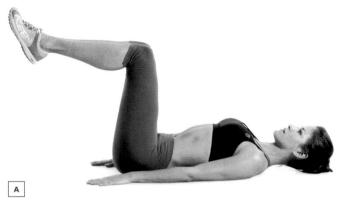

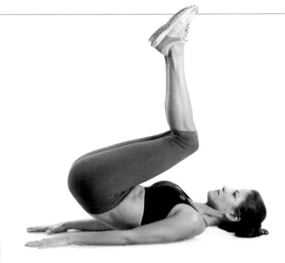

A

- Lie faceup on the floor with your palms facing down.
- Bend your knees 90 degrees.

B

- Raise your hips off the floor and crunch them toward your chest.
- Pause, then slowly lower your legs until your heels nearly touch the floor.

Med Ball Side Rotation •

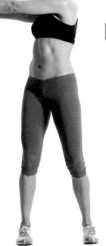

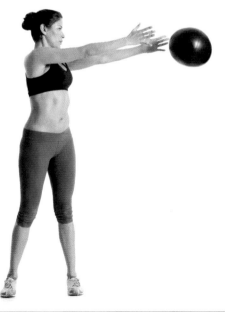

A

- Grab a medicine ball and stand sideways about 3 feet from a brick or concrete wall, with your left side facing the wall.
- Hold the ball at chest level with your arms straight and rotate your torso to your right.

B

- Quickly switch directions and throw as hard as you can against the wall to your left.
- As the ball rebounds off the wall, catch it and repeat the movement.
- Complete the prescribed number of repetitions, then repeat with your right side facing the wall.

Med Ball Slam ●

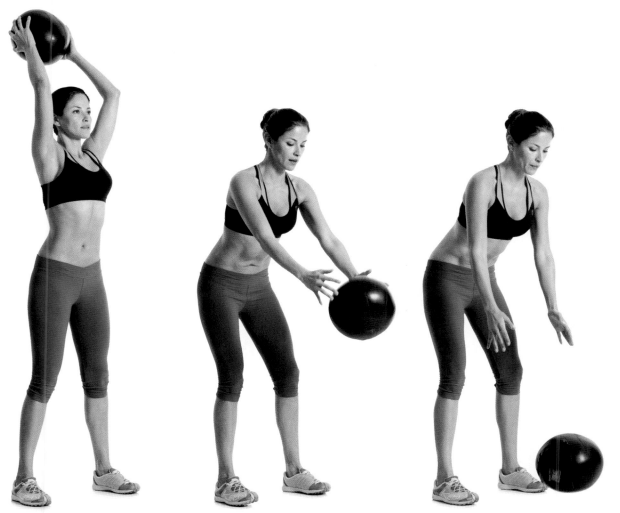

A

- Grab a medicine ball and hold it above your head.
- Your arms should be slightly bent and your feet shoulder-width apart.

B **C**

- Forcefully slam the ball to the floor in front of you as hard as you can.
- Pick the ball up and repeat.

Abs Exercises

Med Ball Russian Twist ●

A

- Sit on the floor with your knees bent and your feet flat.
- Hold a medicine ball, with your arms straight out in front of your chest.
- Lean back so your torso is at a 45-degree angle to the floor.

B

- Brace your core and rotate to the right as far as you can.

C

- Pause, then reverse your movement and twist all the way back to the left as far as you can.

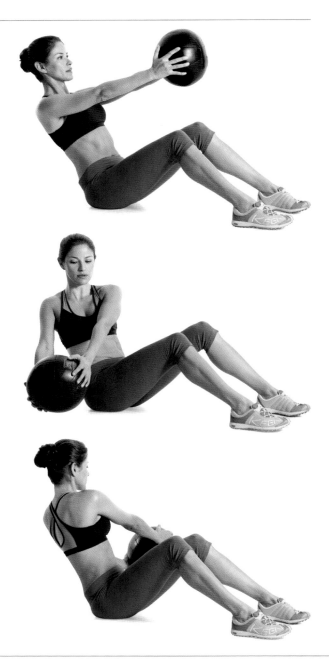

Dead Bugs ●

A

- Lie faceup on the floor with your arms at your sides.
- Raise your legs off the floor so that your hips and knees are bent 90 degrees.

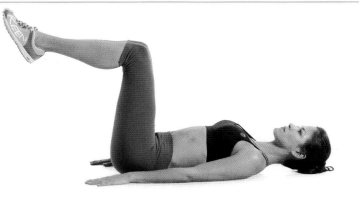

B

- Brace your abs and bring your left knee toward your chest a few inches and your right knee away from your chest a few inches. At the same time, raise your left hand up and over your head.

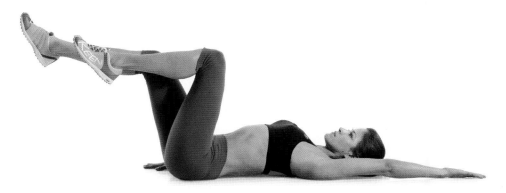

C

- Bring your right knee toward your chest and your left knee away from your chest, as you raise your right arm overhead and lower your left arm back down to your side. That's 1 rep.

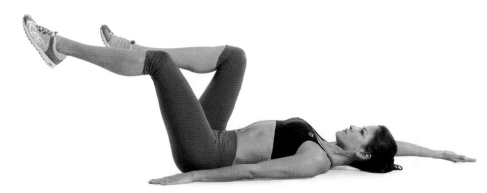

Abs Exercises

Swiss Ball Body Saw ●

A

- Assume a pushup position, but place your elbows and forearms on a Swiss ball. Your body should form a straight line from your shoulders to your ankles.

B

- Squeeze your abs and glutes as tight as you can, then move your forearms forward and backward just a few inches in a sawing motion. That's 1 rep.

Med Ball Side Slams ●

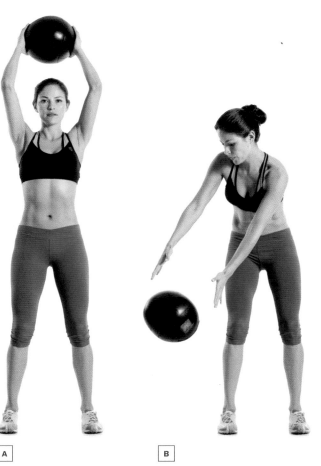

A

- Grab a medicine ball and hold it above your head. Your arms should be slightly bent and your feet shoulder-width apart.

B

- Forcefully slam the ball toward the outside of your left foot as hard as you can.
- Pick the ball up and repeat, this time slamming toward the outside of your right foot. That's 1 rep.

Around the Worlds ●

A

- Place both feet on a bench and assume a pushup position. Your body should form a straight line from your shoulders to your ankles.

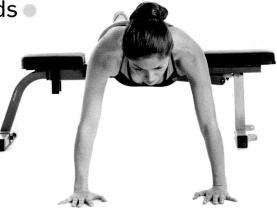

B **C**

- Brace your core and, without dropping your hips or moving your feet, make a full revolution around the bench by "walking" your hands all the way around it. That's 1 rep.

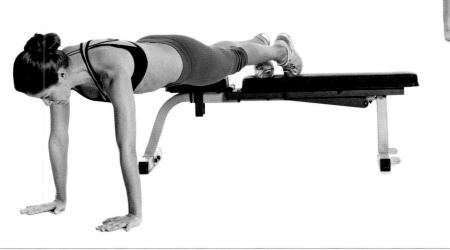

Abs Exercises

Valslide Mountain Climbers ●

A

- Stand with each foot in the middle of the Valslide.
- Lower your body into pushup position, keeping your feet on the Valslide.

B

- With your body in a straight line from your shoulders to your ankles, slide your right knee toward your chest.

C

- Slide back to the start and repeat with your left knee.
- Alternate between both legs until you finish all reps.

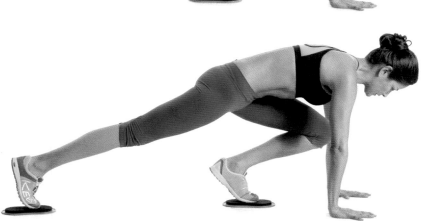

Valslide Body Saw ●

A

- Stand with each foot in the middle of the Valslide.
- Lower your body into pushup position, but place your weight on your elbows and keep your feet on the Valslide.
- Your body should be in a straight line from your shoulders to your ankles.

B

- Squeeze your abs as if you're about to be punched in the stomach, and then slightly slide both of your feet backward.
- Return to the starting position. Your entire body should create a slightly "sawing" motion.

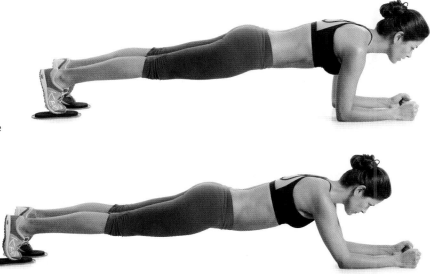

Valslide Upside-Down Angel ●

A

- Stand with each foot in the middle of the Valslide.
- Lower your body into pushup position, but place your weight on your forearms instead of your hands. Make sure your feet remain on the Valslide.

B

- Slide your feet outward without letting your hips drop.
- Pause, then return to the starting position. That's 1 rep.

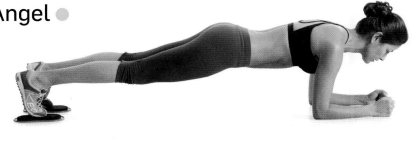

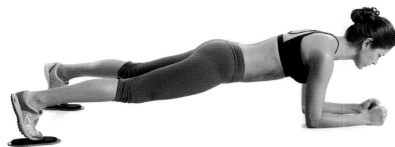

The New Rules of Workouts

ALL EXERCISE ROUTINES ARE NOT CREATED EQUAL.

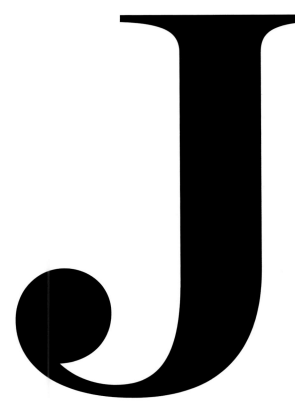

Just as you have good and bad diets, the same could be said about your gym routine. Anyone can put together a bunch of exercises and call it a workout. It's done every day in gyms around the world. But those same programs are what have caused years of fitness frustration. The yelling and screaming of trainers isn't what you need to drop weight fast. There's an art and science to how you design a program. Each exercise needs to serve a purpose to help you reach your goals, and be ordered in a way that keeps you working hard and improving.

That's why we decided to take the guesswork out of exercise so that you could confidently take on any goal and succeed. Whether you want to get ready for the beach, fit into your favorite pair of jeans, or never perform a crunch again (and still lose weight), anything is possible. All you need to do is follow the step-by-step plans and work hard. The results will follow.

But here's the key: Don't change the exercises unless noted by the experts. These workouts were specifically designed to help you get in the best shape of your life. They'll be fun, fast, and effective. But when you reach an exercise that's difficult, don't default back to what you know or avoid the learning curve. Be patient and follow this guide with complete trust. Your faith will be rewarded with reshaped abs, butt, and thighs—and the confidence of knowing that you finally cracked the weight loss code. Your fittest body starts here.

Your Guide to Every Workout

Follow these rules to help simplify your workouts and see results fast

Workout 101

• Exercises will be ordered by number. Perform the exercises in order as listed. That is, do all of the sets of a particular number before moving on to the next one.

• When you see a number and a letter combined, it indicates that the exercises are part of a group (such as 1A, 1B, 1C). That is, do 1 set of the first exercise (1A), 1 set of the second exercise (1B), and so on. Follow this pattern until you've finished all sets of each exercise with the same number. Do this regardless of how many exercises share the same number. Perform all of these exercises before moving on to the next number (2, 3, and 4).

• Each exercise contains specific guidelines for reps, sets, and rest periods.

• The reps are the number of times you will perform an exercise before taking a break. Sometimes the number of reps will not be a number (like 8), but instead be a period of time (30 seconds). In these instances, perform as many reps as you can in the time specified. Or for certain moves, like the plank, hold the exercise until time is up.

• The sets are how many times you will repeat a series of reps.

• The rest periods indicate your breaks after each exercise. Sometimes a rest period will say "0." When this occurs, there is no rest and you should move immediately to the next exercise.

• The acronym AMAP means "as many as possible." When that is listed, you should perform as many reps as you can until your form breaks down.

• Before each workout, perform "The Total Body Jump-Start." It's a warmup designed to prepare your body for each plan.

The Total Body Jump-Start [5–7 minutes]

A GREAT WORKOUT doesn't start with your first rep—it begins with your warmup. After all, a "cold" muscle can end up an injured muscle or can limit your potential results. Your muscles are like a rubber band. When they are cold, they easily snap. But a warm muscle is not only more pliable, it can also generate more force. And a more forceful muscle is one that can shred fat and tone every inch of your body.

This warmup should take 5 to 7 minutes. Perform each of the exercises once, and when you're done, move on to your workout.

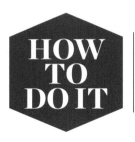

HOW TO DO IT

● Perform each of these exercises as fast and as explosively as possible. The goal is to warm up your muscles and have your body ready to move more weight.

● Try to keep your rest to just 30 seconds after each exercise. If you need more time, take it. If you can use less rest, trim the breaks to just 15 seconds.

● If you find that your body still isn't loose, perform a second set of all exercises.

The Total Body Jump-Start

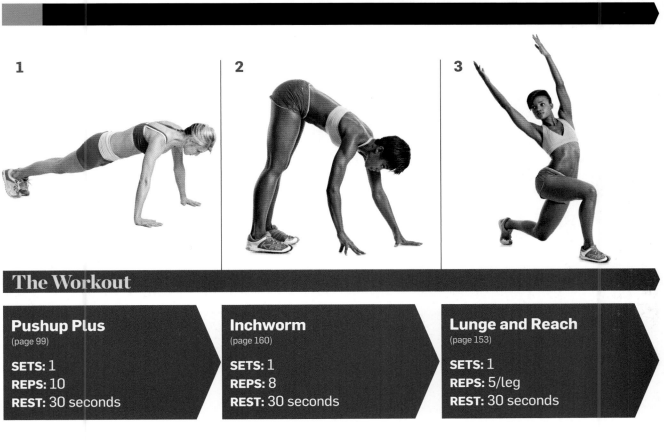

1   **2**   **3**

The Workout

Pushup Plus
(page 99)

SETS: 1
REPS: 10
REST: 30 seconds

Inchworm
(page 160)

SETS: 1
REPS: 8
REST: 30 seconds

Lunge and Reach
(page 153)

SETS: 1
REPS: 5/leg
REST: 30 seconds

The Total Body Jump-Start

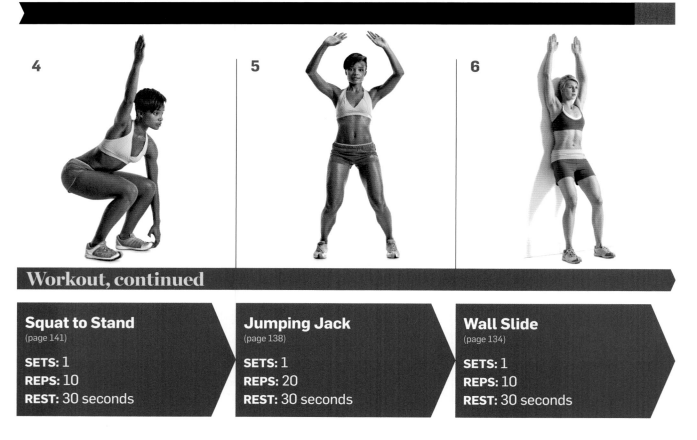

4 **5** **6**

Workout, continued

Squat to Stand
(page 141)

SETS: 1
REPS: 10
REST: 30 seconds

Jumping Jack
(page 138)

SETS: 1
REPS: 20
REST: 30 seconds

Wall Slide
(page 134)

SETS: 1
REPS: 10
REST: 30 seconds

"Physical fitness is not only one of the most important keys to a healthy body, it is the basis of dynamic and creative intellectual activity."
—John F. Kennedy

No-Crunch Abs Workouts

The revolutionary new way to lose weight and tone your body.

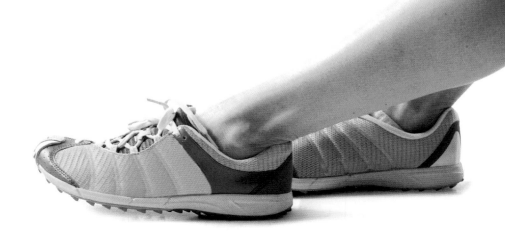

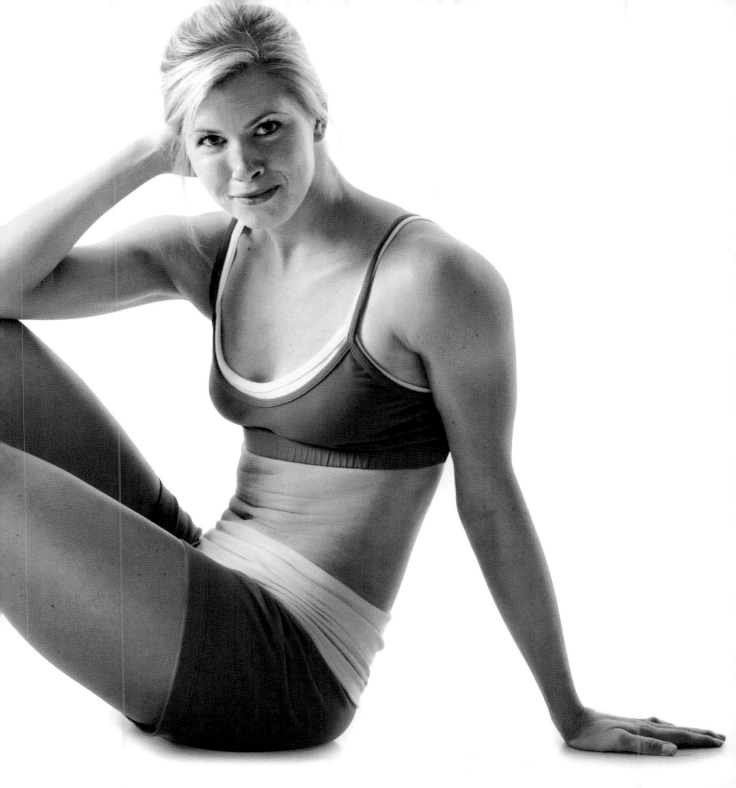

The No-Gym, No-Crunch Workout [30 minutes]

FORGET CRUNCHES, leg lifts, and long, slow pounding on the treadmill. This workout, created by Craig Ballantyne, founder of the Turbulence Training system, will give you stronger, sexier abs and finally make them visible. Unlike traditional abs programs that place a lot of stress on your lower back, these exercises remove pain rather than cause it. And while you'll be working as hard as you would in a high-end, expensive gym, this routine only requires dumbbells and a Swiss ball. Whether you do it in your living room or your backyard, you'll be saying good-bye to the old ineffective exercises and hello to your new trim bod.

ABOUT THE EXPERT

Craig Ballantyne, MSc, CSCS, has been a fitness contributor to *Men's Health* for more than 10 years. Based in Toronto, he is the owner of TurbulenceTraining.com and the editor for *Early to Rise*. His business, CB Athletic Consulting, Inc, has been one of the most popular and effective online training businesses.

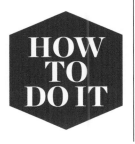

● Perform this workout three times a week. Alternate between Workout A and Workout B three days a week, resting at least a day between each session. That means, you'd perform Workout A on Monday, Workout B on Wednesday, and Workout A again on Friday. The next week you'd perform Workout B on Monday, Workout A on Wednesday, and Workout B on Friday.

● When you see a number with a letter next to it (such as 1A, 1B), that means the exercises are performed as a circuit. For each circuit, do 1 set of each exercise in succession. For example, complete 1 set of exercise 1A, rest as directed, and then perform 1 set of exercise 1B and rest again. Follow this pattern until you've completed all sets of each exercise in the group, and then progress to the next circuit.

The No-Gym, No-Crunch Workout

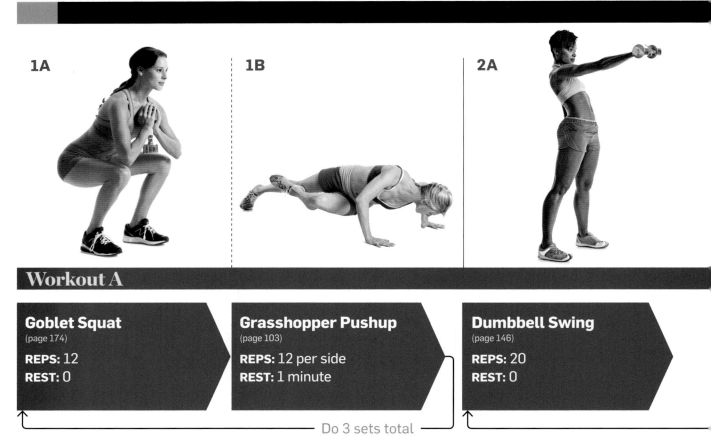

1A

1B

2A

Workout A

Goblet Squat
(page 174)

REPS: 12
REST: 0

Grasshopper Pushup
(page 103)

REPS: 12 per side
REST: 1 minute

Dumbbell Swing
(page 146)

REPS: 20
REST: 0

— Do 3 sets total —

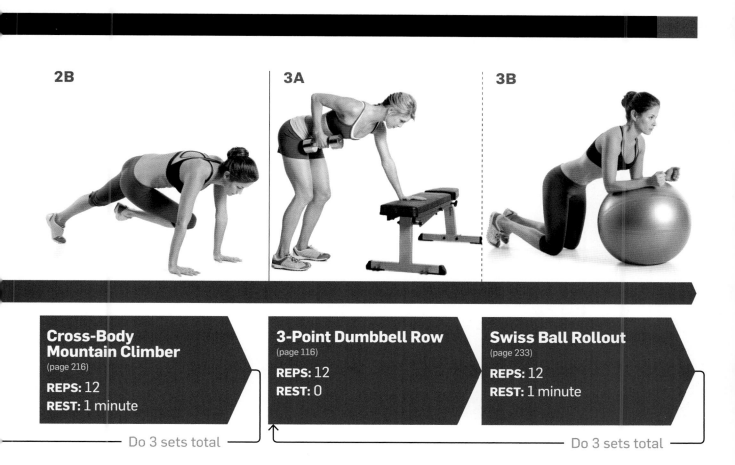

2B

3A

3B

**Cross-Body
Mountain Climber**
(page 216)

REPS: 12
REST: 1 minute

Do 3 sets total

3-Point Dumbbell Row
(page 116)

REPS: 12
REST: 0

Swiss Ball Rollout
(page 233)

REPS: 12
REST: 1 minute

Do 3 sets total

The No-Gym, No-Crunch Workout

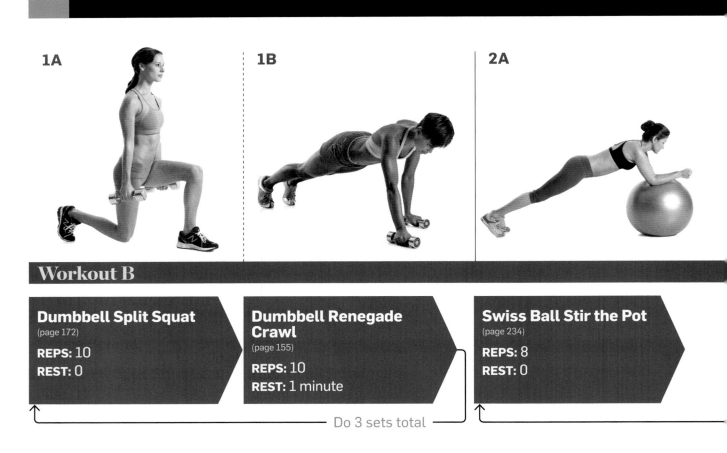

1A

1B

2A

Workout B

Dumbbell Split Squat
(page 172)

REPS: 10
REST: 0

Dumbbell Renegade Crawl
(page 155)

REPS: 10
REST: 1 minute

Swiss Ball Stir the Pot
(page 234)

REPS: 8
REST: 0

— Do 3 sets total —

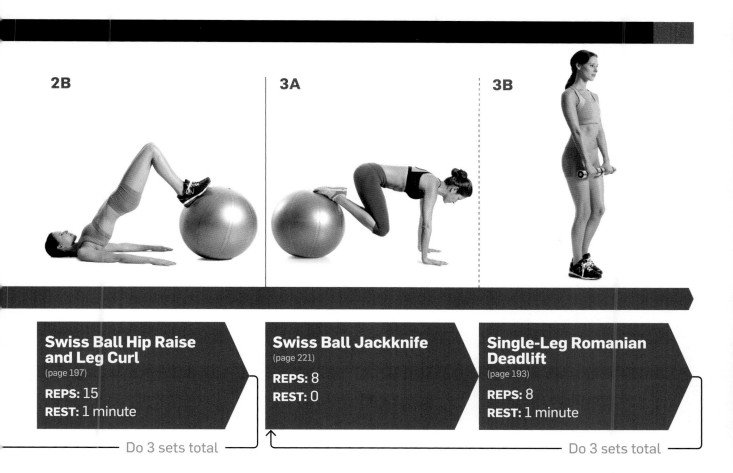

2B

3A

3B

Swiss Ball Hip Raise and Leg Curl
(page 197)

REPS: 15
REST: 1 minute

Do 3 sets total

Swiss Ball Jackknife
(page 221)

REPS: 8
REST: 0

Single-Leg Romanian Deadlift
(page 193)

REPS: 8
REST: 1 minute

Do 3 sets total

The One-Dumbbell Workout [30 minutes]

SOMETIMES THE SIMPLEST workouts are the best ones. This fat-scorching plan was designed by fitness expert Martin Rooney, CSCS, to help you ignite your metabolism as quickly as possible. The entire workout requires only one pair of dumbbells. No more excuses about needing more equipment or taking breaks. After you've finished this plan, you might find yourself canceling your gym membership, and using the extra money to buy a heavier pair of dumbbells and a new wardrobe.

ABOUT THE EXPERT

Martin Rooney is an internationally recognized fitness expert and author, known for training some of the greatest athletes in the world. He has a master's degree in health science and a bachelor's degree in physical therapy from the Medical University of South Carolina, and he also holds a bachelor's degree in exercise science from Furman University. He is the creator of the Training for Warriors system (www.trainingforwarriors.com) and is the COO of the Parisi Speed School, a national franchise.

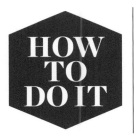

● Do this workout 3 days a week, resting at least a day between each session. So you might lift weights on Monday, Wednesday, and Friday.

● The workout consists of 10 exercises that are broken into two groups (Group 1 and Group 2). Perform 1 set of 10 reps for all of the exercises in Group 1 without any rest. Then, take a 3-minute break and perform 1 set of 10 reps of all the exercises in Group 2. That's one round. Rest 3 more minutes and complete two more rounds.

The One-Dumbbell Workout

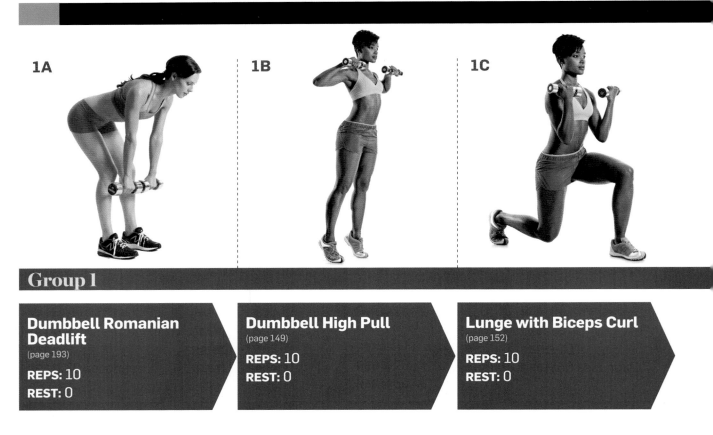

1A

1B

1C

Group 1

Dumbbell Romanian Deadlift
(page 193)
REPS: 10
REST: 0

Dumbbell High Pull
(page 149)
REPS: 10
REST: 0

Lunge with Biceps Curl
(page 152)
REPS: 10
REST: 0

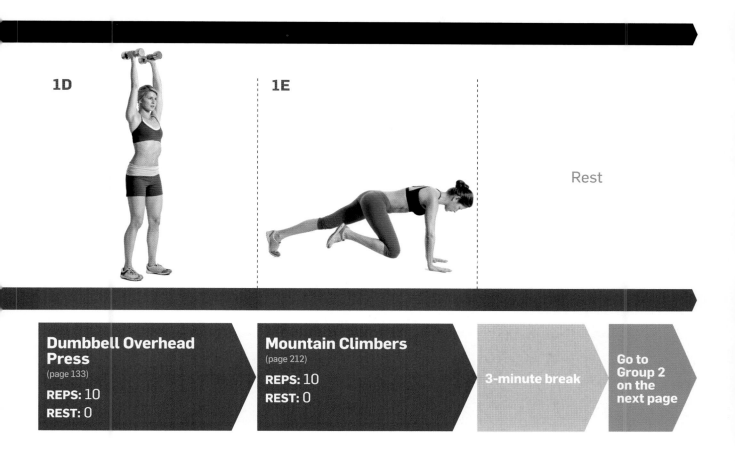

1D

1E

Rest

Dumbbell Overhead Press
(page 133)

REPS: 10
REST: 0

Mountain Climbers
(page 212)

REPS: 10
REST: 0

3-minute break

Go to Group 2 on the next page

The One-Dumbbell Workout

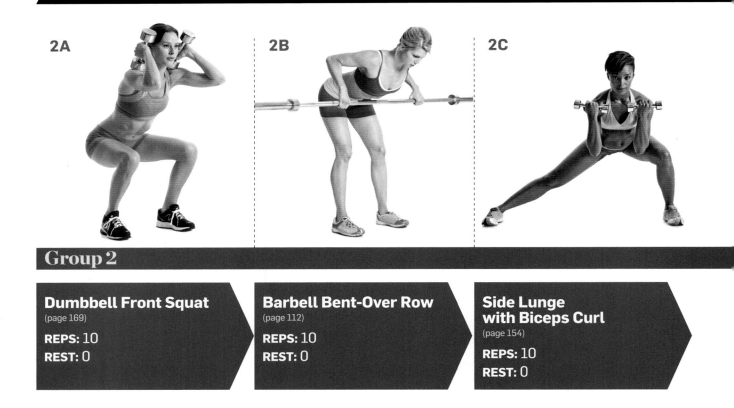

2A

2B

2C

Group 2

Dumbbell Front Squat
(page 169)

REPS: 10
REST: 0

Barbell Bent-Over Row
(page 112)

REPS: 10
REST: 0

**Side Lunge
with Biceps Curl**
(page 154)

REPS: 10
REST: 0

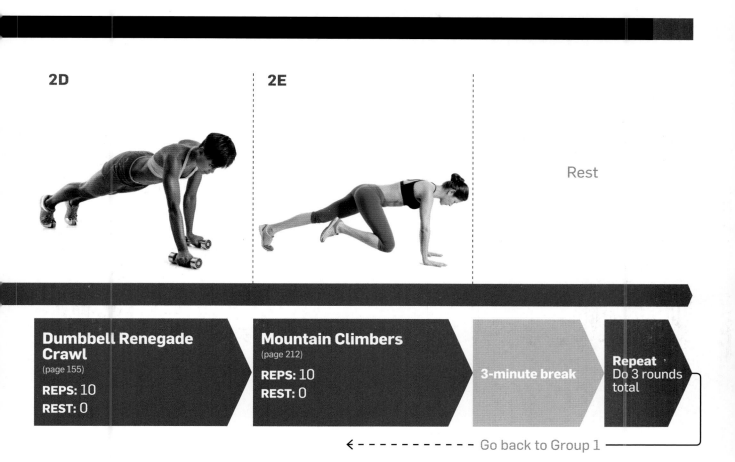

2D

2E

Rest

Dumbbell Renegade Crawl
(page 155)

REPS: 10
REST: 0

Mountain Climbers
(page 212)

REPS: 10
REST: 0

3-minute break

Repeat
Do 3 rounds total

←----------- Go back to Group 1 ————

Fast Track Abs Workouts

Achieve your goals in record time and with less equipment.

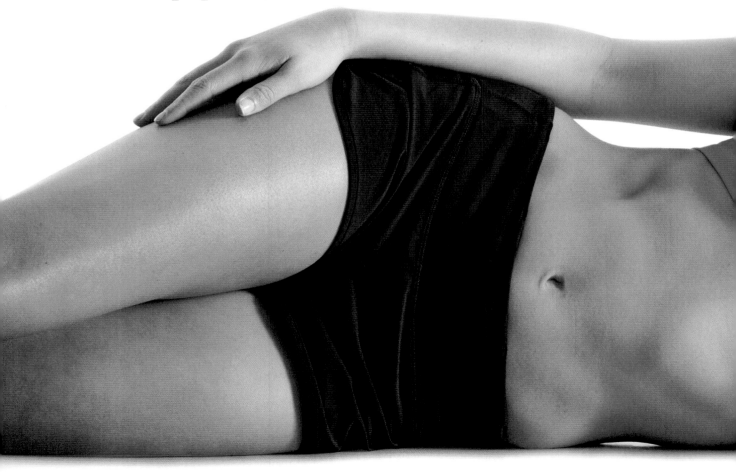

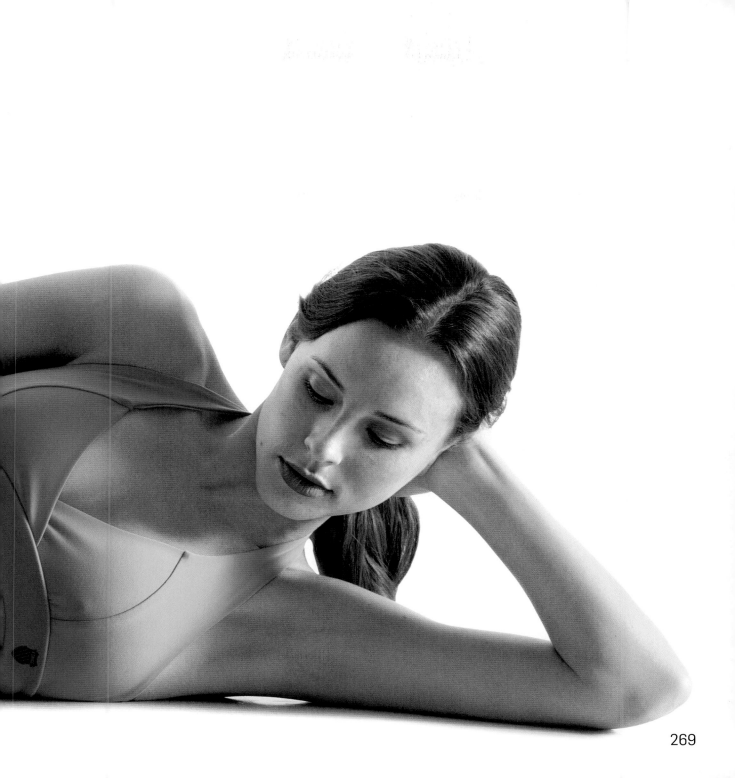

The Fastest Workout Ever Created [10 minutes]

SOMETIME IT SEEMS that the only way to stay in shape is to add 2 hours to your day. After all, your busy schedule conspires against your lean belly dreams and keeps you running around to seeminutegly every place but the gym. While we can't make your wishes for a 26-hour day come true, we can provide the type of workouts that will fit into any schedule and still give you the gorgeous body you want.

This workout takes you out of your normal comfort zone and into fat-burning paradise. Meet the three-exercise workout. It's so simple it'll appear almost too good to be true. But it's been proven to challenge any woman—from beginners to experts—and is the fastest way to help you blast stubborn ab flab.

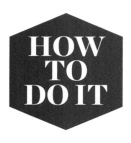

HOW TO DO IT

- Perform these three exercises three times a week, resting at least a day between each session. For example, you could work out on Monday, Wednesday, and Friday.

- To begin, select a weight that enables you to do 10 repetitions using very good form. Set a timer for 10 minutes and perform 5 reps of each exercise (using the same weight) in order. That's one round.

- Once you perform all three exercises, repeat the entire process again. Try to complete as many rounds as possible within 10 minutes without any rest.

- As you progress, you can either add more weight or set the timer for a longer period of time (15 or 20 minutes).

ABOUT THE EXPERT

David Jack is a performance coach and director of Teamworks Fitness/CATZ Sports in Acton, Massachusetts. In addition to coaching, he is regularly involved in consulting, media, and speaking roles in the fitness industry. He is a Men's Health/Rodale national advisor, global spokesman for Reebok Fitness and Training, and an expert advisor to the International Youth Conditioning Association.

The Fastest Workout Ever Created

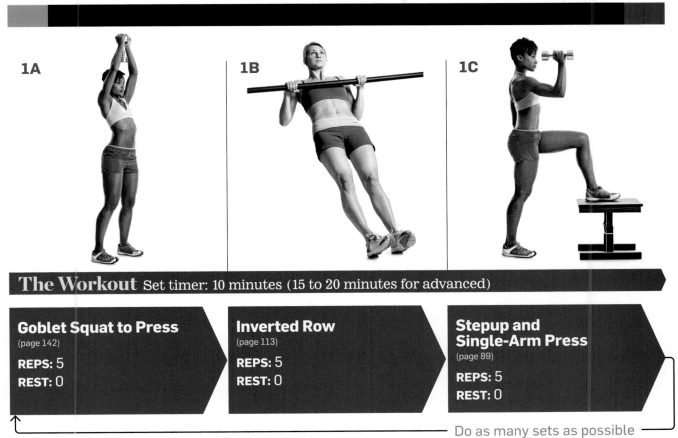

1A   1B   1C

The Workout Set timer: 10 minutes (15 to 20 minutes for advanced)

Goblet Squat to Press
(page 142)

REPS: 5
REST: 0

Inverted Row
(page 113)

REPS: 5
REST: 0

Stepup and Single-Arm Press
(page 89)

REPS: 5
REST: 0

Do as many sets as possible

Revitalize Your Core [25 minutes]

IF YOU WANT to see your abs, the first thing you need to do is stop thinking that certain exercises target individual muscles. Your body is smarter than that. If it weren't, then every late-night TV abs device would do the trick. You see, the layer of fat on your belly has no connection to the muscle beneath your sexy stomach. This workout, created by Craig Rasmussen, CSCS, is the ultimate fat-eliminuteating routine because it targets your metabolism. You'll activate more muscle, burn hundreds of calories, and work all of your core muscles with every exercise.

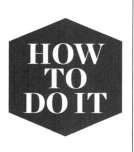

HOW TO DO IT

● Perform this workout three times a week. Alternate between Workout A and Workout B three days a week, resting at least a day between each session. That means, you'd perform Workout A on Monday, Workout B on Wednesday, and Workout A again on Friday. The next week you'd perform Workout B on Monday, Workout A on Wednesday, and Workout B on Friday.

● When you see a number with a letter next to it (such as 1A, 1B), that means the exercises are performed as a circuit. For each circuit, do 1 set of each exercise in succession. For example, complete 1 set of exercise 1A, rest as directed, and then perform 1 set of exercise 1B and rest again. Follow this pattern until you've completed all sets of each exercise in the group, and then progress to the next circuit.

ABOUT THE EXPERT

Craig Rasmussen is a program designer and performance coach at Results Fitness in Newhall, California. He has worked with a wide variety of clientele from all walks of life and has authored several articles that have appeared online and in print media. Craig is a competitive powerlifter and a Certified Strength and Conditioning Specialist through the National Strength and Conditioning Association.

Revitalize Your Core

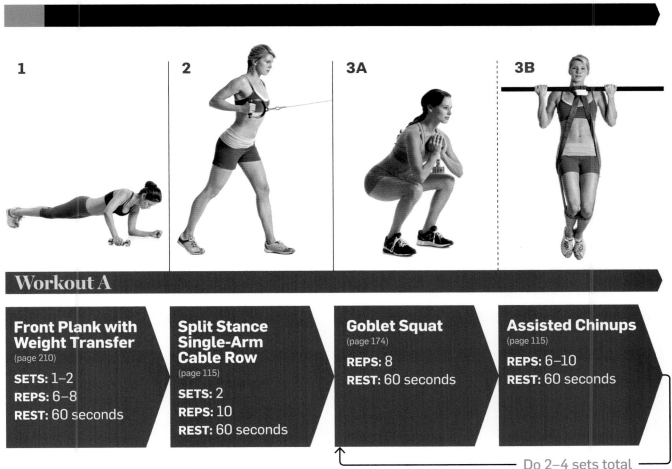

1   **2**   **3A**   **3B**

Workout A

Front Plank with Weight Transfer
(page 210)

SETS: 1–2
REPS: 6–8
REST: 60 seconds

Split Stance Single-Arm Cable Row
(page 115)

SETS: 2
REPS: 10
REST: 60 seconds

Goblet Squat
(page 174)

REPS: 8
REST: 60 seconds

Assisted Chinups
(page 115)

REPS: 6–10
REST: 60 seconds

Do 2–4 sets total

273

Revitalize Your Core

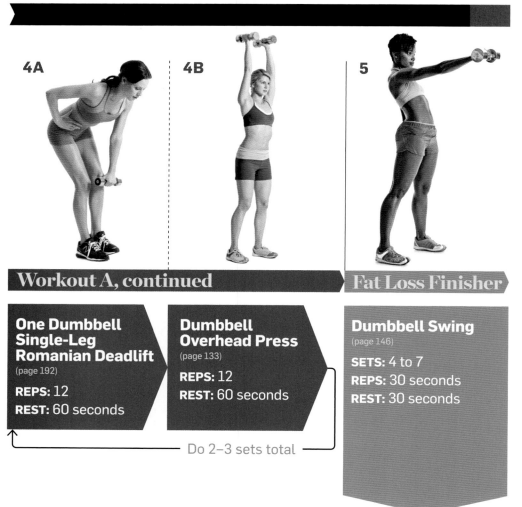

4A

4B

5

Workout A, continued

Fat Loss Finisher

**One Dumbbell
Single-Leg
Romanian Deadlift**
(page 192)

REPS: 12
REST: 60 seconds

**Dumbbell
Overhead Press**
(page 133)

REPS: 12
REST: 60 seconds

Do 2–3 sets total

Dumbbell Swing
(page 146)

SETS: 4 to 7
REPS: 30 seconds
REST: 30 seconds

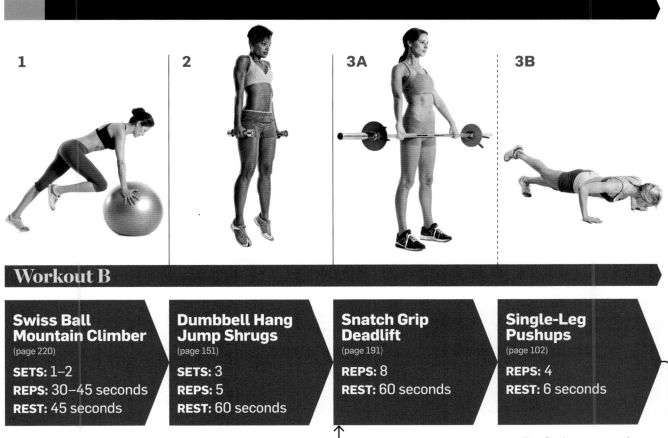

1

2

3A

3B

Workout B

Swiss Ball Mountain Climber
(page 220)

SETS: 1–2
REPS: 30–45 seconds
REST: 45 seconds

Dumbbell Hang Jump Shrugs
(page 151)

SETS: 3
REPS: 5
REST: 60 seconds

Snatch Grip Deadlift
(page 191)

REPS: 8
REST: 60 seconds

Single-Leg Pushups
(page 102)

REPS: 4
REST: 6 seconds

— Do 2–4 sets total

Revitalize Your Core

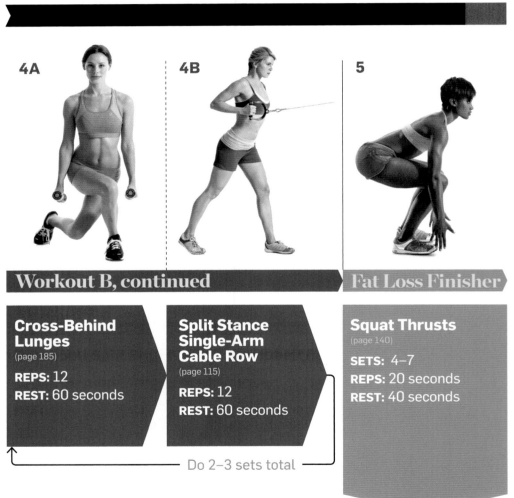

4A

4B

5

Workout B, continued

Fat Loss Finisher

Cross-Behind Lunges
(page 185)

REPS: 12
REST: 60 seconds

Split Stance Single-Arm Cable Row
(page 115)

REPS: 12
REST: 60 seconds

— Do 2–3 sets total —

Squat Thrusts
(page 140)

SETS: 4–7
REPS: 20 seconds
REST: 40 seconds

"The higher your energy level,
the more efficient your body.
The more efficient your body,
the better you feel and the more
you will use your talent
to produce outstanding results."
—Anthony Robbins

THE WORKOUTS

The Secret Abs Workout [45 minutes]

DUMBBELLS AND BARBELLS are great, but you can outsmart fat and blast cellulite using just your bodyweight. This versatile workout requires only one piece of equipment: you. The secondsret to this program is movements that require you to utilize your entire body and balance several muscles at the same time. These exercises not only increase the intensity of your workout, but also fire up your metabolism and shorten the time you spend working out.

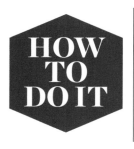

HOW TO DO IT

- Do this workout 3 days a week, resting at least a day between each session. So you might lift weights on Monday, Wednesday, and Friday.
- Each workout consists of four phases: a dynamic warm-up, bodyweight exercises, core movements, and then a cool down.
- Perform all of the exercises as straight sets. That is, do all of the required sets and reps of an exercise before moving on to the next movement.
- Do your best to follow the recommended rest periods, as that will help provide the best results.
- If you want to make any of the exercise more difficult, wear a weighted vest to add resistance.

ABOUT THE EXPERT

Jim Smith, CSCS, is a highly respected, world-renowned strength and conditioning specialist who has been called one of the most innovative strength coaches in the fitness industry. Training athletes, fitness enthusiasts, and weekend warriors, Jim has dedicated himself to helping them reach "beyond their potential." He holds multiple national fitness certifications and is a consultant and lecturer, giving seminutears all over the country. You can find his work at dieselsc.com.

The Secret Abs Workout

WEEK 1

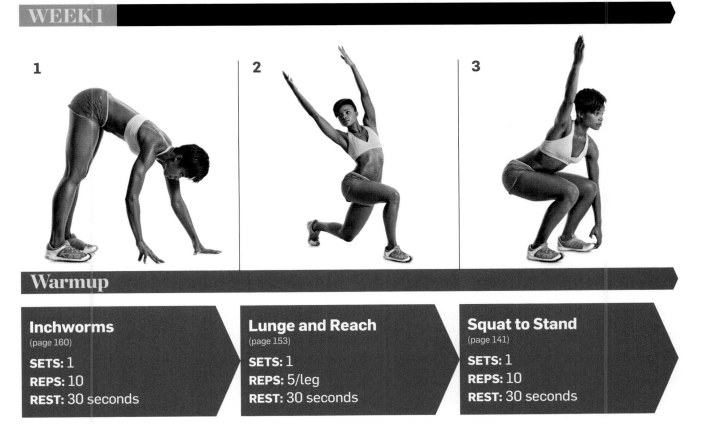

1

2

3

Warmup

Inchworms
(page 160)
SETS: 1
REPS: 10
REST: 30 seconds

Lunge and Reach
(page 153)
SETS: 1
REPS: 5/leg
REST: 30 seconds

Squat to Stand
(page 141)
SETS: 1
REPS: 10
REST: 30 seconds

The Secret Abs Workout

WEEK 1, continued

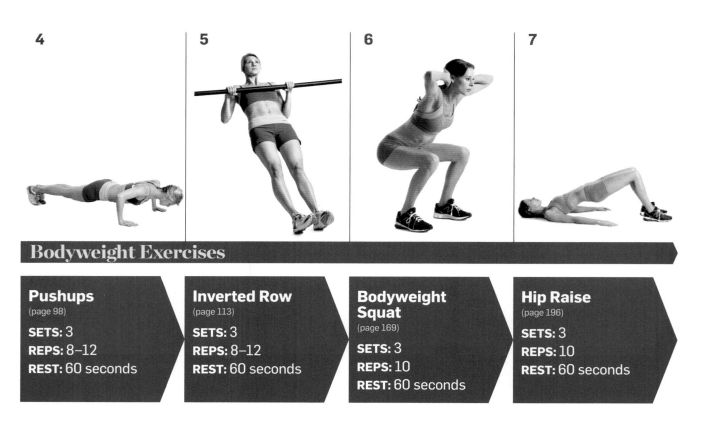

4 **5** **6** **7**

Bodyweight Exercises

Pushups
(page 98)

SETS: 3
REPS: 8–12
REST: 60 seconds

Inverted Row
(page 113)

SETS: 3
REPS: 8–12
REST: 60 seconds

Bodyweight Squat
(page 169)

SETS: 3
REPS: 10
REST: 60 seconds

Hip Raise
(page 196)

SETS: 3
REPS: 10
REST: 60 seconds

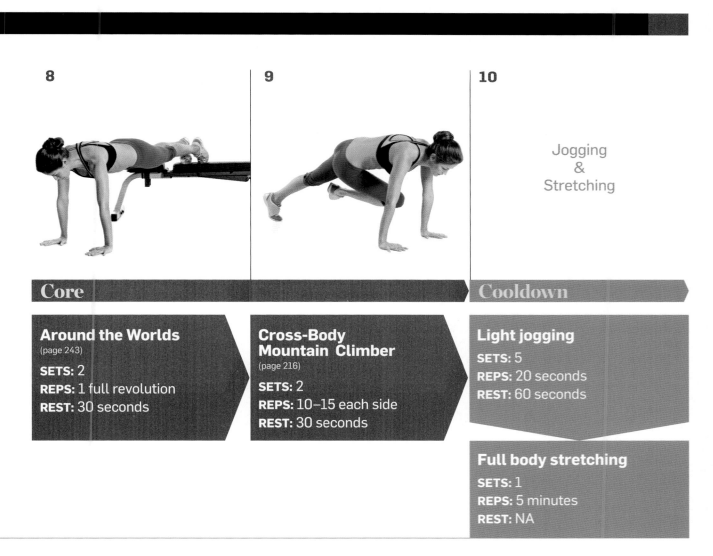

8

9

10

Jogging
&
Stretching

Core

Cooldown

Around the Worlds
(page 243)

SETS: 2
REPS: 1 full revolution
REST: 30 seconds

**Cross-Body
Mountain Climber**
(page 216)

SETS: 2
REPS: 10–15 each side
REST: 30 seconds

Light jogging

SETS: 5
REPS: 20 seconds
REST: 60 seconds

Full body stretching

SETS: 1
REPS: 5 minutes
REST: NA

The Secret Abs Workout

WEEK 2

1

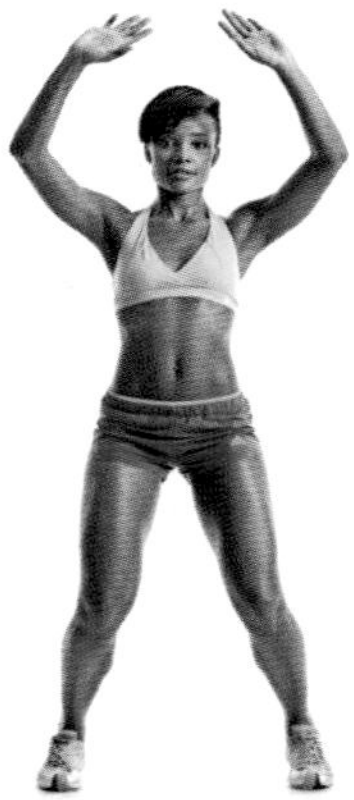

2

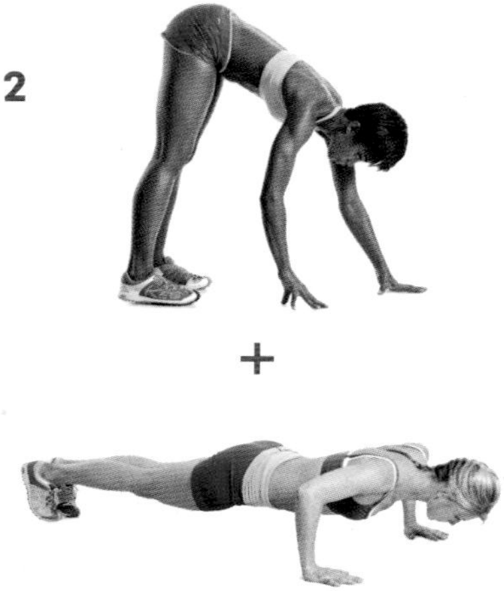

+

3

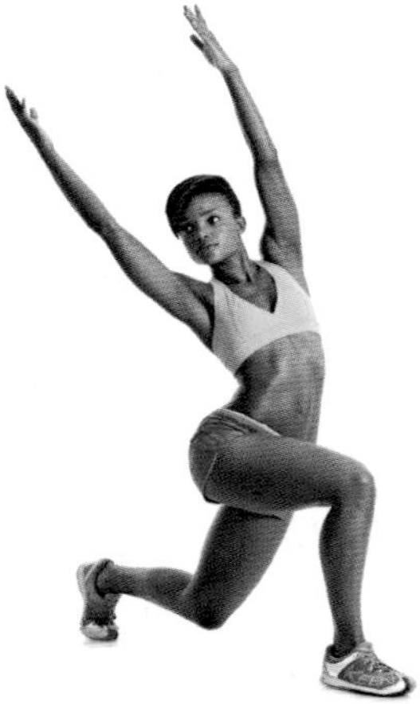

Warmup

Jumping Jack
(page 138)

SETS: 1
REPS: 1–2 minutes, 20
REST: 30 seconds

Inchworm + Pushups
(page 160)   (page 98)

SETS: 1
REPS: 5
REST: 30 seconds

Lunge and Reach
(page 153)

SETS: 1
REPS: 5 each leg
REST: 30 seconds

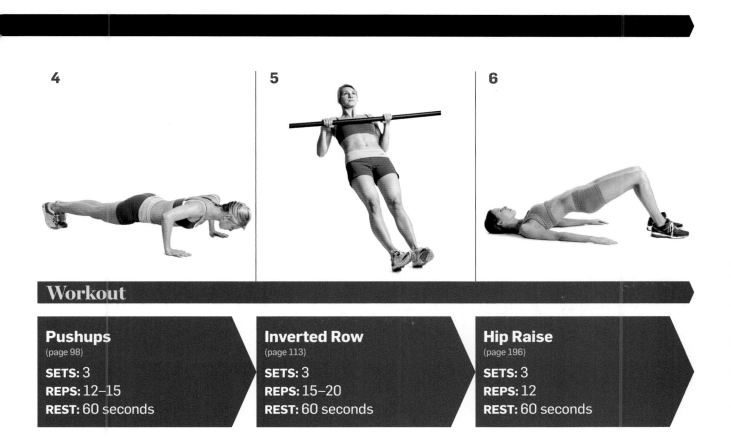

4

5

6

Workout

Pushups
(page 98)

SETS: 3
REPS: 12–15
REST: 60 seconds

Inverted Row
(page 113)

SETS: 3
REPS: 15–20
REST: 60 seconds

Hip Raise
(page 196)

SETS: 3
REPS: 12
REST: 60 seconds

The Secret Abs Workout

WEEK 2, continued

7

8

9

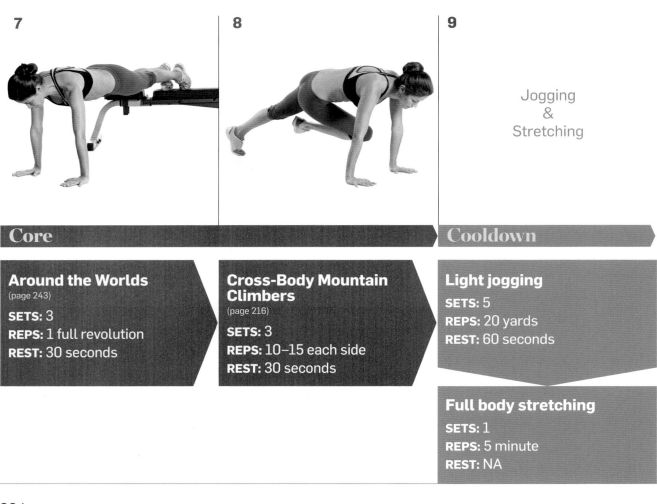

Jogging
&
Stretching

Core

Cooldown

Around the Worlds
(page 243)

SETS: 3
REPS: 1 full revolution
REST: 30 seconds

Cross-Body Mountain Climbers
(page 216)

SETS: 3
REPS: 10–15 each side
REST: 30 seconds

Light jogging

SETS: 5
REPS: 20 yards
REST: 60 seconds

Full body stretching

SETS: 1
REPS: 5 minute
REST: NA

WEEK 3

1   **2**   **3**   **4**

Warmup

Pushups (page 98)	**Inchworm** (page 160)	**Lunge and Reach** (page 153)	**Squat to Stand** (page 141)
SETS: 1	**SETS:** 1	**SETS:** 1	**SETS:** 1
REPS: 15	**REPS:** 10	**REPS:** 6 each leg	**REPS:** 12
REST: 30 seconds	**REST:** 30 seconds	**REST:** 30 seconds	**REST:** 30 seconds

The Secret Abs Workout

WEEK 3, continued

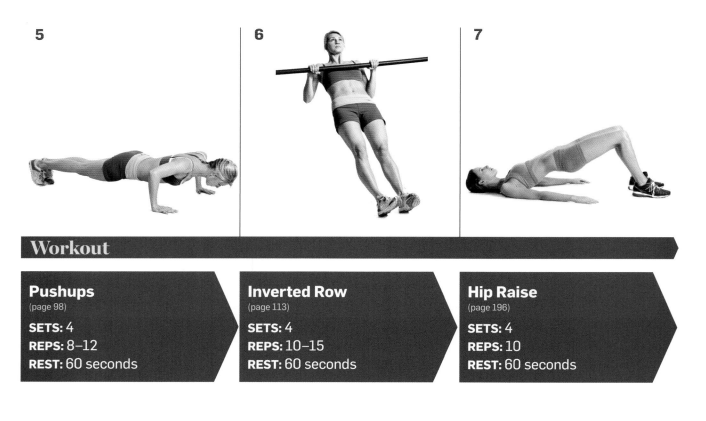

5

6

7

Workout

Pushups
(page 98)

SETS: 4
REPS: 8–12
REST: 60 seconds

Inverted Row
(page 113)

SETS: 4
REPS: 10–15
REST: 60 seconds

Hip Raise
(page 196)

SETS: 4
REPS: 10
REST: 60 seconds

8

9

10

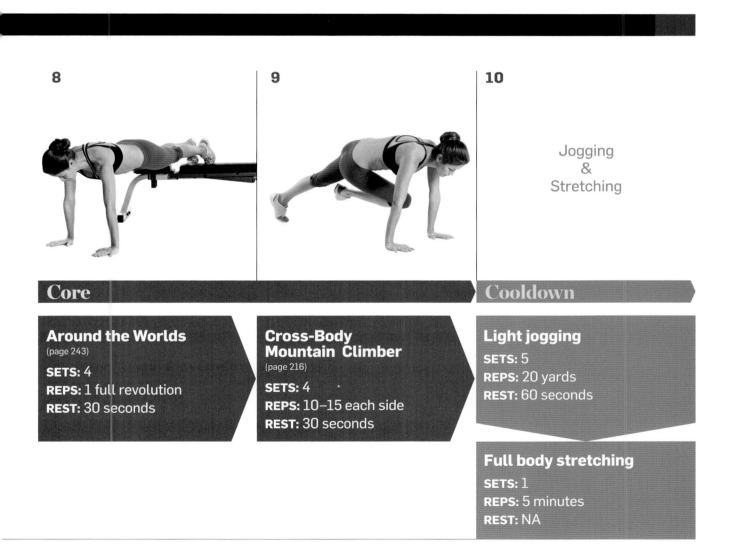

Jogging
&
Stretching

Core

Cooldown

Around the Worlds
(page 243)

SETS: 4
REPS: 1 full revolution
REST: 30 seconds

Cross-Body Mountain Climber
(page 216)

SETS: 4
REPS: 10–15 each side
REST: 30 seconds

Light jogging
SETS: 5
REPS: 20 yards
REST: 60 seconds

Full body stretching
SETS: 1
REPS: 5 minutes
REST: NA

The Secret Abs Workout

WEEK 4

1

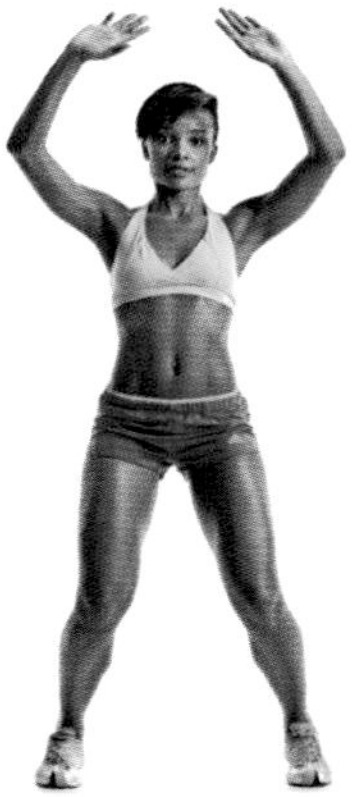

2

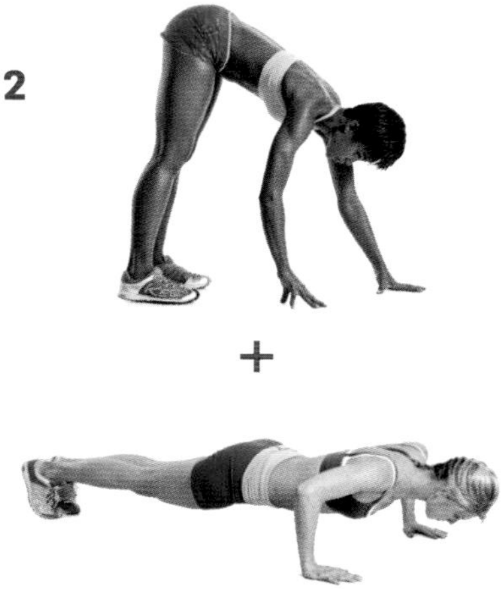

+

3

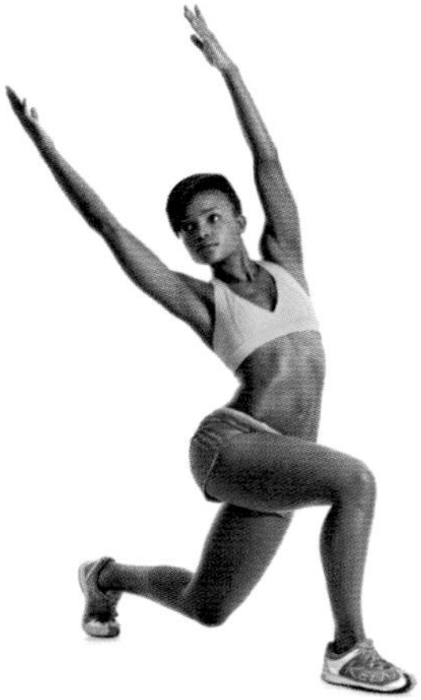

Warmup

Jumping Jack
(page 138)

SETS: 1
REPS: 2–3 minutes, 20
REST: 30 seconds

Inchworm + Pushups
(page 160)   (page 98)

SETS: 1
REPS: 8
REST: 30 seconds

Lunge and Reach
(page 153)

SETS: 1
REPS: 6 each leg
REST: 30 seconds

4

5

6

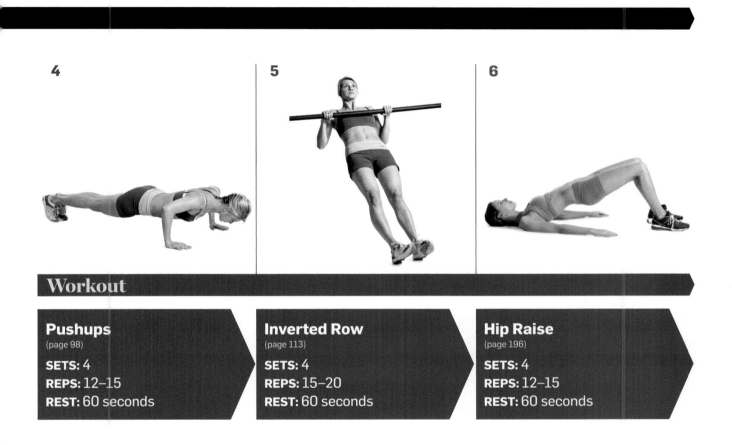

Workout

Pushups (page 98)	**Inverted Row** (page 113)	**Hip Raise** (page 196)
SETS: 4	**SETS:** 4	**SETS:** 4
REPS: 12–15	**REPS:** 15–20	**REPS:** 12–15
REST: 60 seconds	**REST:** 60 seconds	**REST:** 60 seconds

The Secret Abs Workout

WEEK 4, continued

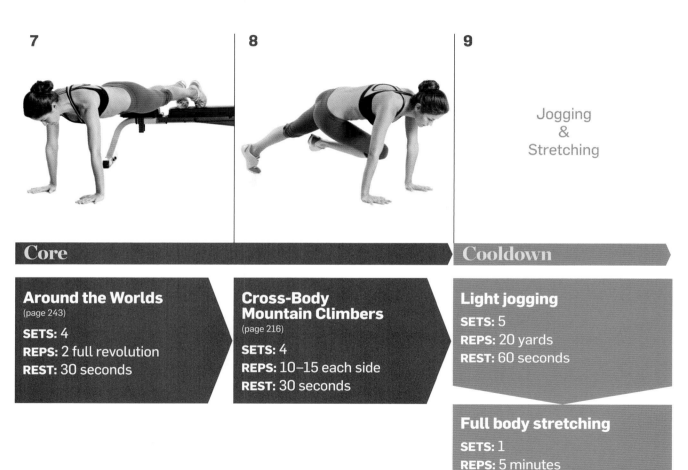

7

8

9

Jogging
&
Stretching

Core

Cooldown

Around the Worlds
(page 243)

SETS: 4
REPS: 2 full revolution
REST: 30 seconds

Cross-Body Mountain Climbers
(page 216)

SETS: 4
REPS: 10–15 each side
REST: 30 seconds

Light jogging

SETS: 5
REPS: 20 yards
REST: 60 seconds

Full body stretching

SETS: 1
REPS: 5 minutes
REST: NA

"Enter every activity
without giving mental recognition
to the possibility of defeat.
Concentrate on your strengths
instead of your weaknesses,
on your powers
instead of your problems."
—Paul J. Meyer

The Travelers Workout [45 minutes]

THE GYM CAN feel like a big waste of time. Whether you're waiting for your equipment or switching from one machine to another, the last thing you need is a crowded facility. That's why going on the road is one of the best opportunities to get a better workout by creating a more efficient plan that requires less setup. This program, developed by BJ Gaddour, CSCS, will guarantee that your next business trip or family vacation won't sabotage your hard work. In fact, you might find yourself in better shape than before you left.

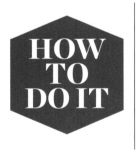

HOW TO DO IT

● Do this workout 3 days a week, resting at least a day between each session. So you might lift weights on Monday, Wednesday, and Friday.

● The workout consists of five groups of three exercises. For each group, perform 1 set of each exercise in the order listed. You will not have a goal number of reps. Instead, do as many reps as you can in 30 seconds and, without resting, move to the next exercise. Once you have completed all exercises in the first group, rest 30 to 60 seconds. That's 1 set. Perform a total of 5 sets of Group 1 and then move on to Group 2. Continue this pattern until you finish all five groups.

● As you improve, you can increase the number of sets you perform.

ABOUT THE EXPERT

BJ Gaddour, CSCS, is an internationally recognized fitness boot camp and metabolic training expert. He is the CEO and fitness director for StreamFIT (streamfit.com), a provider of unlimited streamg follow-along workouts. He is also the co-creator and fitness director for Workout Muse (workoutmuse.com), a company specializing in fitness boot camp music and training systems.

The Travelers Workout

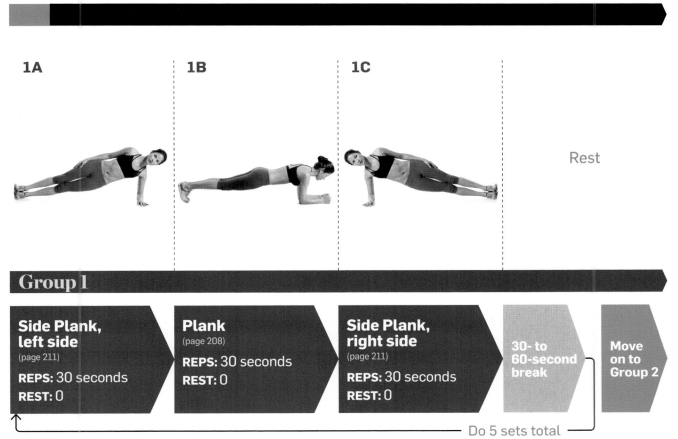

1A **1B** **1C** Rest

Group 1

Side Plank, left side
(page 211)

REPS: 30 seconds
REST: 0

Plank
(page 208)

REPS: 30 seconds
REST: 0

Side Plank, right side
(page 211)

REPS: 30 seconds
REST: 0

30- to 60-second break

Move on to Group 2

Do 5 sets total

The Travelers Workout

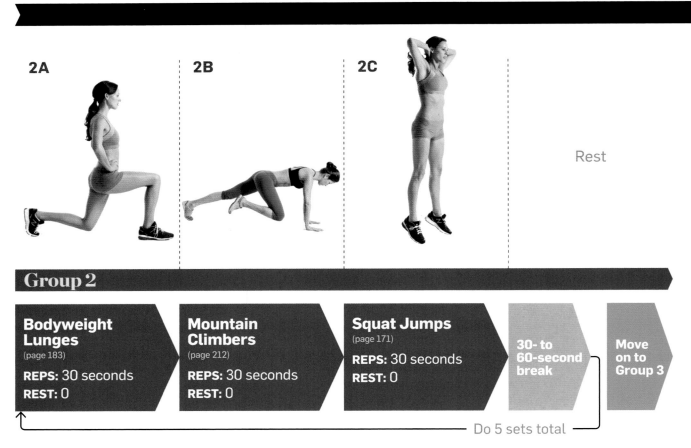

2A　　　**2B**　　　**2C**　　　Rest

Group 2

Bodyweight Lunges
(page 183)

REPS: 30 seconds
REST: 0

Mountain Climbers
(page 212)

REPS: 30 seconds
REST: 0

Squat Jumps
(page 171)

REPS: 30 seconds
REST: 0

30- to 60-second break

Move on to Group 3

Do 5 sets total

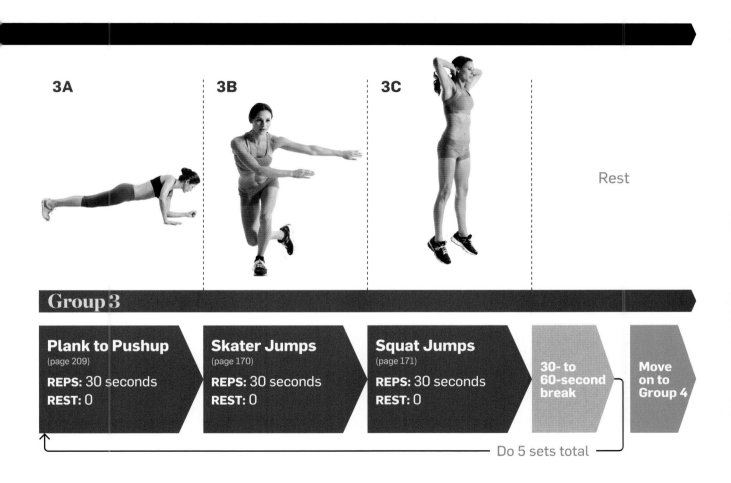

3A

3B

3C

Rest

Group 3

| **Plank to Pushup** (page 209) **REPS:** 30 seconds **REST:** 0 | **Skater Jumps** (page 170) **REPS:** 30 seconds **REST:** 0 | **Squat Jumps** (page 171) **REPS:** 30 seconds **REST:** 0 | **30- to 60-second break** | **Move on to Group 4** |

— Do 5 sets total —

The Travelers Workout

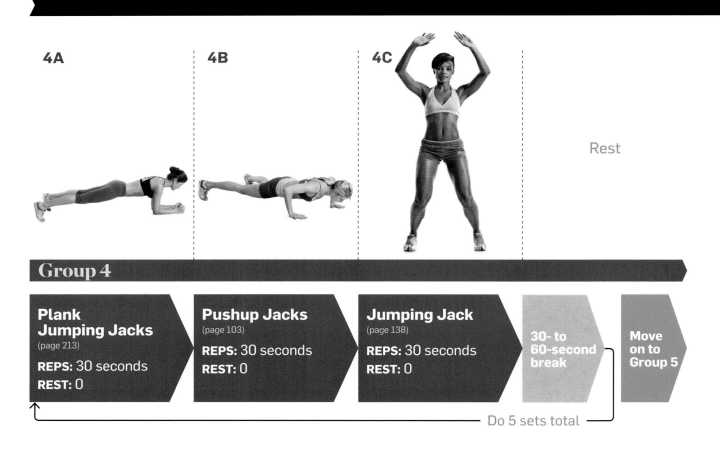

4A

4B

4C

Rest

Group 4

Plank Jumping Jacks
(page 213)
REPS: 30 seconds
REST: 0

Pushup Jacks
(page 103)
REPS: 30 seconds
REST: 0

Jumping Jack
(page 138)
REPS: 30 seconds
REST: 0

30- to 60-second break

Move on to Group 5

— Do 5 sets total —

5A　　　　　　**5B**　　　　　　**5C**

Stationary
Running

Rest

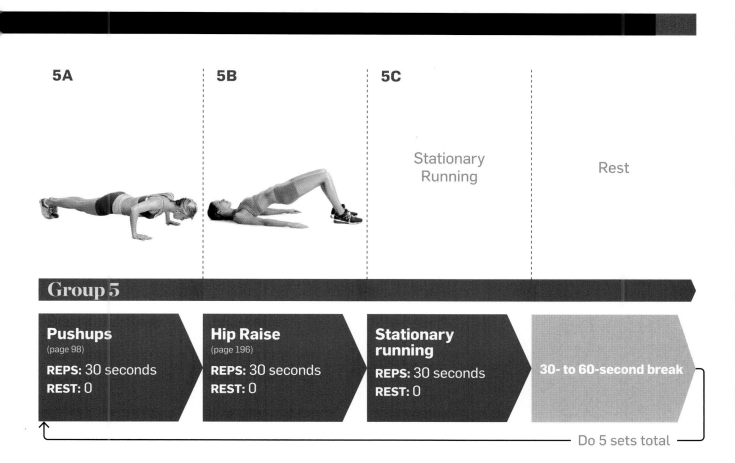

Group 5

| **Pushups**
(page 98)
REPS: 30 seconds
REST: 0 | **Hip Raise**
(page 196)
REPS: 30 seconds
REST: 0 | **Stationary running**
REPS: 30 seconds
REST: 0 | **30- to 60-second break** |

Do 5 sets total

Last-Minute Beach Vacation Workout [45 minutes]

THE BEST BEACH workouts are the ones you can create yourself. This plan will have you ready for bikini season in no time by allowing you to select your favorite exercises. Just follow the template and choose the routine you want to melt pounds and trim inches in 4 weeks.

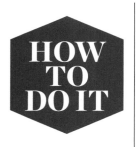

HOW TO DO IT

● Do this workout 3 days a week, resting at least a day between each session. So you might lift weights on Monday, Wednesday, and Friday.

● The workout consists of two groups of three exercises. For each group, select the exercise you want, and perform 1 set of each exercise in the order listed. You will not have a goal number of reps. Instead, do as many reps as you can in 45 seconds, rest 10 seconds, and move to the next exercise. Once you have completed all exercises in the first group, rest 30 to 60 seconds. That's 1 set. Perform a total of 6 sets of Group 1, and then move on to Group 2. Continue this pattern for the second group.

● As you improve, you can increase the number of sets you perform.

3 WAYS TO MAKE YOUR ABS WORK HARDER

1 **Load one side at a time:** Perform asymmetrically loaded exercises like the One-Arm Overhead Press (page 138), squats, or lunges.

2 **Decrease your base of support:** Move from a wide to narrow stance, from a parallel to a staggered or split stance, or from two legs to one leg.

3 **Lengthen your center of gravity:** Perform exercises like squats and lunges while holding the dumbbells overhead instead of at your sides.

Build-Your-Own Dumbbell Complexes

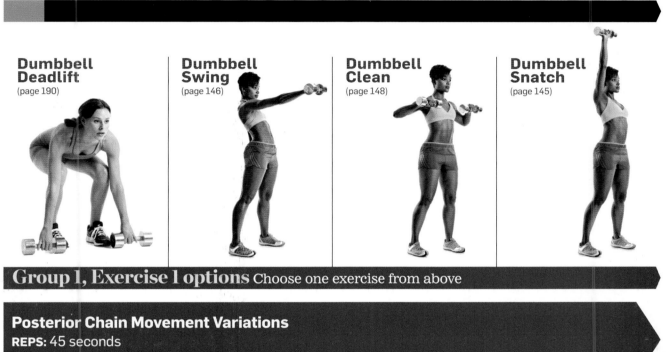

Dumbbell Deadlift (page 190)

Dumbbell Swing (page 146)

Dumbbell Clean (page 148)

Dumbbell Snatch (page 145)

Group 1, Exercise 1 options Choose one exercise from above

Posterior Chain Movement Variations
REPS: 45 seconds
REST: 10 seconds

Build-Your-Own Dumbbell Complexes

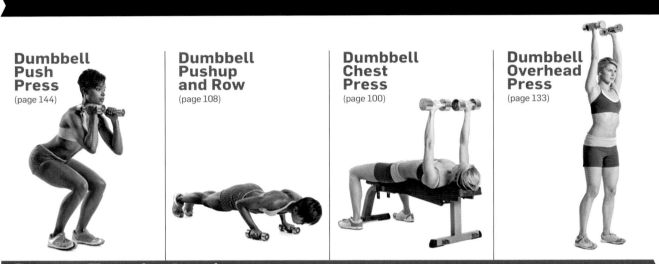

Dumbbell Push Press
(page 144)

Dumbbell Pushup and Row
(page 108)

Dumbbell Chest Press
(page 100)

Dumbbell Overhead Press
(page 133)

Group 1, Exercise 2 options Choose one exercise from above

Pushing Movement
REPS: 45 seconds
REST: 10 seconds

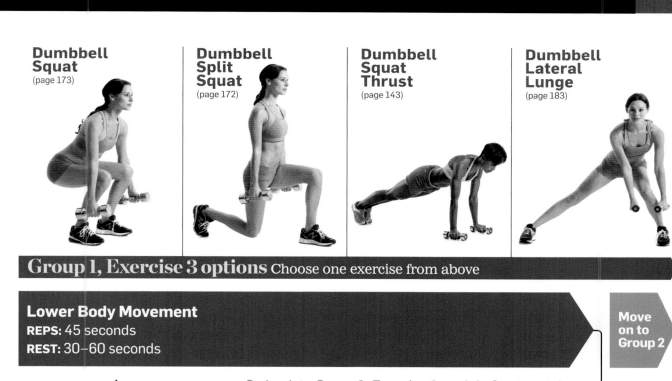

Dumbbell Squat (page 173)

Dumbbell Split Squat (page 172)

Dumbbell Squat Thrust (page 143)

Dumbbell Lateral Lunge (page 183)

Group 1, Exercise 3 options Choose one exercise from above

Lower Body Movement
REPS: 45 seconds
REST: 30–60 seconds

Move on to Group 2

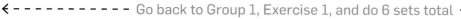

← ‑ ‑ ‑ ‑ ‑ ‑ ‑ ‑ ‑ ‑ ‑ Go back to Group 1, Exercise 1, and do 6 sets total

Build-Your-Own Dumbbell Complexes

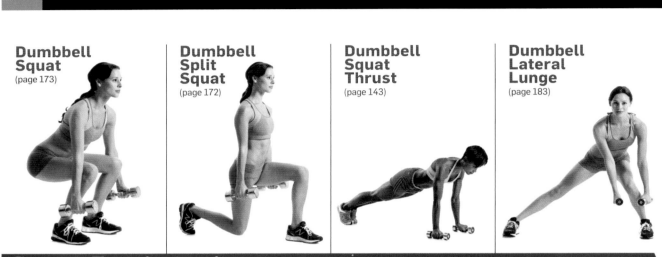

Dumbbell Squat
(page 173)

Dumbbell Split Squat
(page 172)

Dumbbell Squat Thrust
(page 143)

Dumbbell Lateral Lunge
(page 183)

Group 2, Exercise 1 options Choose one exercise from above

Lower Body Movement
REPS: 45 seconds
REST: 10 seconds

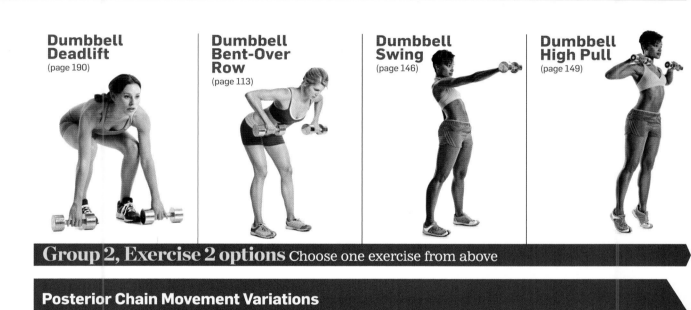

Dumbbell Deadlift
(page 190)

Dumbbell Bent-Over Row
(page 113)

Dumbbell Swing
(page 146)

Dumbbell High Pull
(page 149)

Group 2, Exercise 2 options Choose one exercise from above

Posterior Chain Movement Variations
REPS: 45 seconds
REST: 10 seconds

Build-Your-Own Dumbbell Complexes

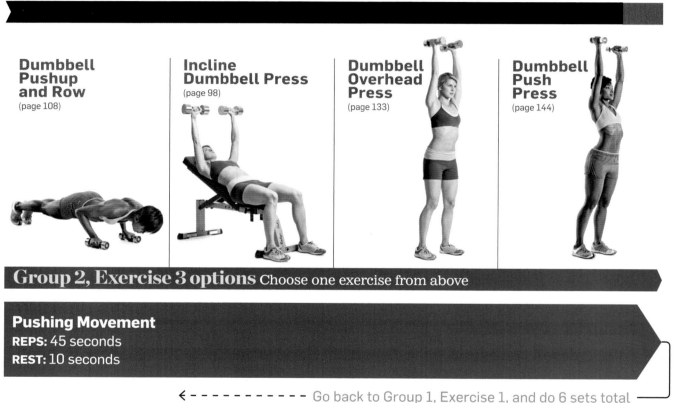

Dumbbell Pushup and Row
(page 108)

Incline Dumbbell Press
(page 98)

Dumbbell Overhead Press
(page 133)

Dumbbell Push Press
(page 144)

Group 2, Exercise 3 options Choose one exercise from above

Pushing Movement
REPS: 45 seconds
REST: 10 seconds

← – – – – – – – – – – – Go back to Group 1, Exercise 1, and do 6 sets total

"If you always put limits
on everything you do, physical or
anything else, it will spread
into your work and into your life.
There are no limits.
There are only plateaus, and you
must not stay there,
you must go beyond them."
—Bruce Lee

Hot Body Workouts

Whether you want to train
like a celeb or have a beach body year-round,
these routines have you covered.

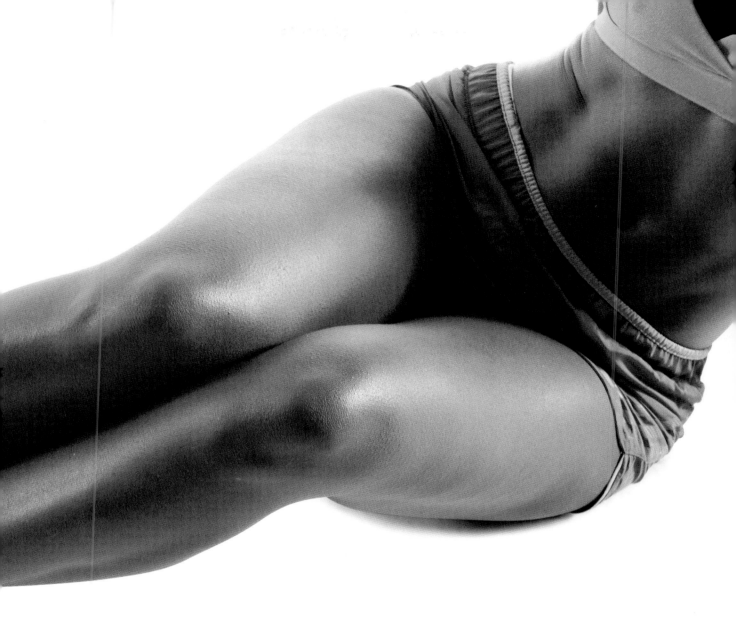

Skinny Jeans Abs Workout [30 minutes]

FORGET FITTING INTO your old pair of jeans. Save up because you're going to need a new wardrobe when you're finished with this 6-week plan. Created by Nick Tumminuteello, founder of Performance University, this workout was created to help you burn more calories and target your abs. You'll outsmart the fat on your body and have the tight, toned look that once seemed impossible.

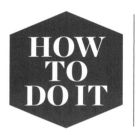

HOW TO DO IT

● Do each weight workout (Workout A, Workout B, Workout C) once a week, resting for at least a day after each session. So you might do Workout A on Monday, Workout B on Wednesday, and Workout C on Friday.

● When you see a number with a letter next to it (such as 1A, 1B), perform them back-to-back without any rest. After you complete the second exercise in the pairing, rest for 60 seconds, and repeat. Once you finish all sets in each group, then move on.

● For accelerated fat loss, add 20 minutes of the cardio of your choice at the end of the workout.

ABOUT THE EXPERT

Nick Tumminuteello is the founder of Performance University, which focuses on training and educating fitness professionals, exercise enthusiasts, and athletes. He has produced educational fitness DVDs and appeared in multiple publications as a fitness expert. You can learn more about him at nicktumminuteello.com.

Skinny Jeans Abs Workout

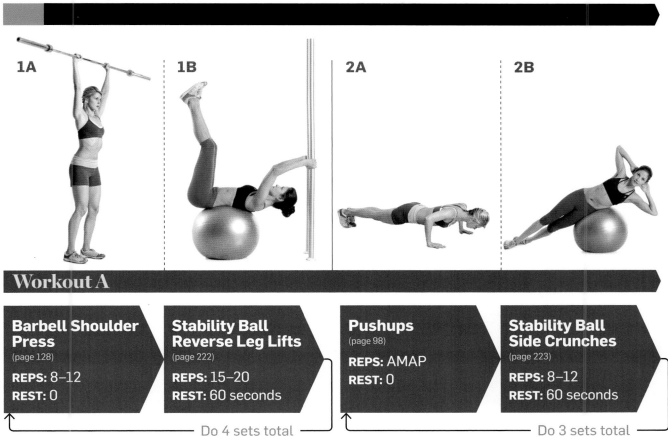

1A

1B

2A

2B

Workout A

Barbell Shoulder Press
(page 128)
REPS: 8–12
REST: 0

Stability Ball Reverse Leg Lifts
(page 222)
REPS: 15–20
REST: 60 seconds

— Do 4 sets total —

Pushups
(page 98)
REPS: AMAP
REST: 0

Stability Ball Side Crunches
(page 223)
REPS: 8–12
REST: 60 seconds

— Do 3 sets total —

Skinny Jeans Abs Workout

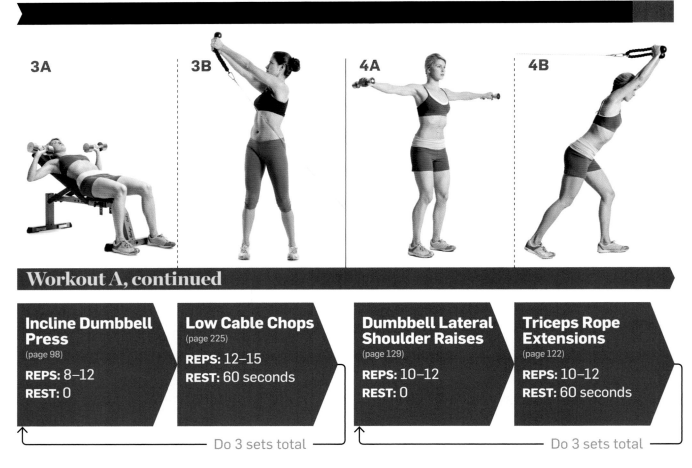

3A   **3B**   **4A**   **4B**

Workout A, continued

Incline Dumbbell Press
(page 98)
REPS: 8–12
REST: 0

Low Cable Chops
(page 225)
REPS: 12–15
REST: 60 seconds

Do 3 sets total

Dumbbell Lateral Shoulder Raises
(page 129)
REPS: 10–12
REST: 0

Triceps Rope Extensions
(page 122)
REPS: 10–12
REST: 60 seconds

Do 3 sets total

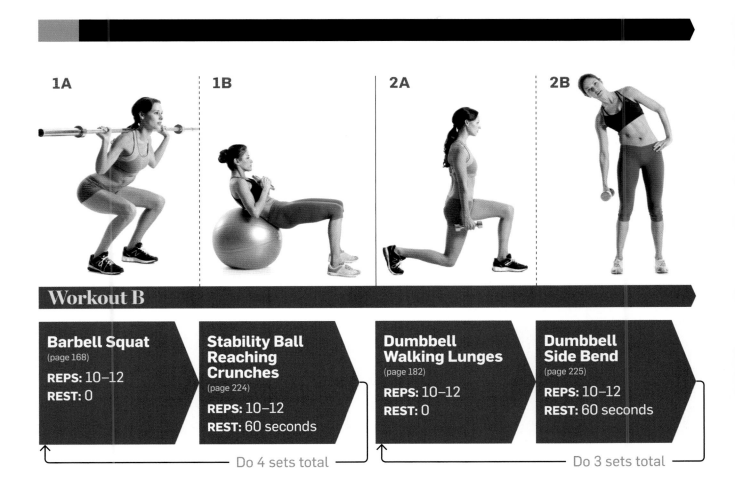

1A

1B

2A

2B

Workout B

Barbell Squat
(page 168)

REPS: 10–12
REST: 0

Stability Ball Reaching Crunches
(page 224)

REPS: 10–12
REST: 60 seconds

— Do 4 sets total —

Dumbbell Walking Lunges
(page 182)

REPS: 10–12
REST: 0

Dumbbell Side Bend
(page 225)

REPS: 10–12
REST: 60 seconds

— Do 3 sets total —

Skinny Jeans Abs Workout

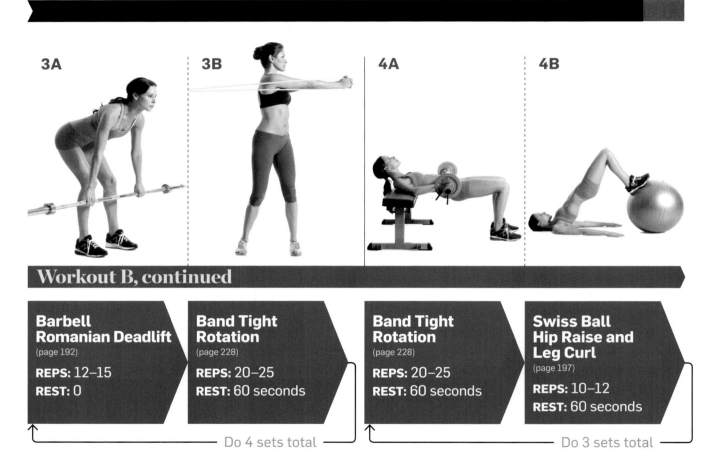

3A

3B

4A

4B

Workout B, continued

Barbell Romanian Deadlift
(page 192)

REPS: 12–15
REST: 0

Band Tight Rotation
(page 228)

REPS: 20–25
REST: 60 seconds

Do 4 sets total

Band Tight Rotation
(page 228)

REPS: 20–25
REST: 60 seconds

Swiss Ball Hip Raise and Leg Curl
(page 197)

REPS: 10–12
REST: 60 seconds

Do 3 sets total

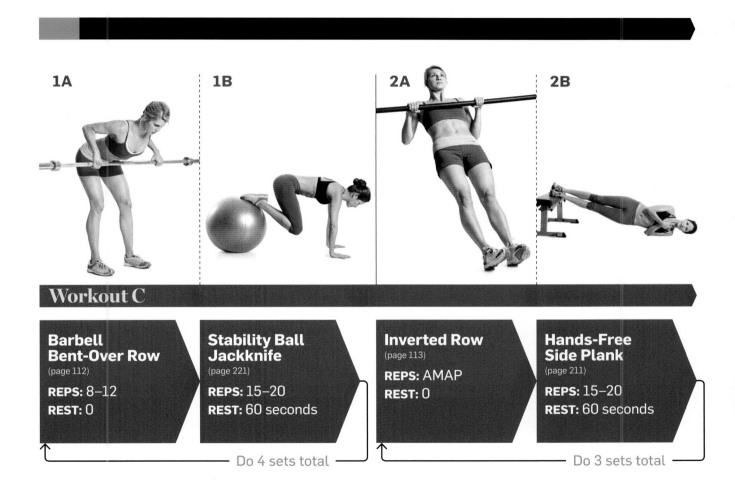

1A

1B

2A

2B

Workout C

**Barbell
Bent-Over Row**
(page 112)

REPS: 8–12
REST: 0

**Stability Ball
Jackknife**
(page 221)

REPS: 15–20
REST: 60 seconds

Do 4 sets total

Inverted Row
(page 113)

REPS: AMAP
REST: 0

**Hands-Free
Side Plank**
(page 211)

REPS: 15–20
REST: 60 seconds

Do 3 sets total

Skinny Jeans Abs Workout

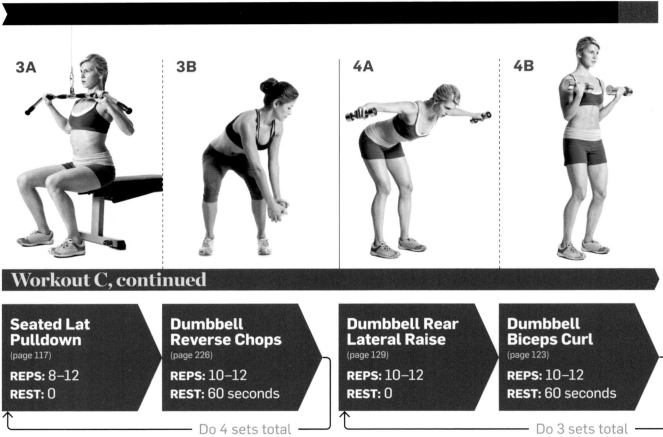

3A

3B

4A

4B

Workout C, continued

Seated Lat Pulldown
(page 117)

REPS: 8–12
REST: 0

Dumbbell Reverse Chops
(page 226)

REPS: 10–12
REST: 60 seconds

Do 4 sets total

Dumbbell Rear Lateral Raise
(page 129)

REPS: 10–12
REST: 0

Dumbbell Biceps Curl
(page 123)

REPS: 10–12
REST: 60 seconds

Do 3 sets total

"No matter who you are,
no matter what you do,
you absolutely, positively
do have the power to change."
—Bill Phillips

The Tight Tush Workout [20 minutes]

YOUR ABS AREN'T the only body part you might want to improve. Take a poll of a thousand women on what else they want to improve, and "butt" will always make the top three (trust us, we've done the research). The results should come as no surprise. After all, few body parts are more important to making you look great in a pair of jeans or an evening gown. That's why this workout, designed by Bret Contreras, CSCS, was developed with you in minuted. Next time you take a body survey, your booty (and your abs, shoulders, and thighs) will be the last concern on your minuted.

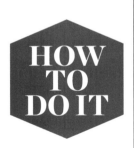

HOW TO DO IT

● Perform this workout three times a week. Do each workout (Workout A, Workout B, Workout C) once a week, resting for at least a day after each session. So you might do Workout A on Monday, Workout B on Wednesday, and Workout C on Friday. All of the exercises are performed as straight sets. That is, do 1 set of the exercises, rest for the prescribed amount of time, and then follow with another set. Finish each set of exercises before moving on to the next.

● If you want to burn additional calories, feel free to add your preferred form of cardio at the end of each session.

ABOUT THE EXPERT

Bret Contreras received a master's degree from Arizona State University and CSCS certification from the National Strength and Conditioning Association. He is currently studying to receive his doctorate at the Sport and Recreation Institute of New Zealand (SPRINZ) at AUT University in Auckland, New Zealand, and maintains a popular blog at bretcontreras.com.

The Tight Tush Workout

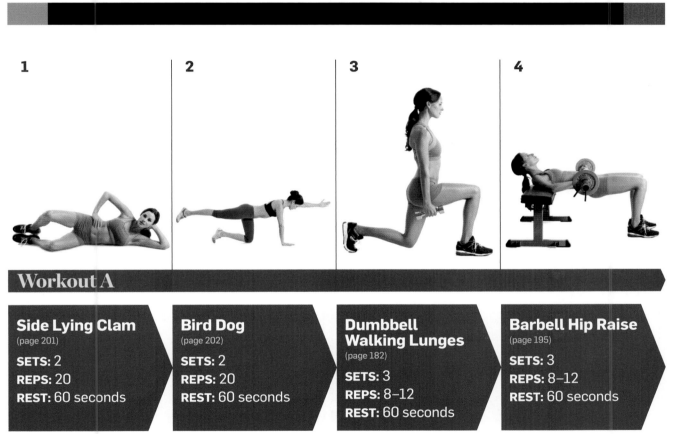

1   **2**   **3**   **4**

Workout A

Side Lying Clam
(page 201)

SETS: 2
REPS: 20
REST: 60 seconds

Bird Dog
(page 202)

SETS: 2
REPS: 20
REST: 60 seconds

Dumbbell Walking Lunges
(page 182)

SETS: 3
REPS: 8–12
REST: 60 seconds

Barbell Hip Raise
(page 195)

SETS: 3
REPS: 8–12
REST: 60 seconds

The Tight Tush Workout

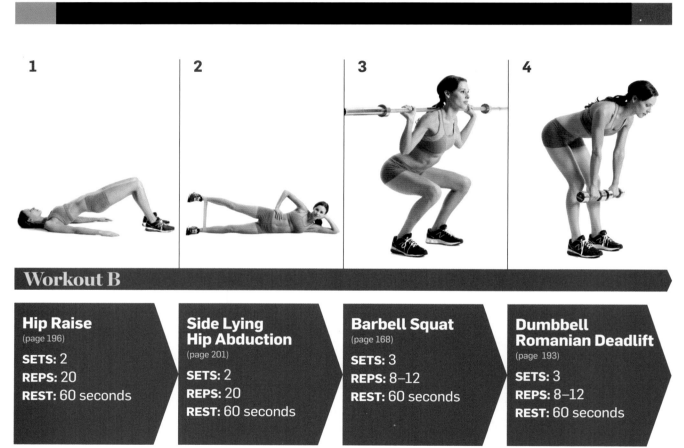

1 **2** **3** **4**

Workout B

Hip Raise
(page 196)

SETS: 2
REPS: 20
REST: 60 seconds

Side Lying Hip Abduction
(page 201)

SETS: 2
REPS: 20
REST: 60 seconds

Barbell Squat
(page 168)

SETS: 3
REPS: 8–12
REST: 60 seconds

Dumbbell Romanian Deadlift
(page 193)

SETS: 3
REPS: 8–12
REST: 60 seconds

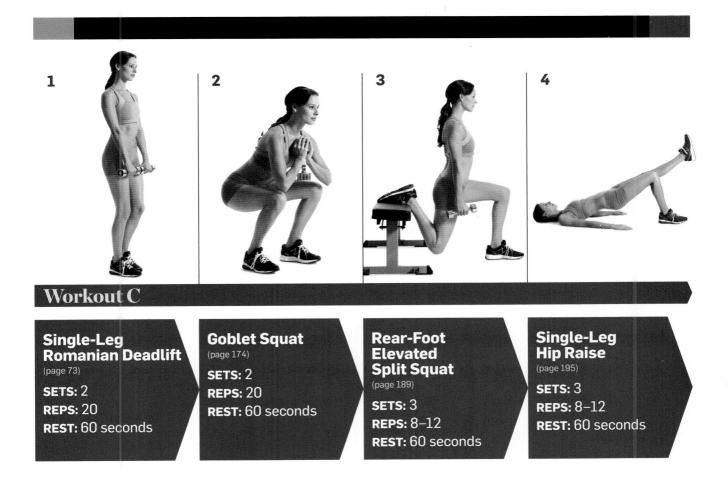

Workout C

1 **Single-Leg Romanian Deadlift**
(page 73)
SETS: 2
REPS: 20
REST: 60 seconds

2 **Goblet Squat**
(page 174)
SETS: 2
REPS: 20
REST: 60 seconds

3 **Rear-Foot Elevated Split Squat**
(page 189)
SETS: 3
REPS: 8–12
REST: 60 seconds

4 **Single-Leg Hip Raise**
(page 195)
SETS: 3
REPS: 8–12
REST: 60 seconds

The Hollywood Workout [60 minutes]

JENNIFER GARNER. Jessica Biel. Poppy Montgomery. Reese Witherspoon. What do all of these women have in common? Valerie Waters. Considered the ultimate Hollywood trainer, Val knows how to transform people—including you— into the best shape of their life. While your lifestyle might differ from a celeb's, your goals are similar: You want to be lean, sexy, and strong but achieve that in the shortest time possible. This workout is designed for just that purpose and to have you looking red-carpet ready in just 4 weeks!

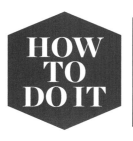

HOW TO DO IT

● Perform this workout three times a week. For instance, you could do this on Monday, Wednesday, and Friday.

● Each workout consists of three circuits. Perform 1 set of all of the exercises in the first circuit, resting 30 seconds between each move. Once you have finished all exercises in the circuit, repeat the process. After you complete all sets in the circuit, then you can move on to the next group of exercises.

ABOUT THE EXPERT

Valerie Waters is one of Hollywood's most sought-after trainers. She is the creator of the Red Carpet Ready program, where you can experience her fitness and diet tips, and learn all of her body transformation secrets. She also created the Valslide. Visit redcarpetready.com, Valeriewaters.com, or valslide.com for more information.

The Hollywood Workout

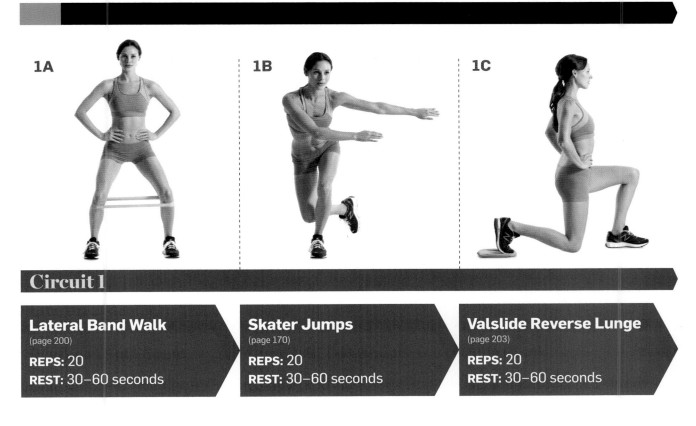

1A **1B** **1C**

Circuit 1

Lateral Band Walk
(page 200)
REPS: 20
REST: 30–60 seconds

Skater Jumps
(page 170)
REPS: 20
REST: 30–60 seconds

Valslide Reverse Lunge
(page 203)
REPS: 20
REST: 30–60 seconds

The Hollywood Workout

1D **1E** **1F**

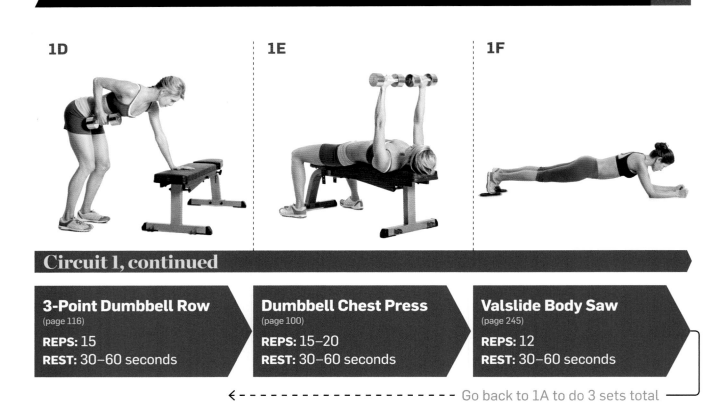

Circuit 1, continued

3-Point Dumbbell Row
(page 116)

REPS: 15
REST: 30–60 seconds

Dumbbell Chest Press
(page 100)

REPS: 15–20
REST: 30–60 seconds

Valslide Body Saw
(page 245)

REPS: 12
REST: 30–60 seconds

← ------------------------------------ Go back to 1A to do 3 sets total

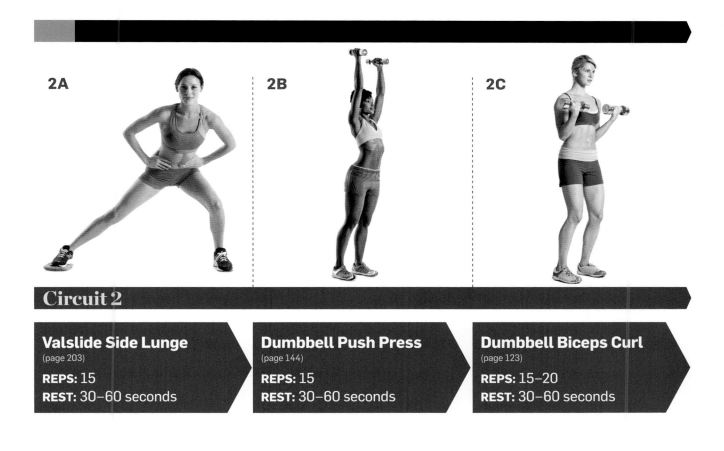

2A

2B

2C

Circuit 2

Valslide Side Lunge
(page 203)
REPS: 15
REST: 30–60 seconds

Dumbbell Push Press
(page 144)
REPS: 15
REST: 30–60 seconds

Dumbbell Biceps Curl
(page 123)
REPS: 15–20
REST: 30–60 seconds

The Hollywood Workout

2D

2E

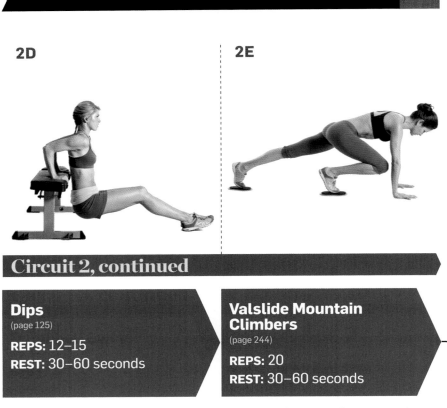

Circuit 2, continued

Dips
(page 125)

REPS: 12–15
REST: 30–60 seconds

Valslide Mountain Climbers
(page 244)

REPS: 20
REST: 30–60 seconds

← – – – – – – – – – – – Go back to 2A to do 3 sets total

3A **3B** **3C** **3D**

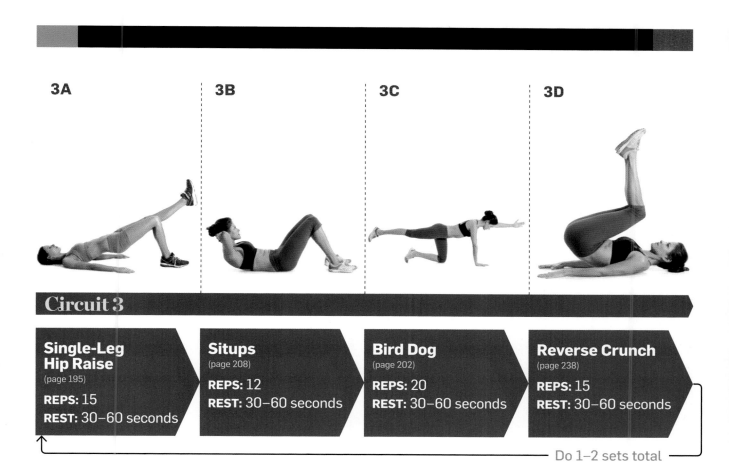

Circuit 3

Single-Leg Hip Raise
(page 195)
REPS: 15
REST: 30–60 seconds

Situps
(page 208)
REPS: 12
REST: 30–60 seconds

Bird Dog
(page 202)
REPS: 20
REST: 30–60 seconds

Reverse Crunch
(page 238)
REPS: 15
REST: 30–60 seconds

Do 1–2 sets total

The Look-Hot-on-Top Workout [10–15 minutes]

IF YOU WANT a tight upper body that would make even Rihanna jealous, you need something different than crunches or situps. In fact, you require exercises that have never been seen before. This workout by Tony Gentilcore, CSCS, might be created by a man, but it's designed to make you a sexier woman. Try out these unique exercises, and then try to tell us we're wrong.

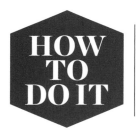

HOW TO DO IT

● Add this exercise routine twice a week on scheduled nonworkout days. That is, if you normally exercise Monday, Wednesday, and Friday, you should do this workout on Tuesday and Thursday. Perform these exercises in circuit fashion with as little rest as possible between exercises. That is, do 1 set of the first exercise and then move to the next exercise as soon as possible. Continue this process until you complete 1 set of all four exercises. That's one round. Rest for 2 minutes, and then perform an additional three rounds.

ABOUT THE EXPERT

Tony Gentilcore is a Certified Strength and Conditioning Specialist through the National Strength and Conditioning Association. Tony is also one of the co-founders of Cressey Performance, one of the premiere strength and conditioning facilities in the country, located just outside of Boston, Massachusetts. For more information, check out his Web site at tonygentilcore.com.

The Look-Hot-on-Top Workout

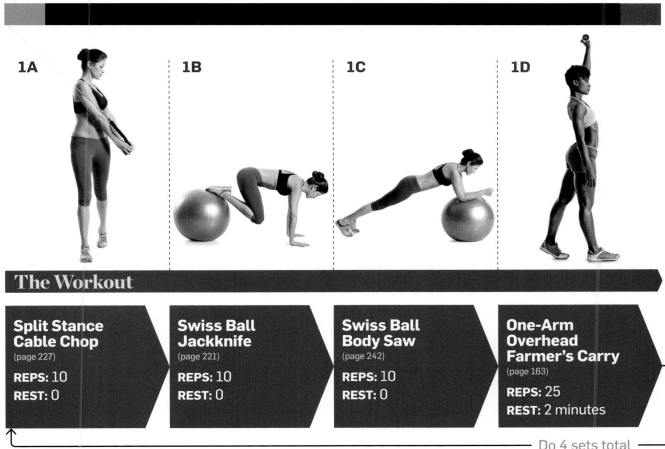

1A **1B** **1C** **1D**

The Workout

Split Stance Cable Chop
(page 227)

REPS: 10
REST: 0

Swiss Ball Jackknife
(page 221)

REPS: 10
REST: 0

Swiss Ball Body Saw
(page 242)

REPS: 10
REST: 0

One-Arm Overhead Farmer's Carry
(page 163)

REPS: 25
REST: 2 minutes

Do 4 sets total

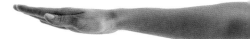

Abs and Your Hormones

Defy your genetics and the aging process to look your best at any age.

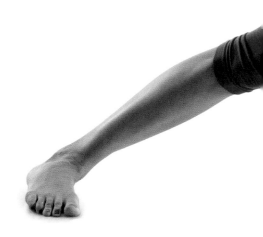

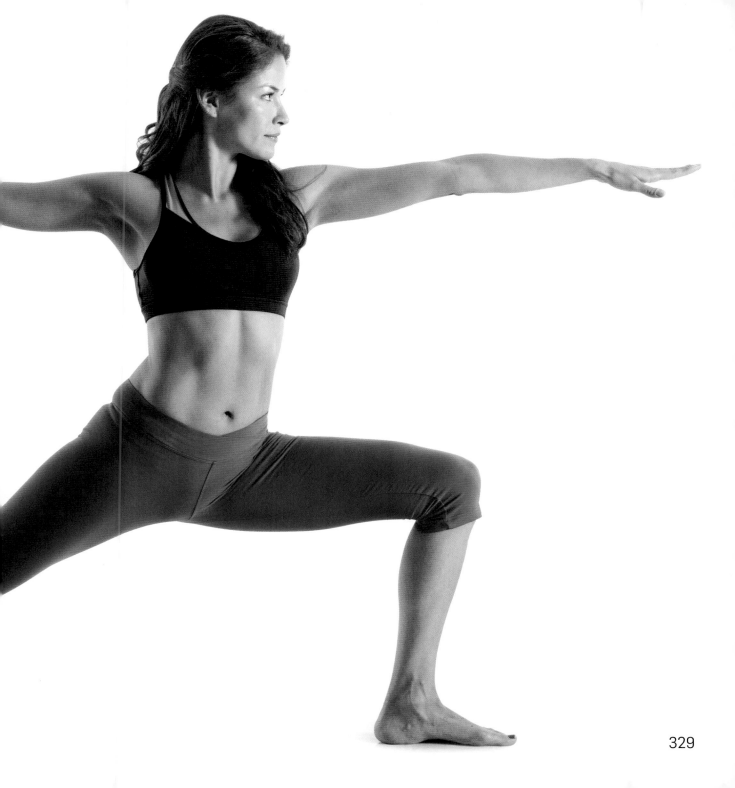

The Bloat-Banishing Workout [30 minutes]

Water weight. That time of month. The bloat. No matter what you call it, it's always a drag when your body is looking and feeling puffy. You can fight it with this workout, designed by personal trainer Anna Renderer, which will strengthen all of the muscles in your core. The results: Your abdominuteal wall will tighten and your entire midsecondstion will be pulled inward. So no matter how your body reacts to your hormones, you'll still have the thinner, sleeker look you want.

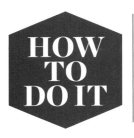

HOW TO DO IT

● Do this workout 3 days a week, resting at least a day between each session. So you might lift weights on Monday, Wednesday, and Friday.

● The workout consists of 10 exercises that will be performed as a circuit. That is, perform 1 set of each exercise in the order listed, resting 30 seconds between each move. Once you have completed all 10, rest for 60 seconds and then repeat the circuit two more times.

ABOUT THE EXPERT

Anna Renderer, MS, is a certified personal trainer with the American Council on Exercise, a certified youth fitness specialist with the International Youth and Conditioning Association, and a performance expert for Gatorade's "Inside Edge." Anna is the founder of SHED IT NOW fitness, specializing in weight loss and optimal performance, Sheditnow.com. She is also the co-founder and CEO of KFIT Health, creating stronger and healthier kids.

The Bloat-Banishing Workout

1A **1B** **1C** **1D**

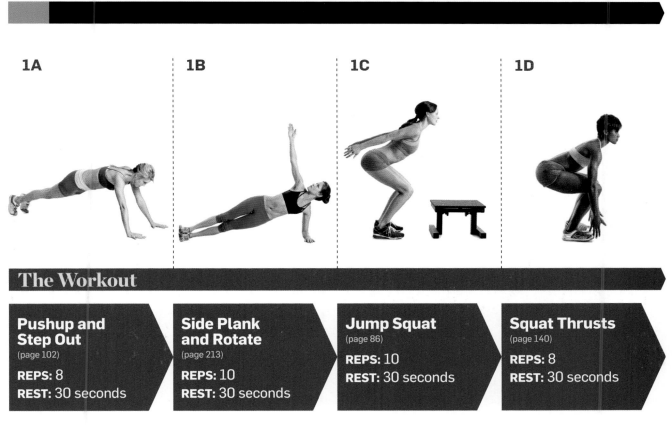

The Workout

Pushup and Step Out
(page 102)

REPS: 8
REST: 30 seconds

Side Plank and Rotate
(page 213)

REPS: 10
REST: 30 seconds

Jump Squat
(page 86)

REPS: 10
REST: 30 seconds

Squat Thrusts
(page 140)

REPS: 8
REST: 30 seconds

The Bloat-Banishing Workout

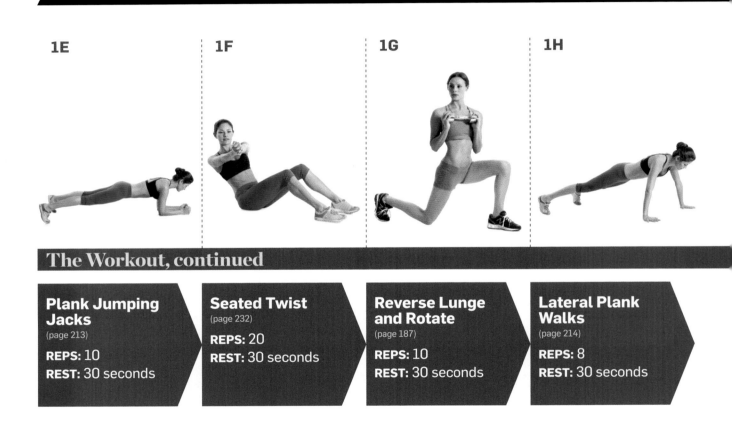

1E

1F

1G

1H

The Workout, continued

Plank Jumping Jacks
(page 213)

REPS: 10
REST: 30 seconds

Seated Twist
(page 232)

REPS: 20
REST: 30 seconds

Reverse Lunge and Rotate
(page 187)

REPS: 10
REST: 30 seconds

Lateral Plank Walks
(page 214)

REPS: 8
REST: 30 seconds

1I

1J

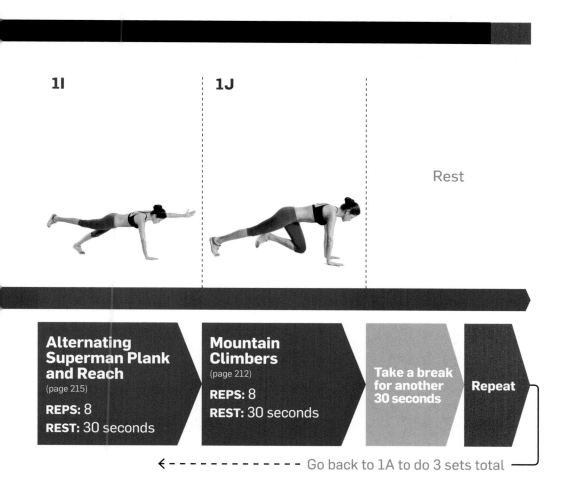

Rest

Alternating Superman Plank and Reach
(page 215)

REPS: 8
REST: 30 seconds

Mountain Climbers
(page 212)

REPS: 8
REST: 30 seconds

Take a break for another 30 seconds

Repeat

← – – – – – – – – – – – – – Go back to 1A to do 3 sets total –

Manage Menopause Workout [60 minutes]

AS YOU AGE, your body naturally loses muscle, and its ability to burn calories is decreased. The good news: Research has shown that the right combination of resistance training movements is the key to discovering your own weight loss fountain of youth. To offset the aging process, you'll combine metabolic boosters that will keep you burning calories 24 hours a day and strength training movements that will be easy on your joints but hard on your fat cells. Once you start this workout, your body—and the aging process—won't stand a chance.

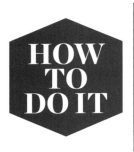

HOW TO DO IT

■ Perform this workout 3 days a week on nonconsecutive days (Monday, Wednesday, and Friday for example). The program consists of six 7-minute circuits. We'll call the circuits groups. Do all of the exercises and sets within a group before moving on to the next circuit. When you see a number with a letter next to it (such as 1A, 1B), that means the exercise is done as part of the group of exercises. Do 1 set of the first exercise, rest as directed, and then move on to the next exercise in the group. Repeat this process until you complete all of your sets for each exercise. Then, rest 1 to 3 minutes and move on to the next group. Based on your level of fitness, try to complete as many sets as possible in each group within 7 minutes.

ABOUT THE EXPERT

Ed Scow, NSCA-CPT, is a fitness and nutrition expert based in Lincoln, Nebraska. He is an expert at creating quick workouts for people lacking free time to devote to exercise, specifically busy parents, as well as cominuteg up with unique ways to rid your life of unhealthy eating habits by focusing solely on the positive. You can learn more about his workouts and nutrition advice at TheFitDadSays.com.

Manage Menopause Workout

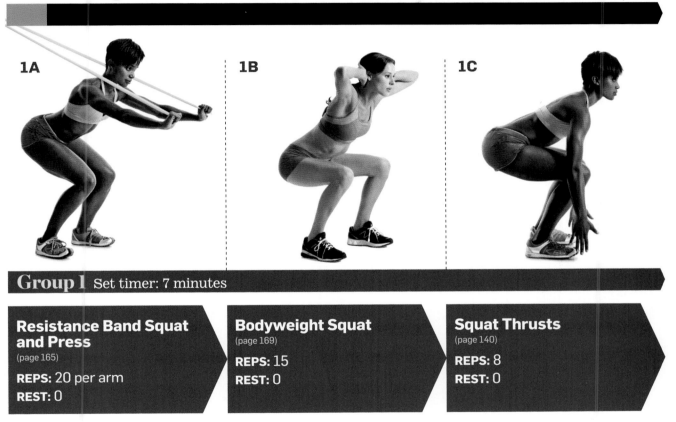

1A   **1B**   **1C**

Group 1 Set timer: 7 minutes

Resistance Band Squat and Press
(page 165)

REPS: 20 per arm
REST: 0

Bodyweight Squat
(page 169)

REPS: 15
REST: 0

Squat Thrusts
(page 140)

REPS: 8
REST: 0

Manage Menopause Workout

1D

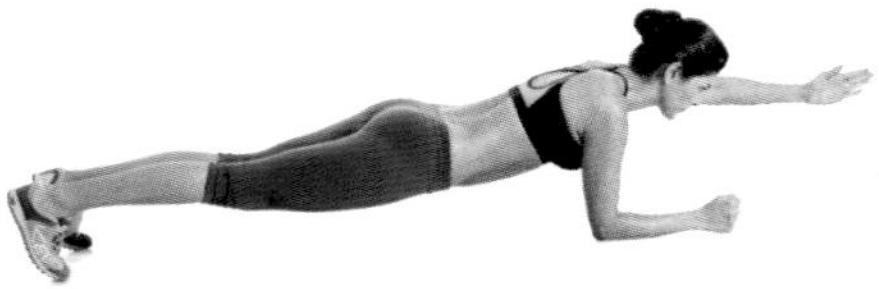

Rest

Circuit 2, continued

Plank with Arm Extension
(page 214)

REPS: 8
REST: 0

Go back to 1A and do as many sets as possible

Rest for 1–3 minutes

Go to Group 2 on the next page

2A   **2B**   **2C**

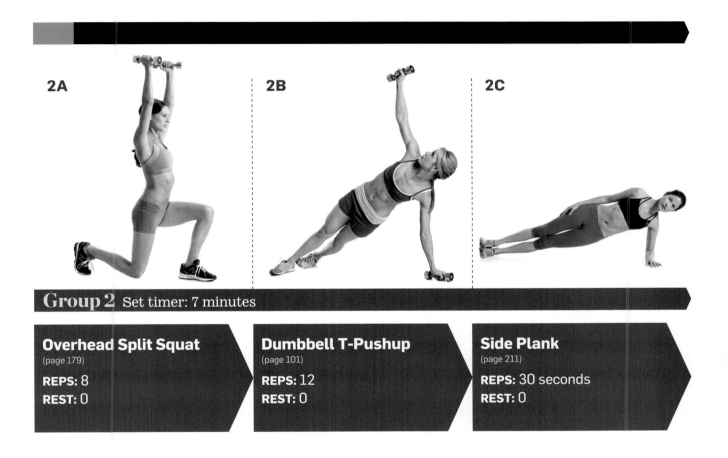

Group 2   Set timer: 7 minutes

Overhead Split Squat
(page 179)

REPS: 8
REST: 0

Dumbbell T-Pushup
(page 101)

REPS: 12
REST: 0

Side Plank
(page 211)

REPS: 30 seconds
REST: 0

Manage Menopause Workout

2D

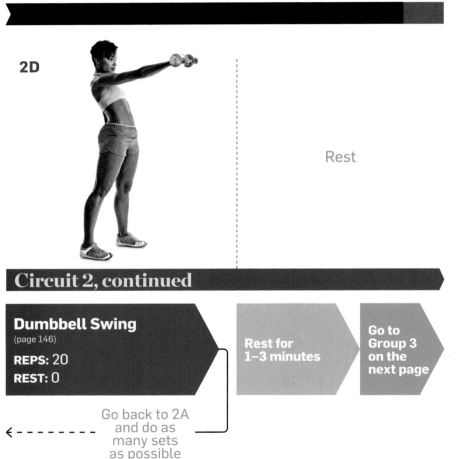

Rest

Circuit 2, continued

Dumbbell Swing
(page 146)

REPS: 20
REST: 0

Rest for
1–3 minutes

Go to
Group 3
on the
next page

Go back to 2A
and do as
many sets
as possible

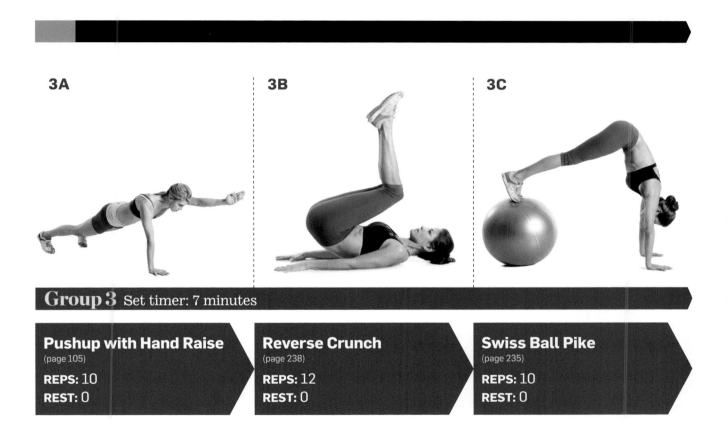

3A

3B

3C

Group 3 Set timer: 7 minutes

Pushup with Hand Raise
(page 105)
REPS: 10
REST: 0

Reverse Crunch
(page 238)
REPS: 12
REST: 0

Swiss Ball Pike
(page 235)
REPS: 10
REST: 0

Manage Menopause Workout

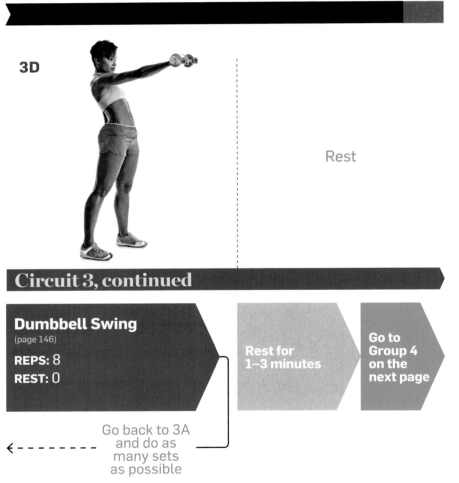

3D

Rest

Circuit 3, continued

Dumbbell Swing
(page 146)

REPS: 8
REST: 0

Rest for 1–3 minutes

Go to Group 4 on the next page

Go back to 3A and do as many sets as possible

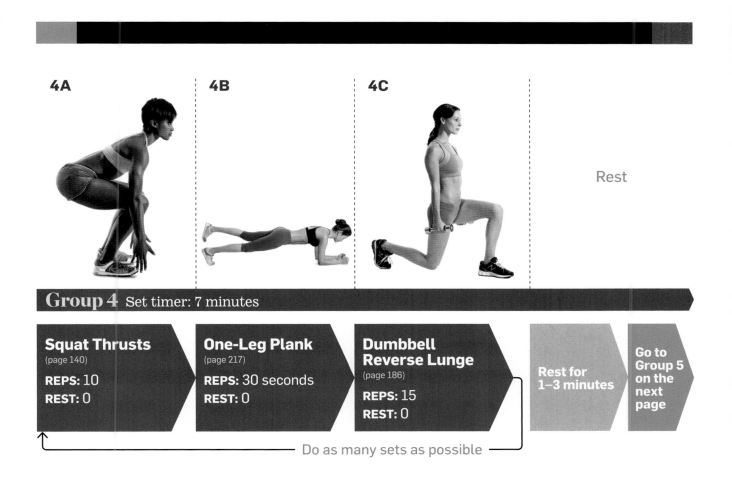

4A

4B

4C

Rest

Group 4 Set timer: 7 minutes

Squat Thrusts
(page 140)

REPS: 10
REST: 0

One-Leg Plank
(page 217)

REPS: 30 seconds
REST: 0

Dumbbell Reverse Lunge
(page 186)

REPS: 15
REST: 0

Rest for 1–3 minutes

Go to Group 5 on the next page

Do as many sets as possible

Manage Menopause Workout

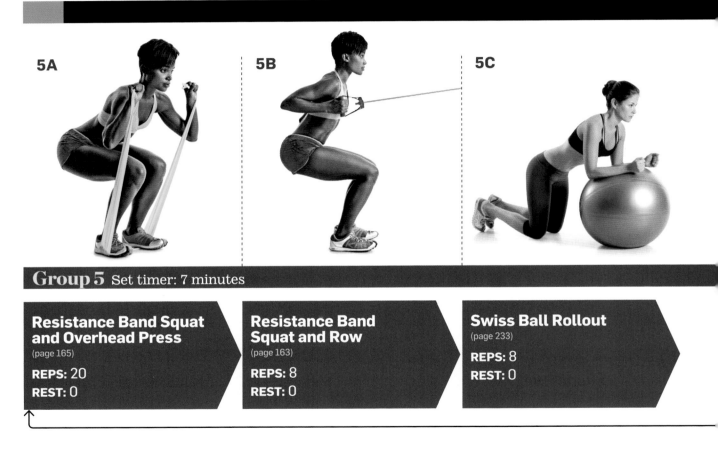

5A

5B

5C

Group 5 Set timer: 7 minutes

Resistance Band Squat and Overhead Press
(page 165)

REPS: 20
REST: 0

Resistance Band Squat and Row
(page 163)

REPS: 8
REST: 0

Swiss Ball Rollout
(page 233)

REPS: 8
REST: 0

5D

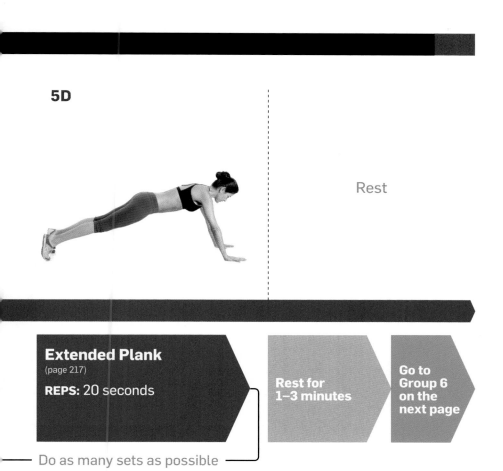

Rest

Extended Plank
(page 217)

REPS: 20 seconds

Rest for
1–3 minutes

Go to
Group 6
on the
next page

— Do as many sets as possible —

Manage Menopause Workout

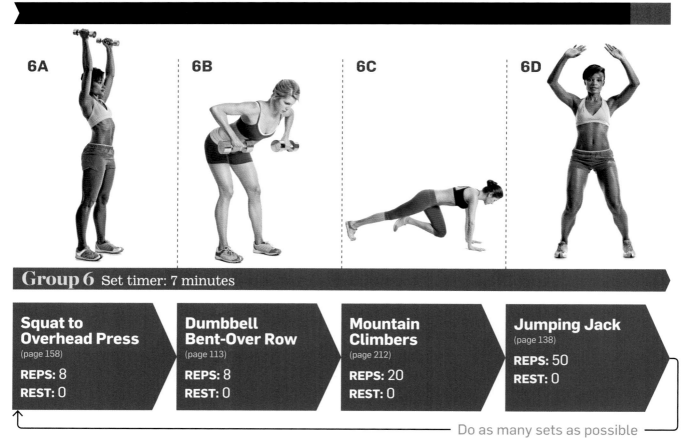

6A   **6B**   **6C**   **6D**

Group 6   Set timer: 7 minutes

Squat to Overhead Press
(page 158)
REPS: 8
REST: 0

Dumbbell Bent-Over Row
(page 113)
REPS: 8
REST: 0

Mountain Climbers
(page 212)
REPS: 20
REST: 0

Jumping Jack
(page 138)
REPS: 50
REST: 0

Do as many sets as possible

"The hardest thing about exercise is to start doing it. Once you are doing exercise regularly, the hardest thing is to stop it."
—Erin Gray

PMS Workout [40 minutes]

MOST WOMEN WOULD rather do just about anything other than workout when it's that time of the month. The idea of running, jumping, or lifting doesn't exactly mesh with feeling heavy, tired, and irritable. But according to celeb trainer Valerie Waters, a little sweat and the right movements are exactly what you need to feel better. This workout was specifically designed for when your body feels most confused. It emphasizes basic movements and avoids anything that might trigger a negative response. Give it a try, and use this as your go-to routine one week every month.

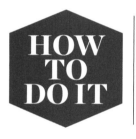

HOW TO DO IT

● Perform this workout three times a week. For instance, you could do this on Monday, Wednesday, and Friday.

● Each workout consists of three circuits. Perform 1 set of all of the exercises in the first circuit, resting 30 seconds between each move. Once you have finished all exercises in the circuit, repeat the process. After you complete all sets in the circuit, you can move on to the next group of exercises.

ABOUT THE EXPERT

Valerie Waters is one of Hollywood's most sought-after trainers. She is the creator of the Red Carpet Ready program, where you can experience her fitness and diet tips, and learn all of her body transformation secrets. She also created the Valslide. Visit redcarpetready.com, Valeriewaters.com, or valslide.com for more information.

PMS Workout

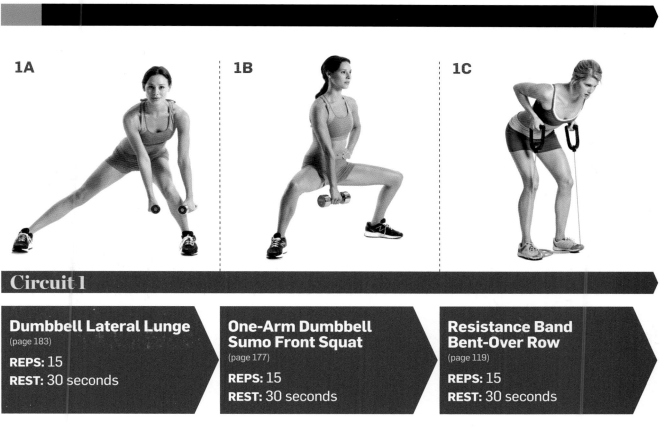

1A

1B

1C

Circuit 1

Dumbbell Lateral Lunge
(page 183)

REPS: 15
REST: 30 seconds

One-Arm Dumbbell Sumo Front Squat
(page 177)

REPS: 15
REST: 30 seconds

Resistance Band Bent-Over Row
(page 119)

REPS: 15
REST: 30 seconds

PMS Workout

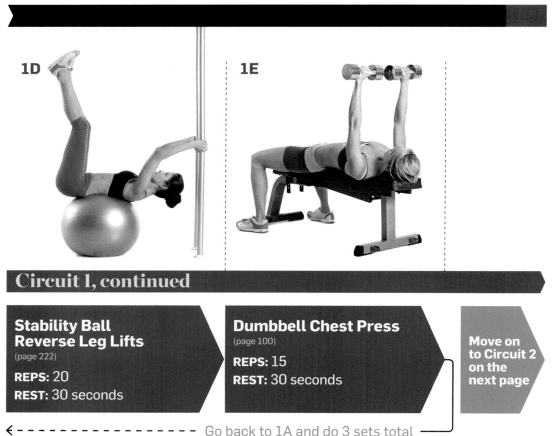

1D

1E

Circuit 1, continued

Stability Ball Reverse Leg Lifts
(page 222)

REPS: 20
REST: 30 seconds

Dumbbell Chest Press
(page 100)

REPS: 15
REST: 30 seconds

Move on to Circuit 2 on the next page

← – – – – – – – – – – – – – – – – – Go back to 1A and do 3 sets total

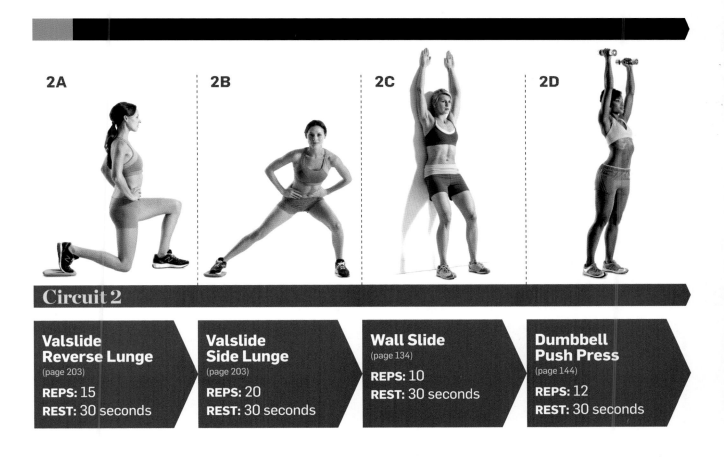

2A

2B

2C

2D

Circuit 2

Valslide Reverse Lunge
(page 203)
REPS: 15
REST: 30 seconds

Valslide Side Lunge
(page 203)
REPS: 20
REST: 30 seconds

Wall Slide
(page 134)
REPS: 10
REST: 30 seconds

Dumbbell Push Press
(page 144)
REPS: 12
REST: 30 seconds

PMS Workout

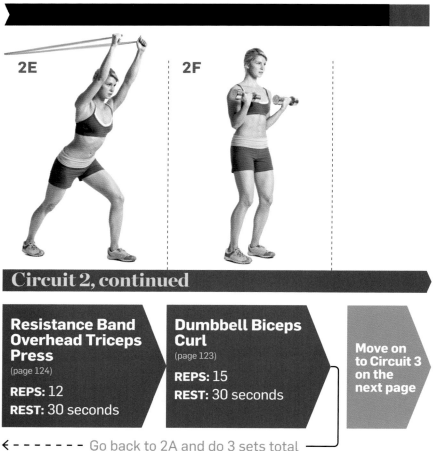

2E

2F

Circuit 2, continued

Resistance Band Overhead Triceps Press
(page 124)

REPS: 12
REST: 30 seconds

Dumbbell Biceps Curl
(page 123)

REPS: 15
REST: 30 seconds

Move on to Circuit 3 on the next page

←- - - - - - - Go back to 2A and do 3 sets total

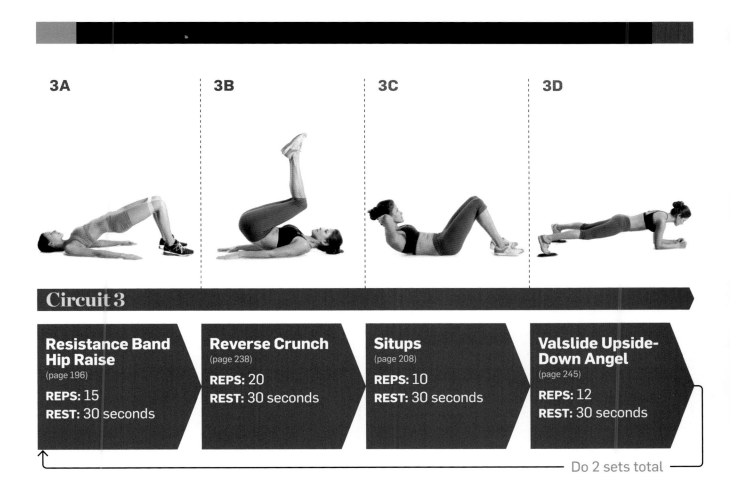

3A

3B

3C

3D

Circuit 3

Resistance Band Hip Raise
(page 196)
REPS: 15
REST: 30 seconds

Reverse Crunch
(page 238)
REPS: 20
REST: 30 seconds

Situps
(page 208)
REPS: 10
REST: 30 seconds

Valslide Upside-Down Angel
(page 245)
REPS: 12
REST: 30 seconds

Do 2 sets total

C H A P T E R   9

Abs For Moms

THE PLANS YOU NEED TO STAY HEALTHY DURING PREGNANCY AND THEN BURN OFF THE BABY WEIGHT.

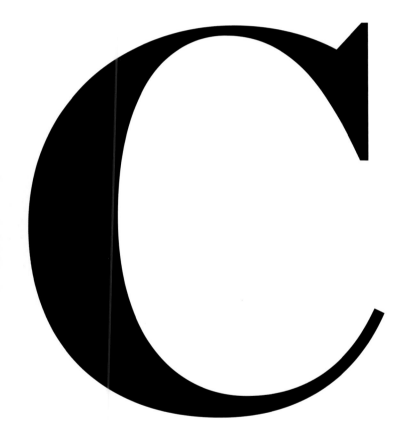

Can I work out when I'm pregnant?"

It's one of the most common questions from expectant mothers. While your body will go through significant changes, you can still stay fit and help prepare your body for a healthy birth. The secret is a three-step approach that was strategically planned for your changing body and considers all the symptoms you're experiencing. By using this specially designed workout, you'll gain less fat, suffer fewer aches and pains, and limit your water retention—all while ensuring that you give birth to a healthy baby.

The Pre-Baby Workout Phase 1: Weeks 1–15 [20 minutes]

PERFORM EACH WORKOUT once a week so that you're exercising 3 days a week. You can switch up the order of workouts or exercises to your preference.

It is best to listen to your body during this phase as you're more likely to be excessively tired, nauseated, or wary about exercising in general. Your workouts are going to involve more rest and less intensity until you get your normal energy back.

Workout A

● Perform as many reps of each of the five exercises in succession for 30 seconds, followed by 30 seconds of rest. Use a timer to keep you on track. Perform these five exercises in succession for four rounds for a 20-minute workout.

Workout B

● Perform as many reps of each of the five exercises in succession for 30 seconds, followed by 30 seconds of rest. Use a timer to keep you on track. Perform these five exercises in succession for four rounds for a 20-minute workout.

Workout C

● Perform as many reps of each of the following six exercises, one after the other, for 30 seconds on and 15 seconds off. Follow with a 90-second rest. Repeat for six total cycles for a 30-minute workout.

The Pregnancy Workout: User's Guide

1 As your belly grows, the pressure on your bladder will increase, making it harder to do "bouncing" exercises like running or jumping.

2 As your abs stretch out, you're going to want to avoid exercises that also stretch your abs, such as hanging leg raises and leg lowering exercises.

3 Your joints will become progressively looser as your pregnancy continues. At this time it is wise to avoid single-leg stability work, like single-leg squats or even reverse lunges.

4 It may get harder to squat and deadlift as your hips widen and your belly increases. Assume a wider stance.

5 While your weight goes up, your total strength will seem to go down. If you were used to doing pushups on your toes, you may be forced into a kneeling position. Same with chinups and pushups; your heavy weight is harder to move.

6 Abdominal crunching exercises are not advised as your pregnancy progresses because they can cause Diastasis recti, splitting of your abdominal wall.

The Pre-Baby Workout: Phase 1, Week 1-15

1A **1B** **1C**

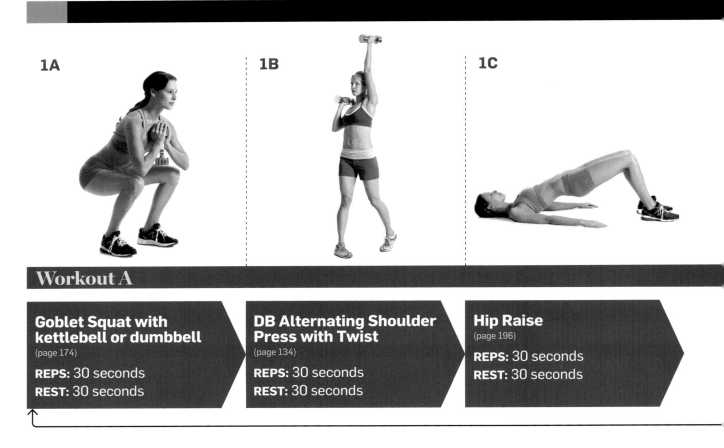

Workout A

Goblet Squat with kettlebell or dumbbell
(page 174)

REPS: 30 seconds
REST: 30 seconds

DB Alternating Shoulder Press with Twist
(page 134)

REPS: 30 seconds
REST: 30 seconds

Hip Raise
(page 196)

REPS: 30 seconds
REST: 30 seconds

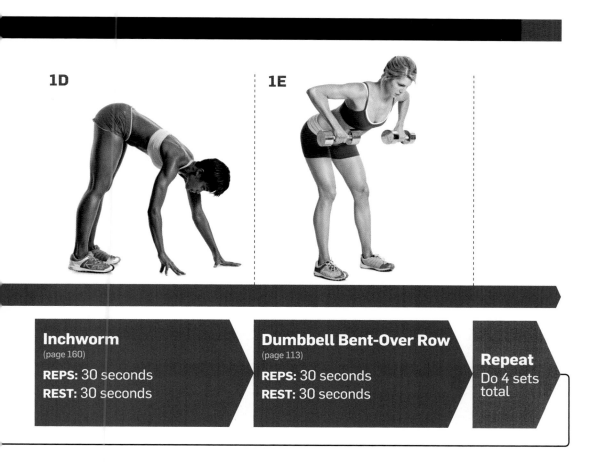

1D

1E

Inchworm
(page 160)

REPS: 30 seconds
REST: 30 seconds

Dumbbell Bent-Over Row
(page 113)

REPS: 30 seconds
REST: 30 seconds

Repeat
Do 4 sets total

THE WORKOUTS

The Pre-Baby Workout: Phase 1, Week 1-15

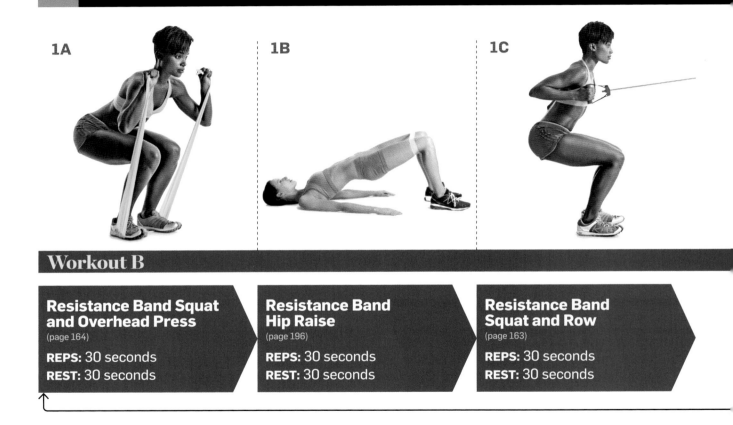

1A 1B 1C

Workout B

Resistance Band Squat and Overhead Press
(page 164)

REPS: 30 seconds
REST: 30 seconds

Resistance Band Hip Raise
(page 196)

REPS: 30 seconds
REST: 30 seconds

Resistance Band Squat and Row
(page 163)

REPS: 30 seconds
REST: 30 seconds

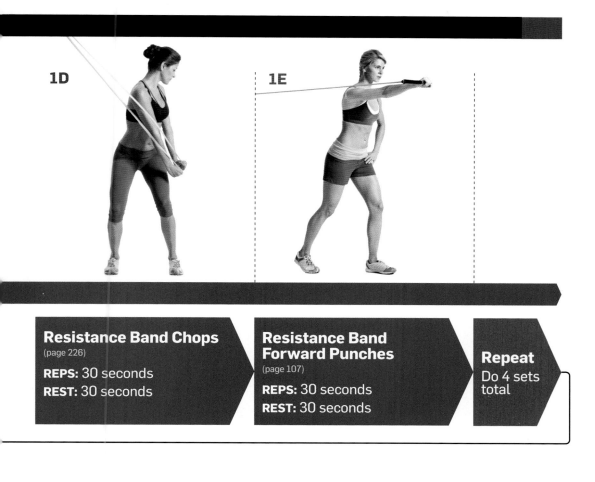

1D

1E

Resistance Band Chops
(page 226)

REPS: 30 seconds
REST: 30 seconds

Resistance Band Forward Punches
(page 107)

REPS: 30 seconds
REST: 30 seconds

Repeat
Do 4 sets total

The Pre-Baby Workout: Phase 1, Week 1-15

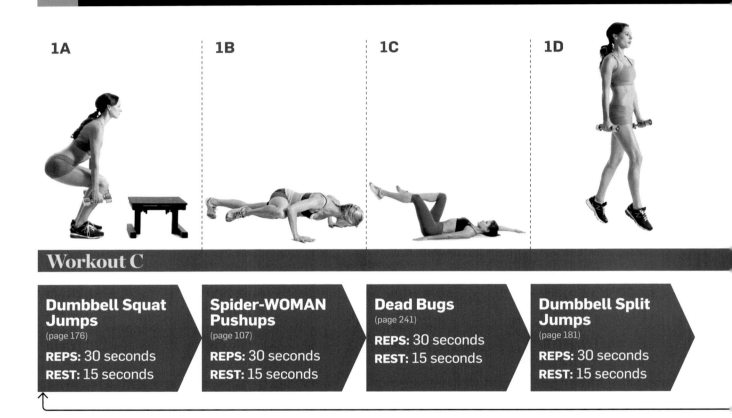

1A **1B** **1C** **1D**

Workout C

Dumbbell Squat Jumps
(page 176)

REPS: 30 seconds
REST: 15 seconds

Spider-WOMAN Pushups
(page 107)

REPS: 30 seconds
REST: 15 seconds

Dead Bugs
(page 241)

REPS: 30 seconds
REST: 15 seconds

Dumbbell Split Jumps
(page 181)

REPS: 30 seconds
REST: 15 seconds

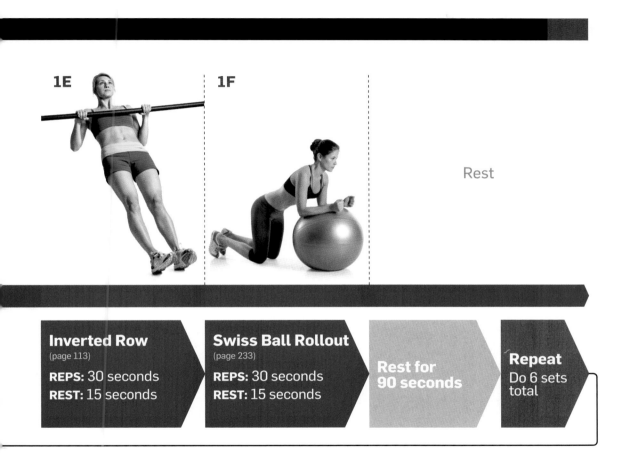

1E

1F

Rest

Inverted Row
(page 113)

REPS: 30 seconds
REST: 15 seconds

Swiss Ball Rollout
(page 233)

REPS: 30 seconds
REST: 15 seconds

Rest for 90 seconds

Repeat
Do 6 sets total

The Pre-Baby Workout Phase 2: Weeks 16–28 [25–30 minutes]

BY THIS POINT, you should really start feeling pregnant. Prior to this, you probably just felt fat. However, now your energy is back and your nausea is gone. So it's time to kick things up a notch and work as hard as your body will let you.

Workout A

● This workout consists of five exercise pairs. Perform as many reps of each set of exercises as you can for 30 seconds and then rest for 15 seconds. Do all sets in a pair (exercise 1A and 1B, for example) before moving on to the next group (2A and 2B).

Workout B

● Perform as many reps of each exercise as you can for 60 seconds followed by 60 seconds of rest. Do 1 set of all seven exercises, rest for 60 seconds, and then repeat for three more rounds (four total rounds). Each exercise is meant to be done at the highest intensity possible.

Workout C

● Perform as many reps of each exercise as you can for 20 seconds followed by 10 seconds of rest. Do 1 set of all seven exercises, rest for 60 seconds, and then repeat for three more rounds (four total rounds). Each exercise is meant to be done at the highest intensity possible.

The Pre-Baby Workout: Phase 2, Week 16-28

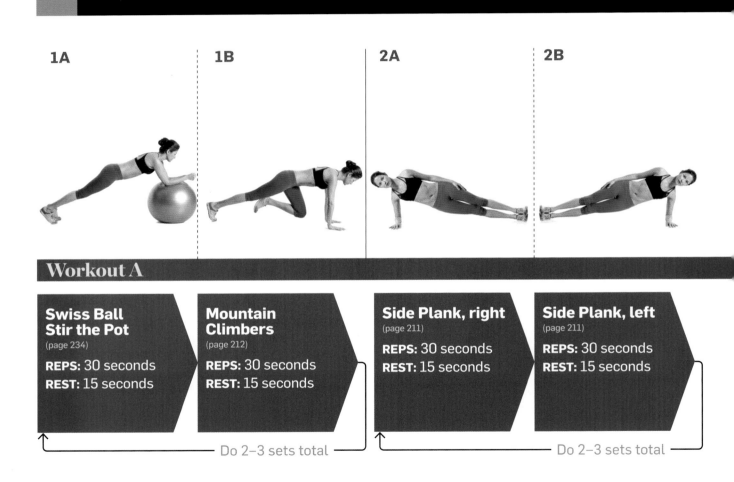

1A **1B** **2A** **2B**

Workout A

Swiss Ball Stir the Pot
(page 234)
REPS: 30 seconds
REST: 15 seconds

Mountain Climbers
(page 212)
REPS: 30 seconds
REST: 15 seconds

— Do 2–3 sets total —

Side Plank, right
(page 211)
REPS: 30 seconds
REST: 15 seconds

Side Plank, left
(page 211)
REPS: 30 seconds
REST: 15 seconds

— Do 2–3 sets total —

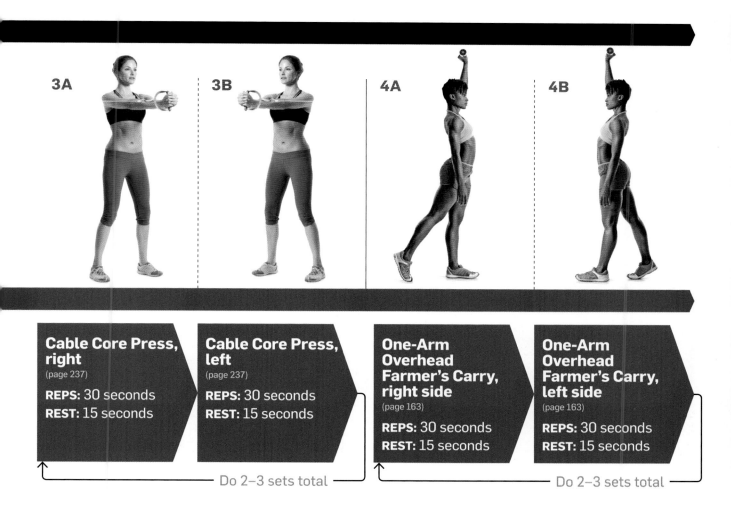

3A

3B

4A

4B

Cable Core Press, right
(page 237)

REPS: 30 seconds
REST: 15 seconds

Cable Core Press, left
(page 237)

REPS: 30 seconds
REST: 15 seconds

One-Arm Overhead Farmer's Carry, right side
(page 163)

REPS: 30 seconds
REST: 15 seconds

One-Arm Overhead Farmer's Carry, left side
(page 163)

REPS: 30 seconds
REST: 15 seconds

Do 2–3 sets total

Do 2–3 sets total

The Pre-Baby Workout: Phase 2, Week 16-28

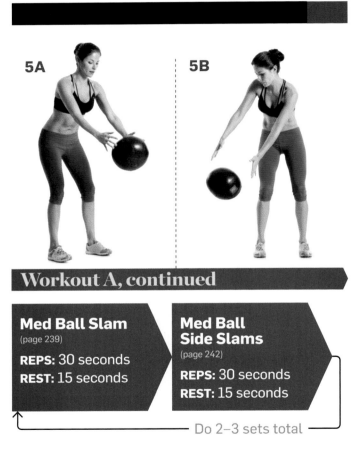

5A

5B

Workout A, continued

Med Ball Slam
(page 239)

REPS: 30 seconds
REST: 15 seconds

Med Ball Side Slams
(page 242)

REPS: 30 seconds
REST: 15 seconds

Do 2–3 sets total

"Lack of activity destroys
the good condition
of every human being,
while movement and methodical
physical exercise
save it and preserve it." —Plato

The Pre-Baby Workout: Phase 2, Week 16-28

1A **1B** **1C** **1D**

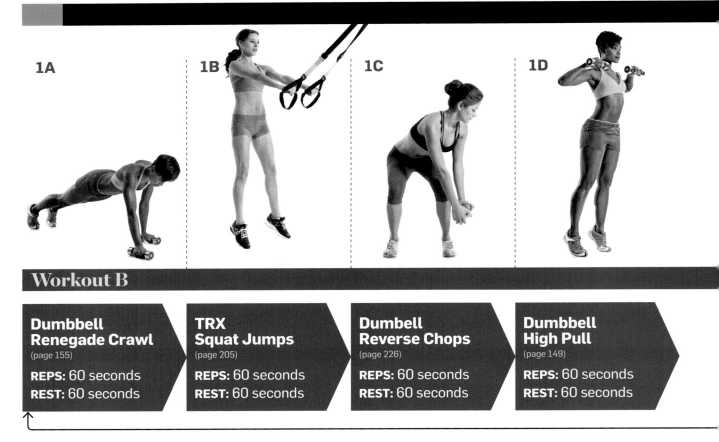

Workout B

Dumbbell Renegade Crawl	TRX Squat Jumps	Dumbell Reverse Chops	Dumbbell High Pull
(page 155)	(page 205)	(page 226)	(page 149)
REPS: 60 seconds	**REPS:** 60 seconds	**REPS:** 60 seconds	**REPS:** 60 seconds
REST: 60 seconds	**REST:** 60 seconds	**REST:** 60 seconds	**REST:** 60 seconds

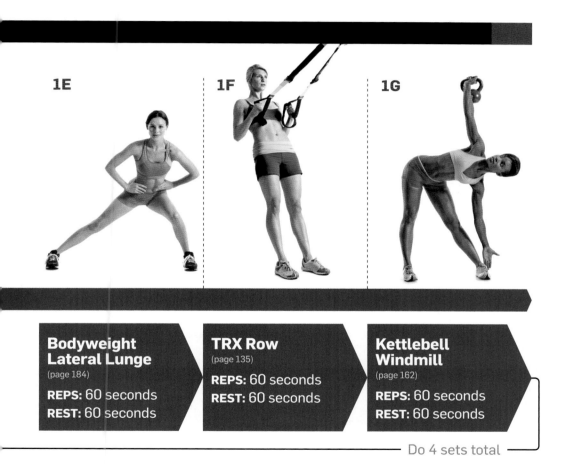

1E

1F

1G

**Bodyweight
Lateral Lunge**
(page 184)

REPS: 60 seconds
REST: 60 seconds

TRX Row
(page 135)

REPS: 60 seconds
REST: 60 seconds

**Kettlebell
Windmill**
(page 162)

REPS: 60 seconds
REST: 60 seconds

Do 4 sets total

The Pre-Baby Workout: Phase 2, Week 16-28

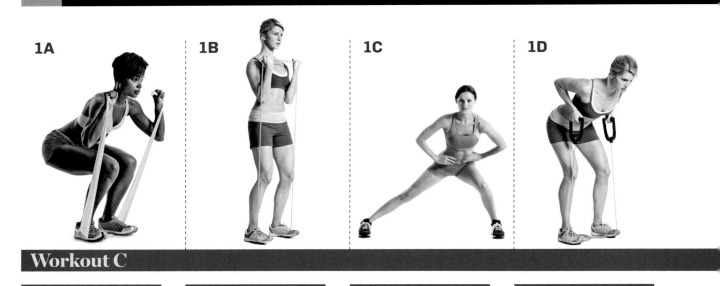

1A   **1B**   **1C**   **1D**

Workout C

Resistance Band Squat and Overhead Press
(page 164)

REPS: 20 seconds
REST: 10 seconds

Resistance Band Biceps Curl hammer curl, or underhand grip
(page 123)

REPS: 20 seconds
REST: 10 seconds

Bodyweight Lateral Lunge
(page 184)

REPS: 20 seconds
REST: 10 seconds

Resistance Band Bent-Over Row
(page 119)

REPS: 20 seconds
REST: 10 seconds

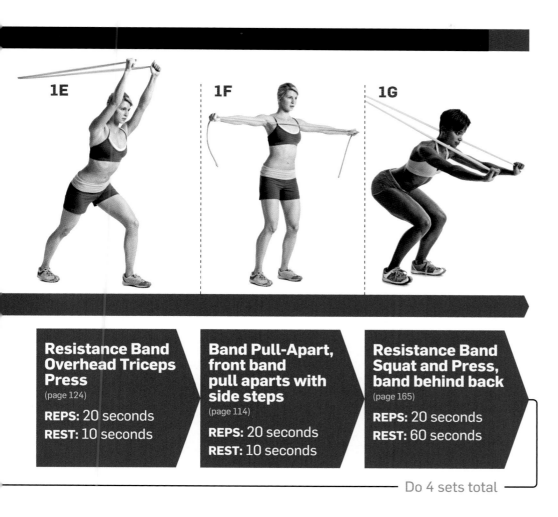

1E

1F

1G

Resistance Band Overhead Triceps Press
(page 124)

REPS: 20 seconds
REST: 10 seconds

Band Pull-Apart, front band pull aparts with side steps
(page 114)

REPS: 20 seconds
REST: 10 seconds

Resistance Band Squat and Press, band behind back
(page 165)

REPS: 20 seconds
REST: 60 seconds

Do 4 sets total

The Pre-Baby Workout Phase 3: Weeks 29–40 [35 minutes]

THIS IS IT—the last of your glory days. The jumping and explosive moves are going to stop, and you will have a harder time moving your body around. You also will probably find yourself squatting wider and enjoying a sumo-style position. But your body is still strong and will amaze you at what it can do.

ABOUT THE EXPERT

Cassandra Forsythe-Pribanic, PhD, RD, CSCS, is the owner and instructor of Fitness Revolution boot camps in Vernon, Connecticut. She is the author of the *The New Rules of Lifting for Women* and *Women's Health Perfect Body Diet*. You can learn more about Cassandra—a mother, wife, and nutrition and women's exercise expert—at cassandraforsythe.com.

Workout A

● Perform this workout as straight sets. That is, do 1 set of the first exercise, rest, and do another set. Continue until you have completed all sets, and then move on to the next exercise. For this workout, you'll perform each exercise for 40 seconds followed by 20 seconds of rest. Complete 5 sets, rest 1 minute, and then move on to the next exercise.

Workout B

● This workout consists of four exercise pairs. Perform as many reps of each set of exercises as you can for 20 seconds and then rest for 10 seconds. Do all sets in a pair (exercise 1A and 1B, for example) before moving on to the next group (2A and 2B).

Workout C

● Perform as many reps of each exercise as you can for 30 seconds followed by 15 seconds of rest. Do 1 set of all six exercises, rest for 90 seconds, and then repeat for five more rounds (six total rounds). Each exercise is meant to be done at the highest intensity possible.

The Pre-Baby Workout: Phase 3, Week 29-40

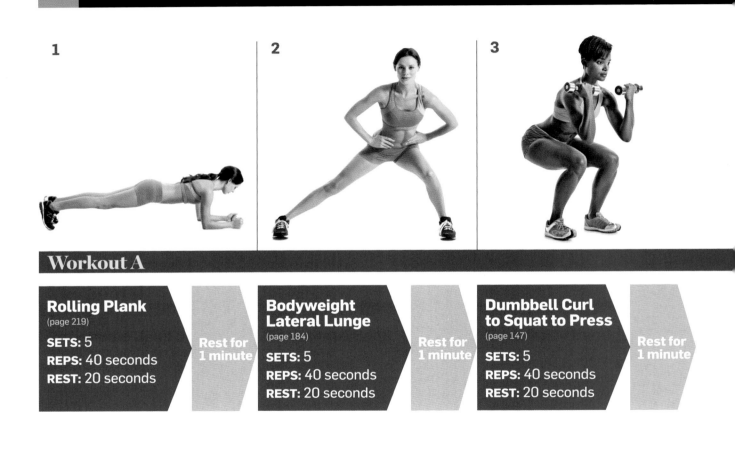

1

2

3

Workout A

Rolling Plank
(page 219)

SETS: 5
REPS: 40 seconds
REST: 20 seconds

Rest for 1 minute

Bodyweight Lateral Lunge
(page 184)

SETS: 5
REPS: 40 seconds
REST: 20 seconds

Rest for 1 minute

Dumbbell Curl to Squat to Press
(page 147)

SETS: 5
REPS: 40 seconds
REST: 20 seconds

Rest for 1 minute

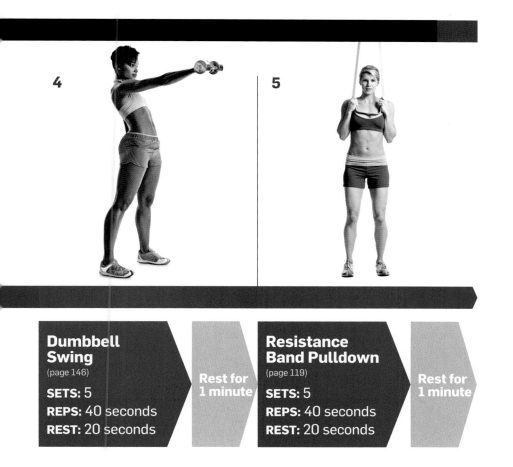

4

5

Dumbbell Swing
(page 146)

SETS: 5
REPS: 40 seconds
REST: 20 seconds

Rest for 1 minute

Resistance Band Pulldown
(page 119)

SETS: 5
REPS: 40 seconds
REST: 20 seconds

Rest for 1 minute

The Pre-Baby Workout: Phase 3, Week 29-40

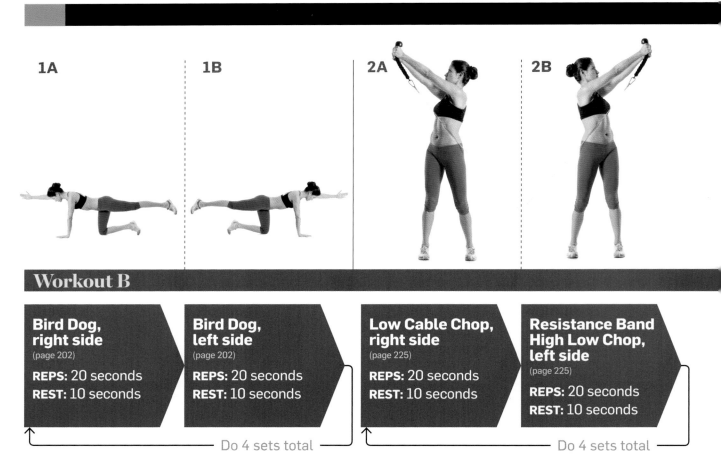

1A **1B** **2A** **2B**

Workout B

Bird Dog, right side
(page 202)
REPS: 20 seconds
REST: 10 seconds

Bird Dog, left side
(page 202)
REPS: 20 seconds
REST: 10 seconds

— Do 4 sets total —

Low Cable Chop, right side
(page 225)
REPS: 20 seconds
REST: 10 seconds

Resistance Band High Low Chop, left side
(page 225)
REPS: 20 seconds
REST: 10 seconds

— Do 4 sets total —

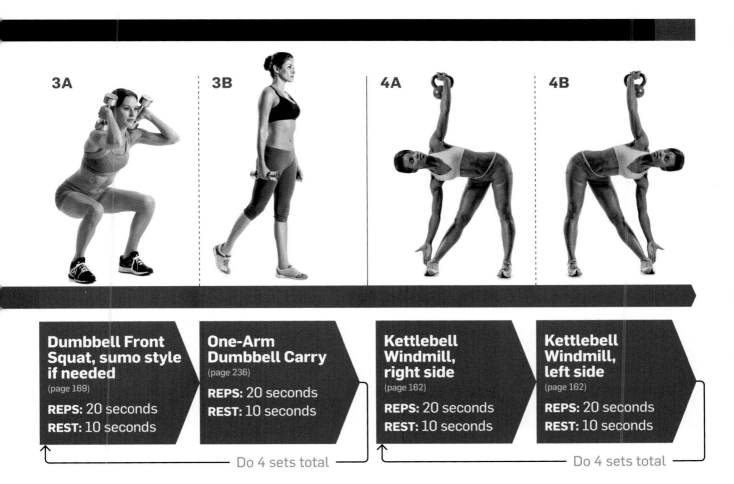

3A

3B

4A

4B

Dumbbell Front Squat, sumo style if needed
(page 169)

REPS: 20 seconds
REST: 10 seconds

One-Arm Dumbbell Carry
(page 236)

REPS: 20 seconds
REST: 10 seconds

— Do 4 sets total —

Kettlebell Windmill, right side
(page 162)

REPS: 20 seconds
REST: 10 seconds

Kettlebell Windmill, left side
(page 162)

REPS: 20 seconds
REST: 10 seconds

— Do 4 sets total —

The Pre-Baby Workout: Phase 3, Week 29-40

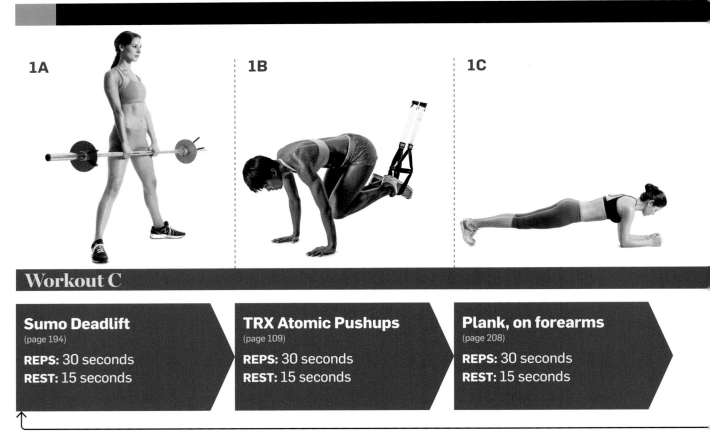

1A

1B

1C

Workout C

Sumo Deadlift
(page 194)

REPS: 30 seconds
REST: 15 seconds

TRX Atomic Pushups
(page 109)

REPS: 30 seconds
REST: 15 seconds

Plank, on forearms
(page 208)

REPS: 30 seconds
REST: 15 seconds

1D

1E

1F

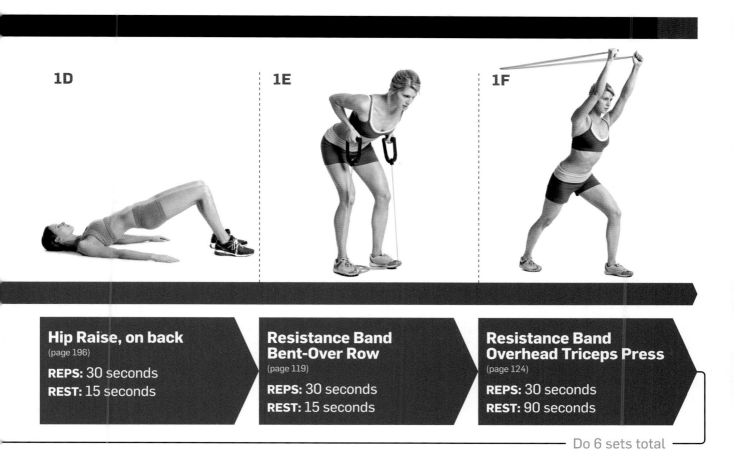

Hip Raise, on back
(page 196)

REPS: 30 seconds
REST: 15 seconds

Resistance Band Bent-Over Row
(page 119)

REPS: 30 seconds
REST: 15 seconds

Resistance Band Overhead Triceps Press
(page 124)

REPS: 30 seconds
REST: 90 seconds

Do 6 sets total

The Lose-the-Baby-Weight Workout [35–40 minutes]

THE EXCESS WEIGHT gained during pregnancy—typically around 15 to 40 pounds—is the nemesis of all new mothers. After your baby is born, you're thrilled with the new addition to your family but not the changes to your wardrobe. If you want the weight gone fast, you can't follow the same program you used for your pre-baby body. That's why Patrick Striet, CSCS, created a routine based on the concept of tri-sets. Each tri-set consists of three exercises: one upper body, one lower body, and one for your core muscles. By rotating through each exercise, you can overload your body, fight off fatigue, and speed up the results in a fraction of the time. Let's make it clear: Tri-sets won't just burn off your baby weight. They'll allow you to drop pounds unlike ever before.

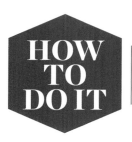

HOW TO DO IT

● Perform this workout 3 days a week on nonconsecutive days (Monday, Wednesday, and Friday for example). For each tri-set, perform a set of exercise A, followed by a set of exercise B, and finally a set of exercise C, resting only 45 seconds between exercises. Once you have completed all of the sets in a group, rest 90 seconds and then move to the next tri-set.

ABOUT THE EXPERT

Patrick "P. J." Striet is a Certified Strength and Conditioning Specialist through the National Strength and Conditioning Association and the owner of FORCE Fitness & Performance in Cincinnati. P. J. serves as the fitness correspondent for 700 WLW radio, and is also a contributor to several popular mainstream magazines and Web sites, including *Men's Health* and Livestrong.com. You can visit his blog at personaltrainerscincinnati.com.

The Lose-the-Baby-Weight Workout

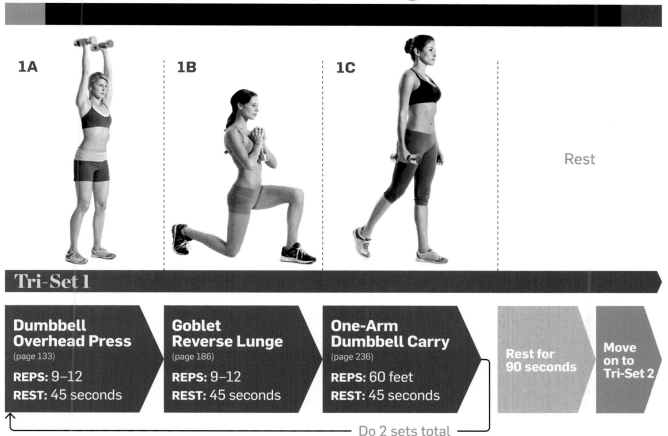

1A

1B

1C

Rest

Tri-Set 1

Dumbbell Overhead Press
(page 133)
REPS: 9–12
REST: 45 seconds

Goblet Reverse Lunge
(page 186)
REPS: 9–12
REST: 45 seconds

One-Arm Dumbbell Carry
(page 236)
REPS: 60 feet
REST: 45 seconds

Rest for 90 seconds

Move on to Tri-Set 2

Do 2 sets total

The Lose-the-Baby-Weight Workout

2A

2B

2C

Rest

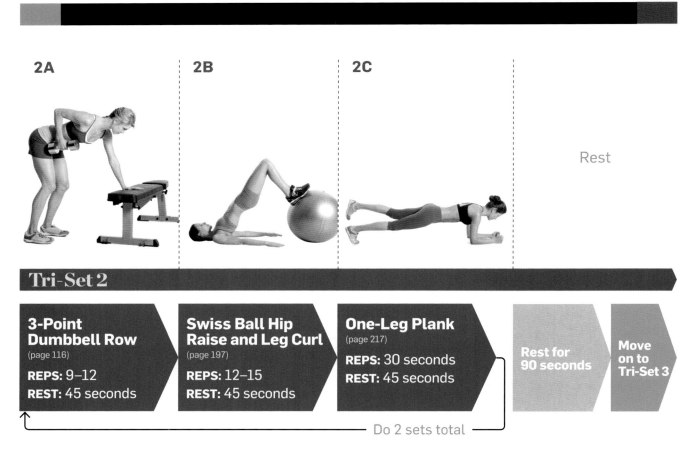

Tri-Set 2

3-Point Dumbbell Row
(page 116)
REPS: 9–12
REST: 45 seconds

Swiss Ball Hip Raise and Leg Curl
(page 197)
REPS: 12–15
REST: 45 seconds

One-Leg Plank
(page 217)
REPS: 30 seconds
REST: 45 seconds

Rest for 90 seconds

Move on to Tri-Set 3

Do 2 sets total

3A

3B

3C

Rest

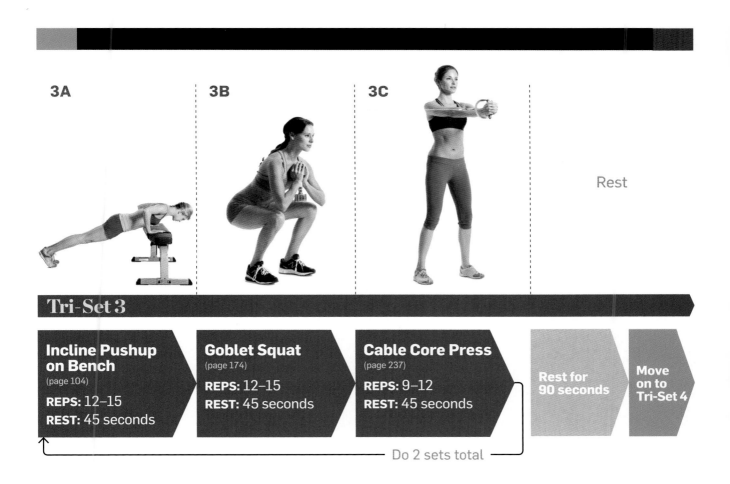

Tri-Set 3

Incline Pushup on Bench
(page 104)
REPS: 12–15
REST: 45 seconds

Goblet Squat
(page 174)
REPS: 12–15
REST: 45 seconds

Cable Core Press
(page 237)
REPS: 9–12
REST: 45 seconds

Rest for 90 seconds

Move on to Tri-Set 4

Do 2 sets total

The Lose-the-Baby-Weight Workout

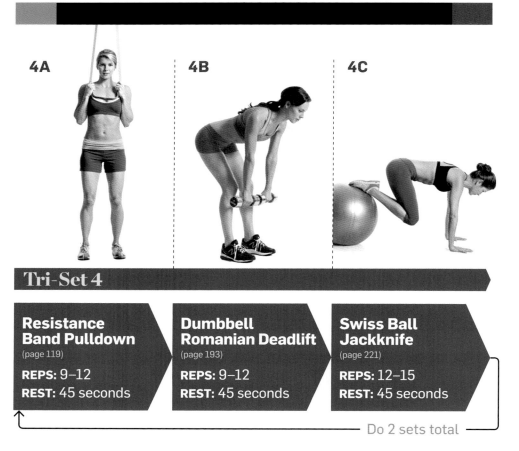

4A

4B

4C

Tri-Set 4

Resistance Band Pulldown
(page 119)

REPS: 9–12

REST: 45 seconds

Dumbbell Romanian Deadlift
(page 193)

REPS: 9–12

REST: 45 seconds

Swiss Ball Jackknife
(page 221)

REPS: 12–15

REST: 45 seconds

Do 2 sets total

"To give anything less
than your best
is to sacrifice the gift."
—Steve Prefontaine

Abs-olutely Delicious Dishes

EAT YOUR WAY THIN WITH GOURMET FLAVORS
THAT ARE ACTUALLY HEALTHY.

There's a variety of

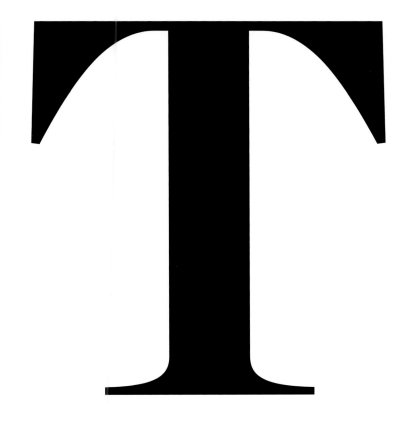

weight loss tricks just waiting for you in your own home. All of them are hiding in your kitchen. While eating out is an enjoyable and convenient experience, cooking your own food is the best way to stay on track. The truth is, most restaurant foods are loaded with calories because they're cooked in a much different way than you ever would. A stick of butter here, an entire bottle of dressing there. Next thing you know, your seemingly healthy salad is loaded with more than 1,000 calories.

But you don't need the extra calories to create a delicious meal. You can enjoy all the benefits of a restaurant and pay less for a meal that won't derail your flat belly dreams. It all starts by reacquainting yourself with your kitchen. We've decided to make

Abs-olutely Delicious Dishes

the process a little bit easier by providing some of the tastiest meals that are also easy to prepare and cook. Many of these options can be made in less than 10 minutes. And if you're in the mood to test your culinary skills, we have some other options that will challenge you and your tastebuds.

Regardless of your cooking experience, anyone can make these meals. They're good for the home, on the go, or even for lunch at work. Try them out, experiment with your own changes, and discover your inner chef. It might be the smallest change you make, but it could be the difference maker that allows you to control your cravings and satisfy your appetite on fewer calories. Each recipe makes one serving unless otherwise noted.

Top Five for a Flat Belly

Some meals pack a little extra nutritional punch. Include any of these on a weekly basis to help improve your mind, skin, energy, and weight loss.

Rainbow Trout

This fish has almost as much eicosapentaenoic acid (EPA) as salmon. This powerful omega-3 fatty acid might help prevent the stress chemical cortisol from boiling over and can help with the health of your skin cells.

Blueberries

No berry is packed with more antioxidants than blueberries. They help counteract aging, reduce inflammation, fight off high blood pressure, and have even been linked with a boost in memory. One cup is all you need for the long list of benefits.

Pumpkin Seeds

They're not just great during Halloween season. Pumpkin seeds contain a boost of magnesium, which can help kick your energy and metabolism into a higher gear. Have them alone or add to eggs, yogurt, or cereal.

Ricotta Cheese

You know those whey protein shakes that come in big jars? This is the food equivalent. It's loaded with amino acids that can help you build muscle, burn fat, and recover faster from your workouts.

Dark Chocolate

Women love dark chocolate, and that's a good thing. According to the *Journal of the American Medical Association*, this healthy treat improves the health of your blood vessels, which helps prevent stress from making your blood pressure surge. Dark chocolate has also been shown to ward off negative moods, meaning it's your best friend after a bad day.

Fat Fighters

Stock up on these foods to help you curb hunger and speed weight loss.

Grapefruit

In a study at the Nutrition and Metabolic Research Center at the Scripps Clinic in San Diego, people who ate half a grapefruit with each meal lost an average of 3.6 pounds in 3 months. The cause might be grapefruit's ability to counter an increase in insulin after you eat and keep your blood sugar lower and your metabolism humming at a faster pace.

Raspberries and Blackberries

Berries are a stealthy source of fiber, which can help you stay full and eat less. Raspberries and blackberries both contain more than 8 grams per cup, which is almost a quarter of your daily allowance. Add them to almost any meal to help slow digestion, reduce your insulin response, and provide an antioxidant boost.

Low-Fat Yogurt

Your fat loss plan requires a double dose of calcium and protein—both of which are found in yogurt. And when you consider that most women are deficient in both nutrients, this food is the perfect way to start your day, boost your afternoon slump, or end your day with dessert.

■

Abs-olutely Delicious Dishes

BREAKFAST

SMOKED SALMON AND SCRAMBLED EGGS ON TOAST

Prep time: 3 minutes
Cook time: 7 minutes

- 1 slice hearty bread, such as sourdough or whole wheat
- 1 egg
- salt
- pepper
- 1 ounce smoked salmon
- 1 red onion, thinly sliced (optional)
- capers (optional)
- fresh dill (optional)
- 1 lemon (optional)

Toast the bread. Meanwhile, in a bowl, whisk the egg with salt and pepper. Pour into a nonstick pan and scramble. Lay the smoked salmon on the toasted bread and top with the scrambled egg. Finish with your choice of red onion, capers, dill, or a squeeze of lemon.

HUEVOS RANCHEROS

Prep time: 5 minutes
Cook time: 2 minutes

- 2 eggs
- 1 scallion, sliced
- 1 tablespoon diced cilantro
- 2 tablespoons shredded Mexican blend cheese
- 2 tablespoons salsa
- 1 medium whole wheat tortilla

In a microwaveable bowl, stir the eggs with a fork until well blended and microwave for 2 minutes. Arrange all the ingredients on the tortilla, fold the ends, then neatly roll.

SPINACH AND FETA FRITTATA

Prep time: 5 minutes
Cook time: 15 minutes

- 3 tablespoons olive oil
- ¼ cup chopped onion
- 2 cloves garlic, minced
- 1 pound baby spinach leaves
- 4 large eggs
- 4 large egg whites
- ¼ cup finely crumbled bread crumbs
- 2 tablespoons fresh basil
- 2 teaspoons grated lemon zest
- ½ teaspoon black pepper
- 1 cup crumbled feta cheese (4 ounces)

1. In a large skillet, heat 1 tablespoon of the oil over medium heat. Add the onion and garlic, and cook for 5 minutes.

2. Add the spinach and stir until wilted. Remove from the skillet and keep warm.

3. In a medium bowl, beat together the whole eggs and egg whites. Beat in the bread crumbs, basil, lemon zest, and pepper.

4. In the same skillet, heat the remaining 2 tablespoons oil over medium heat. Stir the spinach mixture and the feta into the egg mixture, then pour into the skillet. Reduce the heat to low, cover, and cook until the top of the frittata is set.

5. Cut into wedges to serve.

PEANUT BUTTER STRAWBERRY WRAP

Prep time: 5 minutes
Cook time: 0 minutes

- 1 whole wheat tortilla
- 2 tablespoons natural unsalted crunchy peanut butter
- ½ cup sliced strawberries

Lay the tortilla on a work surface. Spread with the peanut butter. Cover with the strawberries. Roll into a tube. Slice on the diagonal into the desired number of pieces.

FLAT GREEN CHILE AND GOAT CHEESE OMELET

Prep time: 5 minutes
Cook time: 25 minutes

2   or more Anaheim green chile peppers (wear plastic gloves when handling)
½   tablespoon butter
1   onion, thinly sliced
½   teaspoon dried oregano (optional)
4   large eggs
½   teaspoon sea salt
¼   cup crumbled goat cheese
    Whole wheat tortillas (optional)

1. Preheat the broiler.

2. Roast the chiles in the flame of a grill or gas burner (or as close as possible to a broiler flame) until the skins are bubbly and charred. Put them in a bowl, cover with a plate, and let them steam for about 10 minutes. Slip off the skins, cut off the stem end, and push out the seeds using the flat side of a knife. Tear or cut the chiles into strips.

3. Heat the butter in an 8" nonstick ovenproof skillet over medium heat. Add the onion and oregano, if desired. Stir and cook gently. If the chile strips are still firm, add them to the skillet. Cook for 12 minutes, or until the onion has softened. Remove the chiles and onion from the skillet and cool slightly.

4. Beat the eggs with the salt. Add the slightly cooled chiles and onion. If desired, add a bit more oregano. The skillet shouldn't need more butter, but if it seems dry, add about a teaspoon and swirl it around the skillet. Add the egg mixture to the skillet and cook over medium-low heat.

5. As the eggs begin to set around the edges, lift them up with the tip of the spatula and let the wet egg flow underneath. Repeat this process until you can't do so easily any longer. Then sprinkle the goat cheese over the top.

6. Once the eggs seem fairly well set, set the pan under the broiler so that the top can finish cooking and become golden. Slide the omelet onto a serving plate and, if desired, dust with extra oregano and serve with warm tortillas, if desired.

EGG AND AVOCADO BREAKFAST SANDWICH

Prep time: 4 minutes
Cook time: 4 minutes

2   large eggs, lightly beaten
1   tablespoon mashed avocado
1   small (3") bagel, halved and toasted

1. Coat a small nonstick skillet with cooking spray and place over medium heat.

2. Add the eggs and cook until set.

3. Spread the avocado on half of the bagel. Top with the eggs and the remaining bagel half.

Abs-olutely Delicious Dishes

LUNCH

SPECIAL SHRIMP SALAD

Prep time: 10 minutes
Cook time: 0 minutes

2¼ tablespoons white wine vinegar
½ teaspoon salt
½ teaspoon chili powder
3 tablespoons extra-virgin olive oil
3 cups butterhead lettuce, torn into pieces
2 grapefruit, cut into segments
2 avocados, peeled and sliced
10 ounces precooked shrimp
1 scallion, including top, thinly sliced
4 teaspoons chopped cilantro

1. Combine the vinegar, salt, and chili powder in a small bowl. Whisk in the oil.

2. Put the lettuce on a serving plate or on 4 individual salad plates. Arrange the grapefruit, avocados, and shrimp over the lettuce. Sprinkle with the scallion and cilantro.

3. Drizzle with the chili dressing.

PERUVIAN SEAFOOD STEW

Prep time: 20 minutes
Cook time: 30 minutes

1 tablespoon olive oil
1 onion, chopped
1 jalapeño chile pepper, seeded and minced (wear plastic gloves when handling)
3 cloves garlic, minced
1 teaspoon ground cumin
1 can (15-ounces) reduced-sodium white beans, rinsed and drained
¾ pound small red potatoes, cut into ¼"-thick slices
½ bunch kale, coarsely chopped
1 bottle (8 ounces) clam juice
3 cups water
½ teaspoon plus ⅛ teaspoon salt
1 pound cod fillets, cut into 1" chunks
1 pound shrimp, peeled, deveined, and cut into 1" pieces
lime wedges
green Salad with Corn (recipe follows)

1. In a soup pot, heat the oil over medium heat. Add the onion and cook, stirring frequently, for 6 minutes, or until golden brown. Stir in the pepper, garlic, and cumin and cook for 1 minute. Add the beans, potatoes, kale, clam juice, water, and ½ teaspoon salt. Bring to a boil. Reduce the heat to low, cover, and simmer for 12 minutes, or until the potatoes are tender.

2. Stir in the cod. Return to a boil, then reduce the heat and simmer, covered, for 2 minutes. Gently stir in the shrimp and simmer, covered, for 2 to 3 minutes, or until the shrimp and cod are cooked through. Serve with the lime wedges.

Green Salad with Corn
In a large bowl, combine 4 cups salad greens and ½ cup fresh or frozen and thawed corn kernels. Drizzle with 1 tablespoon cider vinegar and 1 teaspoon olive oil. Sprinkle with ⅛ teaspoon salt and toss.

Makes 6 servings

TANGY TURKEY CIABATTA

Prep time: 4 minutes
Cook time: 0 minutes

1 tablespoon pesto
1 ciabatta roll
¼ cup baby spinach leaves
2 ounces sliced lean turkey
1 slice part-skim mozzarella cheese
3 pickle slices

Spread the pesto on the ciabatta roll. Layer on the spinach leaves, turkey, cheese, and pickle slices.

GRILLED CHICKEN AND PINEAPPLE SANDWICH

Prep time: 10 minutes
Cook time: 12 minutes

4   boneless, skinless chicken breasts (6 ounces each)
    teriyaki sauce
4   slices Swiss cheese
4   pineapple slices (½" thick)
4   whole wheat buns
    or lettuce wraps
1   red onion, thinly sliced
    Pickled jalapeño chile peppers (wear plastic gloves when handling)

1. Combine the chicken and enough teriyaki sauce to cover in a resealable plastic bag. Marinate in the refrigerator for at least 30 minutes and up to 12 hours.

2. Coat a grill rack with non-stick spray. Preheat the grill. Remove the chicken from the marinade and place on the grill, discarding any remaining marinade. Cook for 4 to 5 minutes on one side. Flip and top each with cheese. Continue cooking until the cheese is melted and the chicken is lightly charred and firm to the touch. Remove and set aside.

3. While the chicken rests, add the pineapple and buns (if using) to the grill. Cook for 2 minutes per side, or until the buns are lightly toasted and the pineapple is soft and caramelized.

4. Top each bun with the chicken, onion, pepper slices, and pineapple.

BERRY GOAT CHEESE SALAD

Prep time: 15 minutes
Cook time: 10 minutes

Dressing
¼   cup sliced strawberries
1   tablespoon fresh orange juice
1½ teaspoons red wine vinegar
½   teaspoon orange zest
½   teaspoon sugar
2   tablespoons fat-free plain Greek yogurt
1   large pinch kosher salt

1. For the dressing: Combine all of the dressing ingredients in a blender or food processor, or whisk together until smooth.

Salad
1   tablespoon pecans
3   cups baby spinach
½   cup halved strawberries
½   cup blueberries
1   yellow tomato, cut into eighths
2   purple radishes, thinly sliced
1   boneless, skinless chicken breast (6 ounces), grilled
1   teaspoon goat cheese crumbles

1. For the salad: Toast the pecans in a 400ºF oven for 2 minutes. Remove from the oven and set aside. In a large bowl, combine the spinach, berries, tomato, and radishes. Drizzle with the dressing. Toss gently.

2. Divide the salad between 2 plates. Place half of the chicken on top of each salad. Sprinkle with the pecans and goat cheese.

BETTER-FOR-YOU EGG SALAD

Prep time: 15 minutes
Cook time: 10 minutes

4   large eggs
8   ounces soft silken tofu
4   teaspoons brown mustard
½   teaspoon salt
⅛   teaspoon hot pepper sauce
⅓   cup minced onion
¼   cup chopped parsley

1. In a medium saucepan, place the eggs in cold water to cover by several inches. Bring to a boil over high heat. Remove from the heat, cover, and let stand for 12 minutes. Run the eggs under cold water until chilled. Peel, halve, and transfer to a large bowl.

2. Add the tofu, mustard, salt, and hot sauce, and mash with a potato masher until some small chunks remain. Fold in the onion and parsley. Cover and chill until serving time.

Abs-olutely Delicious Dishes

DINNER

CHIPOTLE GLAZED STEAK WITH BLACK BEAN SALAD

Prep time: 20 minutes
Cook time: 10 minutes

- 1 can (15 ounces) reduced-sodium black beans, rinsed and drained
- 1 cup frozen and thawed corn kernels
- 2 plum tomatoes, diced
- 1 avocado, diced
- 1 jalapeño chile pepper, seeded and finely chopped (wear plastic gloves when handling)
- 2 tablespoons chopped cilantro
- 2 tablespoons fresh lime juice
- ½ teaspoon salt
- 1½ teaspoons salt-free chipotle seasoning blend
- 1 teaspoon packed brown sugar
- 1 pound sirloin steak, trimmed of visible fat

1. Combine the beans, corn, tomatoes, avocado, pepper, cilantro, lime juice, and ¼ teaspoon salt in a medium bowl.

2. Coat a grill rack with nonstick spray. Preheat a grill or broiler. Mix the seasoning blend, brown sugar, and the remaining salt in a small bowl. Rub the mixture over both sides of the steak. Grill or broil the steak, 4 minutes per side for medium rare, turning once. Let rest for 5 minutes. Thinly slice the steak and serve with the black bean salad.

Makes 4 servings

POLENTA LASAGNA

Prep time: 25 minutes
Cook time: 1 hour

- 1 tablespoon olive oil
- 1 onion, chopped
- 1 carrot, finely chopped
- 3 cloves garlic, minced
- 1 bunch collard greens, coarsely chopped
- ½ cup water
- 1 tube (18 ounces) prepared polenta, thinly sliced
- 1 cup part-skim ricotta cheese
- 1 cup shredded part-skim mozzarella cheese
- 2 cups reduced-sodium marinara sauce
- ½ cup grated Parmesan cheese

1. Preheat the oven to 375°F. Coat a 9" baking pan with nonstick spray.

2. In a large saucepan, heat the oil over medium heat. Add the onion and carrot. Cook for 5 minutes, or until softened. Stir in the garlic. Add the collard greens and water. Bring to a boil, then reduce the heat and cook, stirring frequently, for 10 minutes, or until the greens are tender and the water evaporates.

3. Arrange one-third of the polenta slices on the bottom of the prepared pan. Add half of the collard greens, spreading evenly. With a teaspoon, spoon on half of the ricotta cheese (no need to spread it out). Sprinkle with half of the mozzarella cheese. Spoon on half of the marinara sauce. Repeat the layering once. Top with the remaining polenta slices and sprinkle with the Parmesan cheese.

4. Bake for 35 to 40 minutes, or until hot and bubbly. Let stand 10 minutes before serving.

Mushroom Salad
In a medium bowl, combine 1 tablespoon lemon juice, 1 tablespoon olive oil, ⅛ teaspoon salt, ⅛ teaspoon black pepper, and a pinch of ground red pepper. Add 1 package (8 ounces) sliced mushrooms and 1 rib celery, thinly sliced. Toss to combine. Let stand for 10 minutes before serving.

Makes 6 servings

RICE BOWLS WITH SHRIMP AND BOK CHOY

Prep time: 20 minutes
Cook time: 10 minutes

- 1 cup quick-cooking brown rice blend (brown rice, wild rice, Texmati white, and red rice)
- 3 tablespoons ponzu sauce
- 3 tablespoons unseasoned rice vinegar
- 4 teaspoons dark sesame oil
- 2 teaspoons grated peeled fresh ginger
- 2 teaspoons packed brown sugar
- 1 teaspoon Sriracha sauce
- 1 head bok choy, thinly sliced
- 1 pound cooked shrimp
- 2 carrots, shredded
- 1 cucumber, peeled, halved lengthwise, seeded, and thinly sliced
- ⅓ cup fresh cilantro

1. Cook the rice according to package directions without added salt or fat.

2. In a small bowl, whisk the ponzu sauce, vinegar, 3 teaspoons of the sesame oil, the ginger, brown sugar, and Sriracha sauce.

3. In a large nonstick skillet, heat the remaining sesame oil over medium heat. Add the bok choy and cook 3 to 4 minutes, stirring frequently, or until wilted.

4. Place the rice in the center of 4 bowls. Top with bok choy, shrimp, carrots, and cucumber. Drizzle with the dressing and sprinkle with the cilantro.

Makes 4 servings

CHILI-SPICED FISH TACOS

Prep time: 4 minutes
Cook time: 7 minutes

5 ounces barramundi fillet
   pinch of salt
   pinch of black pepper
   pinch of cumin
   pinch of chili powder
1 teaspoon olive oil
2 corn tortillas
½ cup chopped tomato
½ cup shredded green cabbage
1 tablespoon fresh cilantro
1 teaspoon lime juice

1. Coat a grill rack with non-stick spray. Preheat the grill.

2. Season the fish with the salt, pepper, cumin, and chili powder. Grill (or cook in 1 teaspoon olive oil over medium heat) for 5 minutes. Flip and cook for 2 minutes longer.

3. Divide the fish between the tortillas. Serve with the tomato, cabbage, cilantro, and lime juice.

BEEF, VEGETABLE, AND ALMOND STIR-FRY

Prep time: 10 minutes
Cook time: 15 minutes

½ cup rice
1 pound flank steak, sliced ¼" thick
3 teaspoons reduced-sodium soy sauce
2 teaspoons toasted sesame oil
1 tablespoon grated fresh ginger
2 cloves garlic, minced
2 medium carrots, thinly sliced
1 medium onion, chopped
1 medium red bell pepper, thinly sliced
8 ounces snow peas
3 tablespoons sliced almonds
2 tablespoons hoisin sauce

1. Cook the rice according to package directions.

2. Meanwhile, toss the steak with 2 teaspoons of the soy sauce. Heat 1 teaspoon of the oil in a large nonstick or cast-iron skillet over medium-high heat. Add the ginger and garlic. Cook, stirring, for 30 seconds. Add the steak and cook, stirring occasionally, for 2 to 3 minutes. Transfer to a plate and set aside.

3. Return the skillet to the heat, and add the remaining 1 teaspoon oil, the carrots, onion, and pepper. Cook, stirring occasionally, for 3 minutes, or until the vegetables start to soften. Stir in the snow peas and almonds. Cook, stirring occasionally, for 2 minutes.

4. Add the reserved steak and juices, the hoisin sauce, and the remaining 1 teaspoon soy sauce. Cook, stirring, for 1 minute. Serve over the rice.

ASIAN SALMON BURGERS

Prep time: 12 minutes
Cook time: 11 minutes

1 pound skinless salmon fillet, cut into chunks
¼ cup fresh whole wheat bread crumbs
1 large egg
2 cloves garlic, chopped
2 teaspoons reduced-sodium soy sauce
½ teaspoon dark sesame oil
2 scallions, chopped
4 tablespoons pickled ginger
2 tablespoons toasted sesame seeds
4 whole wheat buns, toasted
¼ cup baby spinach

1. In a food processor, combine the salmon, bread crumbs, egg, garlic, soy sauce, oil, scallions, and 2 tablespoons of the ginger. Pulse until coarsely chopped. Form into 4 equal (3" diameter) patties. Sprinkle the tops with sesame seeds.

2. Heat a large nonstick skillet coated with cooking spray over medium heat. Put the patties sesame-seed side down in the pan. Cook for 5 minutes. Flip and cook for 5 minutes longer, or until done.

3. Place the burgers on the buns. Top with the spinach and the remaining 2 tablespoons ginger.

(continued)

Abs-olutely Delicious Dishes

DINNER cont'd

CHICKEN LETTUCE CUPS

Prep time: 15 minutes
Cook time: 8 minutes

- 2 teaspoons coconut oil
- ½ cup chopped sweet onion
- 1½ cloves garlic, minced
- 1½ cups minced gingerroot
- ½ cup water chestnuts
- 1 cup diced cooked skinless chicken
- 2 tablespoons low-sodium chicken broth
- 1 tablespoon reduced-sodium soy sauce
- 2 tablespoons rice wine vinegar
- 1 pinch black pepper
- 2 cups cooked brown rice
- 2 scallions, thinly sliced
- 4 Bibb lettuce leaves, washed
- 1 teaspoon black sesame seeds

1. Heat the oil in a large skillet over medium-low heat. Add the onion and cook for 3 minutes. Reduce the heat to low. Add the garlic and gingerroot and cook for 1 minute. Add the water chestnuts and cook for 1 minute longer.

2. Add the chicken, broth, soy sauce, vinegar, and pepper and stir well. Add the rice and cook for 3 minutes. Remove from the heat and stir in the scallions.

3. Divide the chicken mixture equally among the lettuce leaves. Sprinkle with the sesame seeds and serve.

PORK GYROS

Prep time: 15 minutes
Cook time: 25 minutes

- 2 tablespoons safflower or olive oil
- 2 tablespoons red wine vinegar
- 1 teaspoon dried oregano
- 4 cloves garlic, minced
- 1 pork tenderloin (1¼ pounds), trimmed
- ½ teaspoon salt
- ¼ teaspoon black pepper
- ⅓ cup fat-free plain Greek yogurt
- 2 tablespoons chopped fresh dill
- 4 whole wheat pitas, halved and toasted if desired
- 2 cups packed baby spinach
- 1 tomato, cut into thin wedges

1. In a large resealable plastic bag, combine 1 tablespoon of the oil, 1 tablespoon of the vinegar, the oregano, and all but ¼ teaspoon of the garlic. Add the pork, seal the bag, and turn to coat the pork with the marinade. Let stand for 30 minutes.

2. Preheat the oven to 425°F. Remove the pork from the marinade and discard the marinade. Season the pork with ¼ teaspoon of the salt and the pepper. Heat the remaining 1 tablespoon oil in a large ovenproof skillet over medium-high heat. Add the pork and cook for 5 minutes, turning occasionally, until browned. Place the skillet in the oven and roast for 15 to 20 minutes, turning once, until a thermometer inserted in the thickest portion registers 155°F and the juices run clear. Remove the pork to a cutting board and let rest for 5 minutes.

3. Meanwhile, in a small bowl, combine the yogurt, dill, the remaining 1 tablespoon vinegar, the remaining ¼ teaspoon garlic, and the remaining ¼ teaspoon salt.

4. Thinly slice the pork. Stuff the pita halves with the pork, spinach, and tomatoes and drizzle with the yogurt sauce.

Watermelon-Cucumber Salad
In a medium bowl, combine 2 cups diced seedless watermelon, ½ peeled, halved, and sliced cucumber, 3 tablespoons crumbled feta cheese, and 1 tablespoon red wine vinegar.

Makes 4 servings

CHICKEN WITH WALNUTS AND SPINACH

Prep time: 16 minutes
Cook time: 39 minutes

- ⅓ cup chopped onion
- 1 tablespoon olive oil
- 1 cup chopped walnut pieces
- 1 cup chopped baby spinach
- ½ cup grated provolone
- 4 thin-sliced boneless, skinless chicken breasts (4 ounces)
- ¼ teaspoon salt
- ¼ teaspoon black pepper

1. Preheat the oven to 375°F. Grease a baking sheet.

2. Heat the oil in a medium skillet over medium-low heat and add the onion. Cook for 5 minutes, or until softened. Add ½ cup of the walnuts and cook for 1 minute. Increase the heat to medium. Add the spinach and cook for 2 minutes, or until wilted. Put the mixture in a bowl and stir in the cheese.

3. Season the chicken with the salt and pepper. Divide the spinach mixture among the chicken slices and roll up to enclose. Coat the chicken with cooking spray and roll in the remaining ½ cup nuts. Place on the baking sheet and bake for 30 to 35 minutes.

HOISIN-ORANGE GLAZED CHICKEN

Prep time: 10 minutes
Cook time: 15 minutes

- 2 navel oranges
- ¼ cup water
- 3 tablespoons hoisin sauce
- 2 tablespoons dry sherry
- 1 tablespoon reduced-sodium soy sauce
- 3 cloves garlic, thinly sliced
- ½ teaspoon five-spice powder
- 4 (5-ounce) boneless, skinless chicken breasts
- 1 bunch asparagus, cut into 2" pieces
- 4 cups broccoli florets
- 1 teaspoon dark sesame oil

1. From one of the oranges, grate ½ teaspoon zest and squeeze ⅓ cup juice. Remove the peel and white pith from the remaining orange, and cut between the membranes to segment the orange.

2. In a large skillet, mix the orange juice, orange zest, water, hoisin sauce, sherry, soy sauce, garlic, and five-spice powder over high heat. Bring to a boil and add the chicken breasts. Reduce the heat and simmer, covered, for 10 to 12 minutes, turning once, or until a thermometer inserted in the thickest portion registers 160°F and the juices run clear.

3. Meanwhile, fill a large saucepan with 1" water and insert a vegetable steaming basket. Add the asparagus and broccoli and bring to a boil. Cover and cook for 3 minutes, or until the vegetables are crisp-tender. Transfer to a bowl and drizzle with the sesame oil.

4. Transfer the chicken to a plate and cover with foil to keep warm. Bring the hoisin mixture to a boil and cook for 1 to 2 minutes, or until thickened and reduced to ½ cup. Cut the chicken on the diagonal into ½"-thick slices. Spoon the sauce over the chicken and top with the orange segments. Serve with the vegetables.

Makes 4 servings

ROAST SALMON WITH WHITE BEAN COMPOTE

Prep time: 15 minutes
Cook time: 20 minutes

- 1 pound wild salmon fillet (in one piece)
- 1 pint grape tomatoes
- 1 tablespoon olive oil
- ½ teaspoon salt
- ¼ teaspoon black pepper
- 1 can (15 ounces) reduced-sodium cannellini beans, rinsed and drained
- ½ cup roasted red and yellow bell peppers, chopped
- ¼ cup pitted kalamata olives, chopped
- 1 tablespoon lemon juice
- ¼ cup chopped fresh basil
- 1 teaspoon balsamic vinegar

1. Preheat the oven to 425°F. Coat a rimmed baking sheet with olive oil nonstick spray.

2. Place the salmon on the prepared baking sheet. Arrange the tomatoes around the salmon. Drizzle the tomatoes with 1 teaspoon of the oil. Sprinkle the salmon and tomatoes with ¼ teaspoon of the salt and ⅛ teaspoon of the pepper. Roast for 12 to 15 minutes, or until the salmon is just opaque in the center and the tomatoes are soft.

3. Meanwhile, in a medium bowl, combine the beans, bell peppers, olives, and lemon juice.

4. Remove the tomatoes to a small bowl and stir in the basil, vinegar, and remaining 2 teaspoons oil, ¼ teaspoon salt, and ⅛ teaspoon pepper. Cut the salmon into 4 pieces, discarding the skin. Serve over the bean compote with the tomato mixture spooned on top.

Sauteed Escarole

In a large nonstick skillet, heat 1 tablespoon olive oil over medium heat. Add 2 cloves garlic, thinly sliced, and cook for 30 seconds. Add 1 bunch escarole, cut into 2" pieces. Cook for 4 to 5 minutes, stirring frequently, or until the escarole is wilted and tender. Stir in ⅛ teaspoon salt.

Makes 4 servings

Abs-olutely Delicious Dishes

SMOOTHIES

MIXED FRUIT BREAKFAST SMOOTHIE

Prep time: 2 minutes
Cook time: 0 minutes

¾ cup soy milk
¼ cup low-fat ricotta cheese
1   scoop vanilla whey protein
½ cup frozen cranberries
⅓ cup frozen mixed fruit

In a blender or food processor, combine the soy milk, ricotta, whey protein, cranberries, and fruit. Blend or process for 1 minute, or until pureed and well blended.

HIGH-PROTEIN BLUEBERRY YOGURT SHAKE

Prep time: 5 minutes
Cook time: 0 minutes

1   cup frozen wild blueberries
½ cup plain Greek yogurt
1   scoop plain or vanilla whey protein powder
1   banana
½ cup pomegranate juice
¼ cup walnut pieces
½ teaspoon vanilla extract

In a blender, combine the blueberries, yogurt, protein powder, banana, pomegranate juice, walnuts, and vanilla extract. Process until smooth.

CHOCOLATE–PEANUT BUTTER SMOOTHIE

Prep time: 3 minutes
Cook time: 0 minutes

1   scoop chocolate protein powder
1   tablespoon cacoa powder
1   tablespoon peanut butter
6   ounces almond milk
4   ice cubes

In a blender, combine the protein powder, cacoa powder, peanut butter, almond milk, milk, and ice cubes. Blend and serve.

STRAWBERRY-BANANA PROTEIN SMOOTHIE

Prep time: 3 minutes
Cook time: 0 minutes

1   whole banana
½ cup strawberries
1   cup almond milk
1½ scoops vanilla whey protein powder
4   ice cubes

In a blender, combine the banana, strawberries, almond milk, protein powder, and ice cubes. Blend and serve.

MINT CHOCOLATE CHIP SMOOTHIE

Prep time: 7 minutes
Cook time: 0 minutes

6 ounces water

1 mint tea bag

6 ice cubes

1 scoop chocolate whey protein powder

½ cup unflavored Greek yogurt

1 tablespoon cacao powder

1 tablespoon cacao nibs or semisweet chocolate chips

Boil the water and let the tea bag steep for 5 to 7 minutes. In a blender, combine the tea, ice cubes, protein powder, yogurt, cacao powder, and cacao nibs or chocolate chips. Blend and serve.

Index

Boldface page references indicate photographs. <u>Underscored</u> references indicate boxed text.